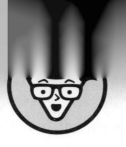

Diabetes Cookbook

5th Edition

by Dr. Simon Poole
Amy Riolo
Authors of *Diabetes For Dummies*
Dr. Alan Rubin

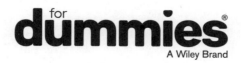

A Wiley Brand

Diabetes Cookbook For Dummies®, 5th Edition

Published by: **John Wiley & Sons, Inc.**, 111 River Street, Hoboken, NJ 07030-5774, www.wiley.com

Copyright © 2024 by John Wiley & Sons, Inc., Hoboken, New Jersey

Published simultaneously in Canada

For general information on our other products and services, please contact our Customer Care Department within the U.S. at 877-762-2974, outside the U.S. at 317-572-3993, or fax 317-572-4002. For technical support, please visit https://hub.wiley.com/community/support/dummies.

Wiley publishes in a variety of print and electronic formats and by print-on-demand. Some material included with standard print versions of this book may not be included in e-books or in print-on-demand. For more information about Wiley products, visit www.wiley.com.

Library of Congress Control Number: 2024933668

ISBN: 978-1-394-24023-4

ISBN 978-1-394-24025-8 (ebk); ISBN 978-1-394-24024-1 (ebk)

SKY10069540_031324

Contents at a Glance

Recipes at a Glance

Small plates on the go

Salads

Starters

Main Dishes

Table of Contents

Introduction

Neither one of us began our career knowing that we'd become so involved in supporting people with diabetes. Our shared passion has always been to help people lead their best lives. We both wanted to support people through illness and lead them to better health. As medical and culinary professionals with decades of experience, we soon realized how healthful lifestyle components that could powerfully and positively influence well-being and prevent illness were often missing from people's lives. On a daily basis, we recommend the Mediterranean diet and lifestyle for people in our care and influence to live better and longer. Fortunately, even though we're based in the United States and England, countless principles of this ancient way of living can still be enjoyed today anywhere on the planet.

According to the American Diabetes Association, 1.4 million Americans are diagnosed with diabetes each year. In 2019, 37.3 million Americans, or 11.3 percent of the population, had diabetes. Many nations around the world aren't far behind. There's a need to offer positive, easy-to-implement practices that can prevent people from developing diabetes in the first place, as well as help them reverse, or at a very minimum, live their best life while dealing with it.

You're reading the fifth edition of *Diabetes Cookbook For Dummies,* and you may be wondering why another edition is necessary. The Centers for Disease Control and Prevention recently suggested that as many as one in three adults in the United States will have diabetes by the year 2050. The International Diabetes Federation reports that 387 million people had diabetes in 2014 and that 552 million will have the disease by 2030 — that's one in every ten people. There has never been a better time to reverse those grim statistics. At the time of writing this book, the amount of free references and information on diabetes, availability of healthful food choices, and information on powerful lifestyle medicine are better than ever. Our intention is to present palatable recipes and meal planning tips that will enable you or your patients or loved ones to live your best lives and enjoy yourself in the process.

Though science and medicine can be complex and sometimes difficult to fully grasp, it's also true that when communicated in a clear and concise way, the stories they tell and the secrets they can reveal may be understood by all. That's the journey on which Amy and I have the privilege to be your guides.

About This Book

This new and revised edition of *Diabetes Cookbook For Dummies* features many new recipes based on the Mediterranean diet that has just been ranked as the best diet in the world for the seventh year in a row by *U.S. News and World Reports*. Many new studies have shown that people who follow a Mediterranean diet have a lower incidence of diabetes. And if they already have diabetes, a Mediterranean diet and lifestyle makes you live your best life despite a diagnosis.

This new and revised edition of *Diabetes Cookbook For Dummies* builds on the widely respected and successful previous editions with a new approach. This cookbook takes a much more holistic look at diabetes, not just as an illness that may have medical treatments but also as it relates to your lives and communities. We also embrace ideas of health being integral to your mind and spirit as well as your bodies and discuss therapies and ways of living that are often omitted from books about medical conditions.

You can use this new edition as an all-purpose cookbook that can help you create delicious and nutritious recipes for breakfast, lunch, dinner, as well as for meals on the go, salads, and desserts. The main feature that distinguishes this book from others is that each of its recipes are complete meals from a nutritional standpoint. That means you don't need to worry about pairing first and second courses or side dishes with mains. We've taken all of that into consideration to make the cooking process as streamlined as possible. With more than 125 chef-driven recipes to please all palates, you can create healthful meals that look as good as good as they are for you.

At the time of writing this book, the recipes were carefully crafted to cost less per person than the price of a meal at a fast-food restaurant. Be sure to take advantage of the many money- and time-saving tips sprinkled throughout the book. If you eat out or travel often, check out the chapters dedicated to eating healthfully away from home.

In addition to ensuring that each recipe (with the exception of the desserts) are complete meals, each recipe was created to maximize bioactive compounds to ensure more nutritional bang for your buck. Both easy and elegant, you'll be able to serve these recipes to guests and enjoy them yourself. You'll also discover how what you eat affects your blood sugar, how to plan meals, and how to make dining a more pleasurable experience.

Here are a few guidelines to keep in mind about the recipes:

>> All eggs are large.

>> All flour is all-purpose unless otherwise specified.

>> All extra-virgin olive oil is the best quality possible.

>> All onions are yellow unless otherwise specified.

>> All pepper is freshly ground black pepper unless otherwise specified.

>> All Greek yogurt is plain and full fat unless otherwise specified.

>> All salt is unrefined sea salt, which contains some raw minerals that help the body digest salt minus any unwanted additives. If you're swapping out regular salt, use an even smaller quantity.

>> All dry ingredient measurements are level — use a dry ingredient measuring cup, fill it using a spoon instead of scooping to the top, and scrape it even with a straight object, such as the flat side of a knife.

>> At the end of many of the recipes we add helpful tips, notes, and ways you can vary the recipe.

>> 🍅 If you need or want vegetarian recipes, scan the list of "Recipes in This Chapter" on the first page of each chapter in Part 2. A little tomato, rather than a triangle, in front of the name of a recipe marks that recipe as vegetarian. (See the tomato to the left of this paragraph.)

This isn't a complete book about diagnosing and treating diabetes and its complications. Check out the most recent editions of *Diabetes For Dummies*, if you need diagnosis and treatment information or *Diabetes Meal Planning and Nutrition For Dummies* (both by John Wiley & Sons, Inc.) if you want a deeper dive into meal planning and nutrition.

Foolish Assumptions

We make the following assumptions about you, our dear reader:

>> You've done some cooking, you're familiar with the right knife to use to slice an onion without cutting your finger, and you can tell one pot from another.

>> You have an interest in diabetes prevention or management — whether for yourself or a loved one.

>> This book also assumes that you know nothing (or very little) about diabetes, nutrition, and cooking for diabetes.

>> You have food intolerances or a healthcare professional has advised you to have a special diet.

>> If you already know a lot about diabetes, you can find more in-depth explanations. No matter your experience level, the recipes in Part 2 are for everyone.

Icons Used in This Book

The icons in this book are like bookmarks, pointing out information that we think is especially important. Here are the icons used in this book:

REMEMBER

This icon points out essential information that you shouldn't forget.

TIP

This icon marks important information that can save you time and energy.

DOCTOR SAYS

This icon marks text (from Simon) with medical advice about the choices you have to optimize your treatment.

TECHNICAL STUFF

This icon gives you technical information or terminology that may be helpful, but not necessary, to your understanding of the topic.

WARNING

This icon warns against potential problems (for example, if you don't treat a complication of diabetes properly).

Beyond the Book

In addition to the content of this book, you can access some related material online. We've posted the Cheat Sheet at www.dummies.com. It contains important information that you may want to refer to on a regular basis. To find the Cheat Sheet, simply visit www.dummies.com and search for "Diabetes Cookbook For Dummies Cheat Sheet."

Where to Go from Here

Where you go from here depends on your needs. Part 1 gives you an introduction to diabetes and its complications as well as an understanding of how to optimize your diet and lifestyle. Part 2 focuses on recipes that can deliver the best results and at the same time be delicious and fun to prepare. All the recipes are nutritious, optimize blood sugar, and are based on the most up-to-date knowledge of what constitutes the healthiest diet for most people with or without diabetes.

You can pick and choose how much you want to know about a subject, but the key points are clearly marked. You may also assume that if you or a loved one has been diagnosed with diabetes that there isn't much you can do about it. Each chapter helps you to develop a positive and proactive approach to living, and flourishing, with diabetes.

1

Flourishing with Diabetes

Discover what you need to know in order to flourish with diabetes.

See the effect food has on your diabetes and your weight.

Plan meals for your weight goal and glucose management.

Understand bioactive compounds and what impact they have on your body.

Choose delicious and healthful ingredients and meals.

Chapter **1**

What It Means to Flourish with Diabetes

Diabetes is one of the most common long-term medical conditions of today's generation, with rates rising dramatically across the globe year on year. Diabetes occurs when problems arise with how blood glucose is regulated; so there's no getting away from the fact that what you eat, combined with modern medicinal therapy is fundamental to its prevention, reversal, avoidance of complications, and optimum long-term management. Of course, that's good news because a greater understanding of how to improve your lifestyle can empower you to take control and help you to live your best life. The even better news is that this journey can be enjoyable, fun, sociable, inspiring, and tasty.

This chapter serves as your entry world into what you need to know about diabetes. Here we discuss the basics about the different types of diabetes and the complications that can arise if blood glucose control is poor. You discover the types of lifestyle changes you can make to make a tangible and measurable difference.

Recognizing Diabetes

With so much diabetes around these days, you may think that recognizing it should be easy. The truth is that it's not easy, because diabetes is defined by blood tests. You can't just look at someone and know the level of glucose — blood sugar — in their blood.

Blood glucose rises and falls depending on what a person is doing — varying with eating, fasting, or exercising. If control of blood glucose levels is compromised and levels rise beyond certain thresholds with risks of complications, then diabetes is diagnosed.

Here we examine what diabetes is, classify the different types of diabetes, discuss the consequences of diabetes, and mention how you can manage it.

Defining diabetes

In 2023 the U.S. Centers for Disease Control and Prevention reported that about 38 million people in the United States have established diabetes and one in five of them don't know they have it.

The level of glucose that means you have diabetes is as follows:

>> A *casual* blood glucose of 200 milligrams per deciliter (mg/dl) or more at any time of day or night, along with symptoms such as fatigue, frequent urination and thirst, slow healing of skin, urinary infections, and vaginal itching in women. A normal casual blood glucose should be between 70 and 139 mg/dl.

>> A *fasting* blood glucose of 126 mg/dl or more after no food for at least eight hours. A normal fasting blood glucose should be less than 100 mg/dl.

>> A blood glucose of 200 mg/dl or greater two hours after consuming 75 grams of glucose.

REMEMBER

A diagnosis of diabetes requires at least two abnormal levels on two different occasions. Don't accept a lifelong diagnosis of diabetes on the basis of a single test.

A fasting blood glucose between 100 and 125 mg/dl or casual blood glucose between 140 and 199 mg/dl is prediabetes. Most people with prediabetes will develop diabetes within ten years unless they make significant lifestyle changes. Although people with prediabetes don't usually develop small blood vessel complications of diabetes like blindness, kidney failure, and nerve damage, they're more prone to large vessel disease like heart attacks and strokes, so you want to get that level of glucose down. In 2019 an estimated 98 million people — that's more than one in three people — in the United States have prediabetes.

The American Diabetes Association has added a new criteria for the definition of diabetes, based around a person's A1C number. *A1C* is a measure of the average blood glucose for the last 60 to 90 days. If the A1C is equal to or greater than 6.5 percent, the person is considered to have diabetes.

REMEMBER

Many countries use different measurements for blood glucose — millimole per liter (mmol/l). The equivalent cut off values for a diagnosis of diabetes are 7.0 mmol/l for a fasting glucose and 11.1 mmol/l for a casual measurement (sometimes called a random blood glucose). The equivalent in mmol/mol for an A1C of 6.5 percent is 48.

Categorizing diabetes

The following list describes the three main types of diabetes:

>> **Type 1 diabetes:** This used to be called *juvenile diabetes* or *insulin-dependent diabetes.* It mostly begins in childhood and results from the body's self-destruction of its own pancreas. The *pancreas* is an organ of the body that sits behind the stomach and makes *insulin,* the chemical or hormone that gets glucose into cells where it can be used. You can't live without insulin, so people with type 1 diabetes must take insulin shots. Type 1 diabetes represents about 10 percent of total diabetes numbers.

>> **Type 2 diabetes:** Once called *adult-onset diabetes,* type 2 used to begin around the age of 40, but it's occurring more often in children, many of whom are getting heavier and heavier and exercising less and less. The problem in type 2 diabetes isn't a total lack of insulin, as occurs in type 1, but a resistance to the insulin, so that the glucose still doesn't get into cells but remains in the blood. It's often associated with being overweight and having a family history of diabetes.

>> **Gestational diabetes:** This type of diabetes is like type 2 diabetes but occurs in women during pregnancy, when a lot of chemicals in the mother's blood oppose the action of insulin. About 4 percent of all pregnancies are complicated by gestational diabetes. If the mother isn't treated to lower the blood glucose, the glucose gets into the baby's bloodstream. The baby produces plenty of insulin and begins to store the excess glucose as fat in all the wrong places. If this happens, the baby may be larger than usual and therefore may be hard to deliver.

When the baby is born, they're cut off from the large sugar supply but are still making lots of insulin, so their blood glucose can drop severely after birth.

The mother is at risk of gestational diabetes in later pregnancies and of type 2 diabetes as she gets older. About 50 percent of women with gestational diabetes develop diabetes at some stage, so regular testing and adopting a healthy lifestyle are both really important after a diagnosis of gestational diabetes. Women should be screened for gestational diabetes at 24 to 28 weeks of the pregnancy.

>> **Other types:** A small group of people with diabetes suffer from one of these much less common varieties of diabetes:

- Latent autoimmune diabetes in adults (LADA), which has characteristics of both type 1 and type 2 diabetes

- Genetic defects of the beta cell, which makes insulin

- Medications that affect insulin action like cortisol or prednisone

- Diseases or conditions that damage the pancreas like pancreatitis or cystic fibrosis

- Genetic defects in insulin action

Knowing the consequences of diabetes

If your blood glucose isn't controlled — that is, kept between 70 and 139 mg/dl after eating or under 100 mg/dl fasting — damage can occur to your body. The damage can be divided into three categories: irritations, short-term complications, and long-term complications.

Irritations

Irritations are mild and reversible but still unpleasant results of high blood glucose levels. The levels aren't so high that the person is in immediate life-threatening danger. The most important of these irritations are the following:

>> Blurred vision

>> Fatigue

>> Frequent urination and thirst

>> Genital itching, especially in females

>> Gum and urinary tract infections

>> Obesity

>> Slow healing of the skin

Short-term complications

These complications can be very serious and lead to death if not treated. They're associated with very high levels of blood glucose — in the 400s and above. The three main short-term complications are the following:

>> **Ketoacidosis:** This complication is found mostly in type 1 diabetes. *Ketoacidosis* is a severe acid condition of the blood that results from lack of insulin. The patient becomes very sick and will die if not treated with large volumes of fluids and large amounts of insulin. After the situation is reversed, however, the patient is fine.

>> **Hyperosmolar syndrome:** This condition is often seen in neglected older people. Their blood glucose rises due to severe dehydration and the fact that the kidneys of the older population can't get rid of glucose the way younger kidneys can. The blood becomes like thick syrup. The person can die if large amounts of fluids aren't restored. They don't need that much insulin to recover. After the condition is reversed, these people can return to a normal state.

>> **Hypoglycemia or low blood glucose:** This complication happens when the patient is on a drug like insulin or a pill that drives the glucose down but isn't getting enough food or is getting too much exercise. After it falls below 70 mg/dl, the patient begins to feel bad. Typical symptoms include sweating, rapid heartbeat, hunger, nervousness, confusion, and coma if the low glucose is prolonged. Glucose by mouth, or by venous injection if the person is unconscious, is the usual treatment. This complication usually causes no permanent damage.

Long-term complications

These problems occur after ten or more years of poorly controlled diabetes or, in the case of the macrovascular complications, after years of prediabetes or diabetes. They can have a substantial impact on quality of life. See the latest edition of our book *Diabetes For Dummies* (John Wiley & Sons, Inc.) for more information on screening for these complications, their prevention, and treatment.

The long-term complications are divided into two groups: *microvascular*, which are due at least in part to small blood vessel damage, and *macrovascular*, associated with damage to large blood vessels.

There is a lot of good news with respect to these complications. Changes to diet and lifestyle, including enjoying the way of life and recipes in Part 2, along with excellent medical treatments to reverse or optimize prediabetes or diabetes can significantly reduce the risk of micro- and macrovascular complications.

MICROVASCULAR COMPLICATIONS

Microvascular complications include the following:

» **Diabetic retinopathy:** Eye damage that leads to blindness if untreated.

» **Diabetic nephropathy:** Kidney damage that can lead to kidney failure.

» **Diabetic neuropathy:** Nerve damage that results in many clinical symptoms, the most common of which are tingling and numbness in the feet. Lack of sensation in the feet can result in severe injury without awareness unless you carefully look at your feet regularly. Such injury can result in infection and even amputation.

MACROVASCULAR COMPLICATIONS

Macrovascular complications also occur in prediabetes and consist of the following:

» **Arteriosclerotic heart disease:** Blockage of the blood vessels of the heart. This is the most common cause of death in diabetes due to a heart attack.

» **Arteriosclerotic cerebrovascular disease:** Blockage of blood vessels to the brain, resulting in a stroke and a common form of dementia.

» **Arteriosclerotic peripheral vascular disease involving the blood vessels of the legs:** These vessels can become clogged and result in amputation of the feet or legs.

Recognizing how you can manage diabetes

Treatment of diabetes involves three essential elements:

» **Diet:** If you follow the recommendations in this book, you can lower your average blood glucose by as much as 30 to 50 mg/dl. Doing so can reduce the complication rate by as much as 33 percent. You can also lower your A1C, prevent or reverse prediabetes, or put type 2 diabetes into remission.

» **Exercise:** Physical activity is crucial to keeping glucose levels in check. We touch on exercise in Chapter 3 and we cover it more extensively in the latest edition of *Diabetes For Dummies* (John Wiley & Sons, Inc.).

» **Medication:** Diabetes medications abound — there are far too many to discuss here, but you can find out about them in *Diabetes For Dummies*.

Understanding Diabetes, Weight, and Chronic Illnesses

You're most likely to flourish when you're feeling fit and well — experiencing good health and free of the burden of chronic diseases. If you do encounter a long-term illness, you can aim, with the support of medical and lifestyle measures, to reduce the symptoms, manage, or even reverse the condition.

Unfortunately, the last 50 years have seen a dramatic rise in the number of people who are living with one or more long-term illness such as diabetes, heart disease, stroke, dementia, kidney disease, and cancer. The World Health Organization (WHO) describes these as *noncommunicable diseases or NCDs.* Prior to good public health measures and antibiotics, infections were the greatest threat to human health, but now NCDs are rising at an alarming rate across the globe, with increased risk of disability or early death.

REMEMBER

This trend can be reversed if people understand and change the modifiable factors — those things that people have some control. Remember the following:

» The dramatic rise in NCDs has occurred with global changes in people's behavior toward a more sedentary lifestyle with increased food portion sizes and greater consumption of high-calorie, high-fat, highly refined, and processed foods with added artificial ingredients including sugars, salt, and preservatives.

» People who are overweight or obese are at an increased risk of developing type 2 diabetes.

» NCDs such as heart disease, stroke, many cancers, and dementia are increased in people who have type 2 diabetes.

» NCDs such as heart disease, stroke, many cancers, and dementia are increased in people who have a poor diet and lifestyle, even if they aren't overweight or obese, and whether they have diabetes or not.

This may seem daunting, but in Part 1 we focus on the flip side where the news is much brighter:

» Most NCDs are preventable or reversible through lifestyle measures such as not smoking, getting regular exercise, improving sleep quality, reducing stress, and having a healthy diet.

» An improved diet and lifestyle can prevent or reverse unhealthy weight gain and obesity.

>> An improved diet and lifestyle can prevent or reverse type 2 diabetes.

>> An improved diet and lifestyle can be key in the better management of type 2 diabetes.

>> An improved diet and lifestyle can prevent or reverse many NCDs with or without type 2 diabetes.

>> If a person is overweight but is maintaining a healthy Mediterranean diet, the risks of developing many NCDs can be lower than a person who is of normal weight but who has a poor diet and lifestyle.

>> An excellent diet can be enjoyable and reduce the risks of developing obesity, type 2 diabetes, and other NCDs.

>> An excellent diet can be enjoyable and reduce the risks or the worsening of NCDs even if they're established with or without type 2 diabetes or obesity.

Getting the Most Nutritional Value from Your Foods

A central tenant is an understanding of nutrition and how and what you eat affects your blood glucose and your general health.

Numerous diets are promoted for people with diabetes, some that have little evidence to back them and many that advocate restricting foods or certain macronutrients. Researchers are learning that the lowfat/high-carbohydrate diets advised by many government agencies may be causing more harm than good. Furthermore, many health professionals are moving away from just using calorie counting and body mass index (BMI) as a measure of food intake and its consequences and moving toward a greater focus on portion sizes, the quality of foods, and their effect on glucose and insulin balance and broader effects of the choices people make.

REMEMBER

An excellent diet:

>> **Provides optimum control of blood glucose.** We explore this more in the chapters in Part 1, which consider the role of good quality carbohydrates and nutrient combinations in foods.

>> **Helps to achieve and maintain a healthy weight.** This is especially important for those people with diabetes who are overweight.

>> **Has been shown to reduce the risk of other diseases, in particular those that are more common as complications of diabetes.** The components for an excellent diet should include not only good quality and healthy carbohydrates, fats, and proteins, but also should be rich in vitamins, micronutrients, and anti-inflammatory and antioxidant bioactive compounds that are protective and support optimum mental and physical health. We consider these in Chapter 4. Processed foods should be kept to a minimum or excluded.

>> **Is sustainable so that its glycemic control, healthy weight, and anti-inflammatory benefits are maintained in the long term.** In other words, it's enjoyable, varied, and tasty, and you can incorporate it into your daily life.

>> **Is ethical and sustainable for the environment.** Human health depends on the health of this beautiful planet.

We consider the three macronutrient groups — carbohydrates, proteins and fats — as well as micronutrients and vitamins in Chapter 2. In Chapter 4 we examine *bioactive compounds* — chemicals from plants found in small amounts in people's diet that may have considerable effects on promoting and maintaining health. We also show how the quality of your foods really matters.

We share detailed information about diabetes, its causes, treatments, and an approach to lifestyle that can empower you to take control of your glucose metabolism, prediabetes, diabetes, and weight, and enjoy excellent health and well-being in the recent editions of our books *Diabetes For Dummies* and *Diabetes Meal Planning and Nutrition For Dummies* (John Wiley & Sons, Inc.).

Exercising and Resting

Exercise is just as important as diet in controlling your blood glucose. A group of people who were expected to develop diabetes because their parents both had diabetes was asked to walk 30 minutes a day. Eighty percent of those individuals who did walk didn't develop the disease. These people didn't necessarily lose weight, but they did exercise.

Too many people complain that they just can't find the time to exercise. But a recent study showed that just 7½ minutes of highly intense exercise a week had a profound effect on the blood glucose. Here are some ways that different amounts of exercise can help you:

>> Thirty minutes of exercise a day gets you in excellent physical shape and reduces your blood glucose substantially.

>> Sixty minutes of exercise a day helps you to maintain weight loss and get you in even better physical shape.

An exercise partner helps ensure that you get out and do your thing. Having someone you can exercise with can be extremely helpful. Choose an activity you enjoy and are likely to maintain.

Here are some more facts about exercise to keep in mind:

>> You don't have to get in all your minutes of exercise in one session. Two 30-minute workouts are just as good as and possibly better than one 60-minute workout.

>> Although walking is excellent exercise, especially for the older population and a great place to start for people who are sedentary, the benefits of more vigorous exercise and for a longer time are greater still.

>> Everything counts when it comes to exercise. Your decision to take the stairs instead of the elevator may not seem like much, but if you do so day after day, it makes a profound difference. Another suggestion that may help over time is to park your car farther from your office or bike to the office.

>> A *pedometer* (a small gadget worn on your belt that counts your steps, or now commonly incorporated into smart watches and mobile devices) may help you to achieve your exercise goals. An objective may be to get up to 10,000 steps a day by increasing your step count every week.

You also want to do something to strengthen your muscles. Larger muscles take in more glucose, providing another way of keeping it under control. You'll be surprised by how much your stamina will increase and how much your blood glucose will fall. Resistance training (weightlifting) may be just as important as aerobic exercise in improving diabetic control. In the Nurses' Health Study, for example, resistance training resulted in a substantial reduction in the occurrence of diabetes.

TIP

Place a daily limit on activities that are completely sedentary, such as watching television or scrolling on TikTok or Instagram. Use the time you might have once spent on these activities to exercise.

Knowing the New Blood Pressure Limits

Keeping your blood pressure in check is particularly important in preventing the macrovascular complications of diabetes. But elevated blood pressure also plays a role in bringing on eye disease, kidney disease, and neuropathy. You should have your blood pressure tested regularly.

REMEMBER

Studies have shown that previous blood pressure goals weren't significantly more beneficial and did raise the risk of low blood pressure, fainting, and dizziness. The new goal is to keep your blood pressure under 140/80 for most adults, however targets might be less tight for older people or alternatively more ambitious for people with diabetes and other conditions such as heart or kidney disease. You may want to get your own blood pressure monitor so that you can check it at home yourself.

The statistics about diabetes and high blood pressure are daunting. Seventy-one percent of people with diabetes have high blood pressure, but almost a third are unaware of it. Almost half of them weren't being treated for high blood pressure. Among the treated patients, less than half were treated in a way that reduced their pressure to lower than 130/80.

TIP

You can do plenty of things to lower your blood pressure, including losing weight, avoiding salt, eating more fruits and vegetables, and, of course, exercising. But if all else fails, your doctor may prescribe medication.

One class of drugs in particular is very useful for people with diabetes with high blood pressure: angiotensin converting enzyme inhibitors (ACE inhibitors), which are especially protective of your kidneys. If kidney damage is detected early, ACE inhibitors can reverse the damage.

SIMON'S JOURNEY TO COMBAT DIABETES

My (Simon) journey to combine medical practice with writing and speaking on the subject of diet and lifestyle began several years ago when emerging evidence began to show how powerfully the way people live affects their chances of becoming ill or flourishing in good health. As physicians, we're generally trained to approach our medical careers with the emphasis on using medicines to reverse established illness. However, I soon realized that the most rewarding approach to medicine was to combine the application of modern medical therapies with a broader paradigm to encourage and inspire people to take control of their health as much as possible through the ways they live their lives.

Many of my patients in Cambridge, England, at first perceived that the journey to an improved lifestyle would be one of pain and misery, but they soon found the opposite to be true. Equipped with a greater understanding of the ways in which exercise and diet (in the form of positive nutrition) can dramatically improve well-being was key to their success. Soon patients who were following a Mediterranean lifestyle were showing powerfully improving results, mirroring as individuals the evidence that was being documented in scientific research. During my career, I've seen rates of obesity, diabetes, and the illnesses associated with these conditions soar. It became clear that a compelling need exists to look after growing numbers of people with diabetes in our communities with the best possible medical care but also to be empowered to choose the route to optimum health and well-being through wise and enjoyable lifestyle decisions.

Enjoying a Healthful Lifestyle

Diabetes is just one part of your life. It can affect the rest of your lifestyle, however, and your lifestyle certainly affects your diabetes. In this section, we take up some of these other parts of your lifestyle, all of which you can alter to the benefit of your health and your diabetes.

Limiting your alcohol intake

A good place to start is with alcohol. A small glass of wine can be a pleasant addition to dinner, and some studies show that alcohol in moderation can lower the risk of a heart attack. In some groups of people, though it can also increase the risk of many types of cancer as well as liver disease, especially in excess. For a person with diabetes, it's especially important that food accompany the wine because alcohol reduces the blood glucose; a complication called hypoglycemia may occur (see the section "Short-term complications," earlier in this chapter).

WARNING

Never drink alcohol without food, especially when you're taking glucose-lowering medication.

The following people shouldn't drink alcohol at all:

>> Pregnant women

>> Women who are breastfeeding

>> Children and adolescents

>> People who take medications that interact with alcohol

>> People with medical conditions that are worsened by alcohol, such as liver disease and certain diseases of the pancreas

AMY'S STORY — HELPING TO NOURISH OTHERS

My entire career was unintentionally based on diabetes. Had it not been for my mother's diagnosis with type 2 diabetes when I was 15, I'd probably have never thought about it. But I had the responsibility of cooking for my mom and our family, and I chose to use it as an opportunity to help heal her while creating delicious meals that the rest of us would enjoy as well. In those days, my actions were a simple labor of love that I never dreamed would lead to a career. I painfully witnessed my mother and others suffer complications from diabetes that I would love to eradicate forever.

For that reason, I decided to dedicate my life to help others nourish not only their bodies but their minds and spirits as well. I am now a Mediterranean Lifestyle Ambassador because I witnessed my family members living in Calabria, Italy, with relatively few major health complications and enjoying their lives much longer than most people do in the United States. It's not only their diet but also their mentality and lifestyle that makes the difference. Nowadays, each of my cookbooks attempts to capture those often unspoken secrets of the Mediterranean diet that make it so successful, while translating them in a manner that could be interpreted and followed anywhere.

My greatest goal is to have my readers enjoy as much "sweetness from life" as possible. I believe spending time with a loved one, having a good laugh, holding someone's hand, sharing hugs, watching sunsets, and whatever your daily pleasures happen to be are the glue that anchors a healthful diet and lifestyle together. These events give us the inspiration to continue and to make positive choices. I created the recipes in Part 2 with a desire to provide as many nutrients, vitamins, and minerals as possible while ensuring flavor and variety as well. I hope they're as fun for you to make as they are delicious to eat.

REMEMBER

Alcohol adds calories without any nutrition. Alcohol has no vitamins or minerals, but you do have to account for the calories in your diet. If you stop drinking alcohol, you may lose a significant amount of weight. For example, a person who has been drinking three drinks a night and stops might lose 26 pounds in a year.

Improving your lifestyle in other ways

Here are major ways you can improve the rest of your lifestyle:

>> Enjoy meditation and other forms of mindfulness activities.

>> Focus on your psychological well-being — seek support when you need it.

>> Develop and maintain a positive approach to life.

>> Discover ways to get healthful sleep.

>> Find ways to spend more time doing what you love.

>> Get out into nature as often as possible.

>> Take naps — even short ones when you can.

>> Avoid tobacco in any form. It is the number-one killer.

>> Avoid illicit drugs.

>> Drive safely.

>> Socialize more! Benefit from relationships and your community.

>> Maintain your sense of humor.

TIP

Try making changes one at a time, and when you think you have that one under control, move on to the next.

» Coping with carbohydrates

» Selecting protein

» Choosing the fat in your diet

» Eating enough micronutrients
(vitamins and minerals)

» Timing your food

Chapter **2**

Identifying Healthful Nutrition That Tastes Great

This chapter focuses on explaining the types of nutrients that your body needs and how the Mediterranean diet and lifestyle help you thrive. You discover how to enjoy satisfying meals that can help you meet your health goals. The essential nutrients you get from the foods in your diet are *macronutrients* (the nutrients you consume in largest quantities — carbohydrates, proteins, and fat), micronutrients (the essential minerals and vitamins that you consume in smaller amounts), and *bioactive compounds* (chemicals produced by plants that play a vital role in promoting and maintaining health — we discuss them in greater detail in Chapter 4).

Foods often contain combinations of macronutrients and micronutrients in varying amounts, though some foods that have a majority of one macronutrient are often reduced to being described as "a carb," "a fat," or "a protein," which isn't helpful when considering the complex characteristics of most foods.

The type of carbohydrates, which can be complex or made up of simple sugars, are of particular importance to people with diabetes because of the lack of, or resistance to, the hormone insulin that regulates blood glucose levels. But, as we describe in the second edition of *Diabetes Meal Planning and Nutrition For Dummies* (John Wiley & Sons, Inc.), having high-quality proteins, healthy fats, and sufficient vitamins and minerals, is important to support health and well-being.

Putting the best macronutrients, micronutrients, and bioactive compounds together in foods to create the optimum diet may seem like rocket science. Fortunately, an existing dietary pattern has evolved over millennia and provides an excellent balance, resulting in a healthy, sustainable, and enjoyable lifestyle.

Switching to a Mediterranean Diet and Lifestyle

The best diet for people with prediabetes and diabetes is one that follows the principles of an excellent diet and that has the evidence to back it up. The Mediterranean diet has been extensively studied and is widely acknowledged as a way of eating that can help to regulate blood glucose and prevent many of the complications of diabetes. The following sections take a closer look at what the Mediterranean diet is, why it's important for people with diabetes and prediabetes, and how you can start to follow it.

Examining the ins and outs of the Mediterranean diet

The Mediterranean diet is a dietary pattern inspired by the traditional eating habits of people living in the Mediterranean region, particularly in countries like Spain, Italy, Greece, and areas of North Africa.

The Mediterranean diet can be described as a plant-based diet because so much of it consists of vegetables, fruits, whole grains, and extra-virgin olive oil (EVOO). In the past, meat has been less available and affordable, so many days might be vegetarian.

It focuses on eating the following:

>> **Natural, local, and seasonal produce:** These include whole grains, vegetables, legumes and beans, fruits, EVOO, nuts, seeds, herbs, and spices.

>> **Dairy products:** They're fermented and eaten in moderation, especially yogurt and cheese.

>> **Meat:** Fish and poultry are consumed more than red meat. Processed foods aren't part of the diet.

>> **Drinks:** They include water, herbal teas, coffee, and in some cultures a small amount of alcohol, usually red wine, always with a meal.

TECHNICAL
STUFF

The Mediterranean diet can be traced back thousands of years, and it has evolved over time with the introduction of foods from other parts of the world, including tomatoes and chocolate from the Americas and coffee from Africa.

The Mediterranean diet is more than just a list of ingredients — it's a way of life. In our other books, the most recent editions of *Diabetes For Dummies* and *Diabetes Meal Planning & Nutrition For Dummies* (John Wiley & Sons, Inc.), we discuss the importance of lifestyle beyond simply considering what to eat. UNESCO recognized this broader scope of the Mediterranean diet by its inclusion, describing it as

a set of skills, knowledge, rituals, symbols, and traditions concerning crops, harvesting, fishing, animal husbandry, conservation, processing, cooking, and particularly the sharing and consumption of food. Eating together is the foundation of the cultural identity and continuity of communities throughout the Mediterranean basin. It is a moment of social exchange and communication, an affirmation and renewal of family, group or community identity. The Mediterranean diet emphasizes values of hospitality, neighborliness, intercultural dialogue and creativity, and a way of life guided by respect for diversity.

Noting what the science says

Research shows that the Mediterranean diet is beneficial for people who have diabetes. The evidence also demonstrates the diet reduces the risk of other chronic diseases including heart disease, stroke, many cancers, and dementia.

The American physiologist professor Ancel Keys studied the people of Greece and Southern Italy, having observed the remarkable number who enjoyed healthy aging without the burden of chronic diseases such as heart disease and cancers. His team looked at the diets of those regions and compared them with those of countries like the United States and the Netherlands, concluding that the Mediterranean diet was key.

The first big study of the 21st century confirming the benefits of the Mediterranean diet was published in the *Archives of Internal Medicine* in December 2007. It showed a significant reduction in deaths from all causes. With further evidence mounting, a study called PREDIMED — a Spanish study that stands for PREvención con DIeta MEDiterránea — followed more than 7,000 people over seven years who were either assigned to a lowfat diet or a Mediterranean diet supplemented with EVOO or nuts. The findings showed a reduction in many diseases and mortality over the period.

Numerous other outcomes from PREDIMED have been published, including findings published in The *Annals of Internal Medicine* in January 2014 showing that patients who followed a Mediterranean diet supplemented with EVOO had a significant reduction in the onset of diabetes compared to the control group who were just given advice on a lowfat diet.

Many other studies point to the effectiveness of the Mediterranean diet in preventing or managing diabetes as well as achieving and maintaining a healthy weight. The respected committee of experts who rank dietary patterns each year for *U.S. News & World Report* repeatedly award the top spot overall and for diabetes to the Mediterranean diet.

Recognizing the diet's benefits for you and the planet

The way in which the Mediterranean diet works to promote health so powerfully is a combination of many factors, including the following:

» The Mediterranean diet is composed of high-quality, low glycemic index carbohydrates like vegetables and whole-grains. (Refer to the section "Adding Up Carbohydrates — Precursors of Glucose" later in this chapter for more about carbohydrates.)

» On the Mediterranean diet protein comes from fish, which includes healthy fats or beans and other legumes that are packed full of fiber, vitamins, minerals, and other compounds that support good health. (Check out the section "Eating Enough Quality Protein" later in this chapter for more about protein.)

» On the Mediterranean diet fats are healthy and a high proportion of total fat is in the use of super healthy EVOO for cooking and flavoring. (See the section "Focusing on Fat" later in this chapter for more about fats.)

» The ingredients are rich in a variety of vitamins and minerals as well as protective bioactive compounds.

>> The Mediterranean diet doesn't contain processed or ultraprocessed foods. The way in which natural foods are combined may also have positive effects.

>> The Mediterranean diet has been shown to promote a diverse and beneficial gut. Refer to Chapter 4 where we discuss how the diet benefits the gut micobiome.

Evidence shows the Mediterranean diet is also good for the environment. It emphasizes eating more plants, reducing the consumption of red meat and processed foods, and consuming more local produce with less reliance on intensive, industrial farming methods.

You may be put off eating well because you're concerned that it costs more. Although supermarkets often discount less healthy foods, some data shows that the Mediterranean diet is affordable especially when you cook from scratch. Recent evidence from Rhode Island and Australia have confirmed that even with some ingredients like EEVO costing a little more than cheaper oils, overall, eating the Mediterranean diet isn't cost prohibitive.

Just as important as environmental sustainability is having a diet that's personally sustainable for the long term. Studies have shown that people are able to stick to the Mediterranean diet because it's satisfying, tasty, and enjoyable. If you have any doubt, the delicious recipes in Part 2 prove the point!

The Mediterranean diet is an excellent diet for people who live with prediabetes and diabetes. Furthermore, it's also great for family and loved ones because it is a go-to diet for everyone. It can be adapted for specific medical conditions such as celiac disease. You can also adjust it, if for example, your healthcare professional has advised you to reduce your carbohydrates a little or your blood glucose monitoring has indicated that certain foods have a particular effect on your individual glucose profile. Many people from all parts of the world find that adopting the Mediterranean diet is practical and enjoyable, and evidence supports its beneficial effects in populations living in other regions.

Incorporating the diet into your life

You may be curious how you can get started with the Mediterranean diet without moving to Greece. Here are some suggestions:

>> Make sure that most of your meal and snacks consist of fruits and vegetables, preferably unprocessed and whole. If you eat bread or cereal, make sure it's whole grain. The same is true for rice and pasta.

» Skip butter and use olive oil on bread or pasta instead. *Tahini* (blended sesame seeds) is another great alternative to butter. Other options are peanut, almond, cashew, sunflower, and pumpkin seed butters.

» Eat a handful of almonds, cashews, pistachios, and walnuts for a delicious snack or spread some 100 percent almond or peanut butter on a healthy cracker or whole-grain bread

» Add herbs and spices that we discuss in Chapter 5 to flavor your foods.

» Grill or bake fish with EVOO instead of breading it; especially good for you are tuna, salmon, trout, mackerel, and herring, fresh or in cans.

REMEMBER

If you're allergic to fish and seafood, you can find good omega-3 fats from some plant sources including chia seeds and flaxseeds and green vegetables including Brussels sprouts and spinach. If you're allergic to nuts, good fats are available from EVOO and avocados, with minerals from seeds, vegetables, legumes, and fruits.

» If you eat dairy, opt for good quality fermented products like yogurt and cheese, avoiding processed dairy products and those with added sugars.

» Food has a lot more to it than just the macronutrients, so if you're trying to reduce your carbohydrates, start with reducing the unhealthy added sugars and sweeteners such as high fructose corn syrup.

» Make sure that you're getting enough fiber and other healthy nutrients of Mediterranean-diet carbohydrates. Remember, healthy sourdough and carrots are both carbs, but they're very different from unhealthy sodas and cake.

» In general, eat smaller portions, especially of red meat, and eat consciously, gratefully, and socially if at all possible. Know what's in your food, avoid processed foods with lists of ingredients you don't recognize, and choose quality above quantity.

The way in which the diet works to promote health so powerfully is a combination of many factors. The next few sections of this chapter explore macronutrients. The Mediterranean diet is composed of high-quality, low glycemic index carbohydrates like vegetables and whole grains. Protein can come from fish, which includes healthy fats or beans and other legumes.

WARNING

The food that you find in Italian chain restaurants across the United States is not Mediterranean food. They use a lot of butter, full-fat cheese, cream sauce, meat, and white-flour pasta among other non-Mediterranean foods. So, don't think you're eating Mediterranean just because the restaurant serves pasta. Furthermore, a convenience meal sold in a supermarket may also appear to be

"Mediterranean," but it's most likely full of preservatives such as sodium nitrite and emulsifiers, which are best avoided and come from a factory and certainly not from the Mediterranean.

Adding Up Carbohydrates — Precursors of Glucose

When you eat a meal, the immediate source of glucose in your blood comes from the carbohydrates in that meal. One group of carbohydrates is the starches, such as cereals, grains, pastas, breads, crackers, starchy vegetables, beans, peas, and lentils. Fruits make up a second major source of carbohydrate. Milk and milk products contain not only carbohydrate but also protein and a variable amount of fat, depending on whether the milk is whole, lowfat, or fat-free. Other sources of carbohydrate include cakes, cookies, candies, sweetened beverages, and ice cream. These foods also contain a variable amount of fat.

These sections help you understand the amount of carbohydrates in your diet and their effect on blood glucose.

Determining the amount of carbohydrate: Does it matter?

For decades, the American Diabetes Association (ADA) has been recommending specific percentages of each macronutrient — carbohydrate, protein, and fat — for people with diabetes. After completely reviewing the evidence, the ADA has concluded in its Clinical Practice Recommendations for 2014,

There is not an ideal percentage of calories from carbohydrate, protein, and fat for all people with diabetes; therefore, macronutrient distribution should be based on individualized assessment of current eating patterns, preferences, and metabolic goals.

The Mediterranean diet as it is usually described isn't particularly low in carbohydrate, but we know that it's good for blood glucose control and diabetes management. Some people may find that their diabetes control is improved with a lower carbohydrate intake, but it makes sense to understand the typical Mediterranean diet and follow its principles and adjust it accordingly.

Considering a typical day on the Mediterranean diet

If the ADA recommendations in the previous section appear a little vague to you and you want some more concrete guidelines, here's what a typical day on a Mediterranean diet looks like, along with the breakdown of macronutrients for that day:

- >> **Breakfast:** 1 cup yogurt with ¾ cup berries and 1 slice whole-wheat bread with 2 tablespoons hummus
- >> **Snack:** 1 apple
- >> **Lunch:** 4 ounces salmon with herbs grilled or baked in EVOO with baked kale and ½ cup peas
- >> **Snack:** 6 almonds and ¼ cup grapes
- >> **Dinner:** 4 ounces white-meat chicken with rosemary, ⅓ cup brown rice and broccoli, 1 slice whole-wheat bread, and a glass of red wine
- >> **Snack:** 4 whole-grain crackers with 4 ounces cheese

REMEMBER

This day of a Mediterranean diet is 45 percent carbohydrate, 25 percent protein, and 30 percent fat. You don't have to stick to these percentages — this is just one example of a typical day on the Mediterranean diet.

Understanding why limiting carbs is important

Carbohydrates provide the most readily available source of sugars and contribute most to the *post prandial* increase in blood glucose — the rise seen after eating a meal that's regulated with an effective insulin response.

Many health professionals advise that people with diabetes reduce carbohydrates significantly and adopt a low-carb diet to lose weight and improve diabetes control. Doing so may help some people because there's individual variation in how people (and their gut microbiome) handle the foods they eat.

The Mediterranean diet has been shown to support a healthy weight and reduce the risks of diabetes and its complications despite its relatively high percentage of total carbohydrates because the carbohydrates in the Mediterranean diet are high quality and low glycemic index (refer to the next section for more about the glycemic index).

The Mediterranean diet works in other ways to regulate blood glucose. The combination of EVOO with a carbohydrate, for example with bread or pasta, reduces the speed of absorption of sugars. Compounds called polyphenols (see Chapter 4) in EVOO and other foods of the Mediterranean diet improve blood glucose regulation through increasing the efficiency of insulin and the diversity of the gut microbe.

TIP

There is a lot more to food than just the macronutrients, so if you're trying to reduce your carbohydrates, start with lowering the unhealthy added sugars and sweeteners such as high-fructose corn syrup you consume and make sure that you're getting enough fiber and other healthy nutrients of Mediterranean-diet carbohydrates.

Considering the glycemic index

The various carbohydrate sources differ in the degree to which they raise the blood glucose. This difference is called the *glycemic index* (GI), and it refers to the glucose-raising power of a food compared with white bread.

REMEMBER

In general, choose foods with a lower glycemic index in order to keep the rise in blood glucose to a minimum. Predicting the glycemic index of a mixed meal (one that contains an appetizer, a main dish, and a dessert) is nearly impossible, but you can make some simple substitutions to lower the glycemic index of your diet, as shown in Table 2-1. These substitutions are very much in keeping with the Mediterranean diet.

TABLE 2-1

Simple Diet Substitutions to Lower GI

High GI Foods	Low GI Foods
White bread	Whole, traditional grain bread
Processed breakfast cereal	Unrefined cereals like oats or low GI cereals
Plain cookies and crackers	Cookies made with dried fruits or whole grains like oats and no added ingredients
Cakes and muffins	Cakes and muffins made with fruits, oats, and whole grains and no added ingredients
Tropical fruits like bananas	Temperate-climate fruits like apples and plums
Potatoes	Whole-wheat pasta or legumes
Rice	Basmati, brown rice, long-grain rice, or other low GI rice

Many of these lower GI foods contain a lot of fiber. Fiber is a carbohydrate that can't be broken down by digestive enzymes, so it doesn't raise blood glucose and adds no calories. Fiber has been shown to reduce the risk of coronary heart disease and diabetes while it improves bowel function and supports a healthy and diverse gut microbiome. For the person who has diabetes already, fiber reduces blood glucose levels. The riper the fruit, the higher the GI.

TIP

If a food has a lot of fiber in it (more than 5 grams per serving), you can subtract the grams of fiber from the grams of carbohydrates in that food in determining the calories from carbohydrate.

The best sources of fiber are fruits, whole grains, and vegetables, especially the legumes. Animal food sources don't provide fiber. Doctors recommend that you consume 25 grams of fiber daily. Table 2-2 shows some sources of larger amounts of fiber.

TABLE 2-2

Sources of Fiber

Food, Amount	Fiber (g)	Calories
Navy beans, cooked, ½ cup	9.5	128
Bran cereal, ½ cup	8.8	78
Kidney beans, ½ cup	8.2	109
Split peas, cooked, ½ cup	8.1	116
Lentils, cooked ½ cup	7.8	115
Black beans, cooked, ½ cup	7.5	114
Plain whole-wheat English muffin	4.4	134
Pear, raw, small	4.3	81
Apple, with skin, 1 medium	3.3	72

Fiber can be present in two forms:

>> **Insoluble:** It doesn't dissolve in water but stays in the intestine as *roughage*, which helps to prevent constipation; for example, fiber found in whole-grain breads and cereals, and the skin of fruits and vegetables.

>> **Soluble:** It dissolves in water and enters the blood where it helps lower glucose and cholesterol; for example, fiber found in barley, brown rice, and beans, as well as vegetables and fruits. Soluble fiber also feeds the microbiome and creates short-chain fatty acids and other metabolites that help regulate insulin, glucose, and metabolism.

Eating Enough Quality Protein

Protein comes from meat, fish, poultry, milk, and cheese. It can also be found in beans, peas, and lentils, which we mention in the section "Adding Up Carbohydrates — Precursors of Glucose" earlier in this chapter. Meat sources of protein can be low or very high in fat, depending on the source. Because people with diabetes should be trying to keep the saturated fat content of their diets fairly low, low saturated fat sources of protein, such as skinless white–meat chicken or turkey or fish, are better choices.

Beans, peas, and lentils, which can be very good sources of protein, don't contain fat but do contain carbohydrate. They're also high in fiber and vitamins such as B vitamins, minerals, and other compounds that support good health. These compounds, which are biologically active, are called *bioactive compounds* (refer to Chapter 4 for more detail).

Protein doesn't cause an immediate rise in blood glucose, but it can raise glucose levels several hours later, after your liver processes the protein and converts some of it into glucose. Therefore, protein isn't a good choice if you want to treat low blood glucose, but a snack containing protein at bedtime may help prevent low blood glucose during the night.

Focusing on Fat

Fat comes in many different forms. The one everyone talks about is cholesterol, the type found in the yolk of an egg. However, most of the fat that people eat comes in a chemical form known as *triglyceride*. This term refers to the chemistry of the fat, and we don't have to get into the details of it for you to understand how to handle fat in your diet. In the following sections, we start with a discussion of cholesterol and then turn to other forms of fat.

Zeroing in on cholesterol — a risk for heart disease

These days, just about everyone knows their cholesterol level. You usually find out your total cholesterol level, a combination of so-called good cholesterol and bad cholesterol. If your total is high, much of that cholesterol may be the good kind — *HDL (high-density lipoprotein)* cholesterol. If you're interested in knowing the balance between good and bad cholesterol in your body, talk with your medical practitioner, who may recommend a *lipid panel,* a blood test that delivers more details.

The Framingham Study, an ongoing study of the health of the citizens of Framingham, Massachusetts, has shown that the total cholesterol amount divided by the good cholesterol figure gives a number that's a reasonable measure of the risk of a heart attack. People who had results that were less than 4.5 were at lower risk of heart attacks, while those with results of more that 4.5 were at higher risk. The risk increases as the number rises.

More recently, another component of the total cholesterol in your blood, the so-called bad cholesterol or *LDL-C (low-density lipoprotein cholesterol)* has been found to have an important role in causing heart attacks. For people at high risk of a heart attack, the recommended level for LDL used to be less than 100 mg/dl but has recently been lowered to less than 70 mg/dl.

The following sections examine what the risk factors are to heart disease and explain what healthcare providers give people with this risk, oftentimes people with diabetes.

Recognizing the factors that increase the risk of heart disease

A raised LDL cholesterol is just one of many factors that may increase a person's risk of heart disease. Other factors include the following:

>> Conditions with high levels of inflammation, such as rheumatoid arthritis

>> Diabetes

>> Extent of background inflammation with cholesterol plaques in blood vessels becoming inflamed and then more likely to form blood clots that can trigger a heart attack

>> Family history of heart disease

>> High blood pressure

>> Obesity

>> Poor diet

>> Sedentary lifestyle

>> Smoking

REMEMBER

The risk of heart disease increases with advancing age. You may not be able to modify your chronological age, but your doctor may order tests, take your lifestyle into account, and offer you a heart age that may reflect a better than average risk of heart disease for your age.

In addition, proinflammatory and anti-inflammatory (increasing and decreasing inflammation respectively) factors in a person's diet and lifestyle may affect the risk of a raised LDL cholesterol resulting in a heart attack or stroke.

TIP

Most foods don't contain much cholesterol. People make most cholesterol in the liver to be used in the body for maintaining the outer cell layers. An excess of certain types of saturated fat in the diet can increase the amount of LDL cholesterol to levels associated with an increased risk of heart disease. Naturally occurring cholesterol in foods such as shrimp and eggs contributes a relatively small amount to blood cholesterol levels and are fine to be eaten from time to time.

Understanding why statins are used

When total and bad cholesterol levels are too high, drugs called *statins* are usually given, especially to people with diabetes. Recently, new guidelines have been published by the American Heart Association for the use of statins. The UK's National Institute for Health and Care Excellence has offered similar guidelines. Unless a symptom or reason indicates otherwise, statins are used almost always in people who have existing heart disease. However, their recommended use for people who don't have existing heart disease but who are perceived to be at risk is a little more controversial.

Guidelines work with algorithms that include age, smoking history, a diagnosis of diabetes, a family history of heart disease, height, weight, and cholesterol levels. If the estimated risk of developing heart disease in the next ten years is calculated to be more than a certain percentage (10 percent is used in the UK), then statins may be advised.

The use of statins in recent years has certainly prevented many heart attacks and strokes; however, the calculation has some limitations:

>> If the patient adheres to a Mediterranean diet and regularly exercises with other lifestyle factors, then using statins may reduce the risk. At this point, though, researchers don't know because those factors aren't measured or considered.

>> Deciding to take a statin or to make a lifestyle change is difficult for a patient when the most important measurement predicting risk is one that can't change — a person's age.

>> Most healthcare professionals are unlikely to be able to describe what the original risk might be reduced to — the risk certainly isn't zero. If your risk of developing cardiovascular risk is calculated to be 13.5 percent, the question is how many percentage points of risk reduction a statin will give you.

TIP

Alongside lifestyle measures and diabetes medication where necessary, taking a statin may well be appropriate, but as with all medications it has potential pros and cons. Side effects can occur with statins and taking a statin can interfere with others drugs you're taking. Ask your healthcare professional about the possible benefits and risks of taking medications.

REMEMBER

The guidelines also state that patients on statins no longer need to get LDL cholesterol down to a specific target number, which means that when you're on statins, you rarely, if ever, need to be retested. And the guidelines recommend that adding other cholesterol-lowering drugs isn't necessary because they haven't been shown to reduce heart attack or stroke risk. This may in part reflect the theory that statins not only work by reducing LDL cholesterol levels but also may have a localized anti-inflammatory effect to stabilize cholesterol plaques in blood vessels.

Looking closer at fat

Although cholesterol gets all the press, most of the fat you eat is in the form of triglyceride, the fat you see on fatty meats, contained in whole-fat dairy products, and in many processed foods. Here are the several forms of triglyceride:

>> **Saturated fat** is the kind of fat that comes mainly from animal sources like that big piece of rib-eye steak you ate the other night. Butter, bacon, cream, and cream cheese are other examples. Healthcare professionals used to advise that because most saturated fat increases your bad cholesterol levels, you should avoid it. However not all saturated fats are created equal, and the situation is more complicated.

Although fermented dairy products like yogurt and cheeses contain high levels of saturated fat, no convincing evidence demonstrates that they increase the risk of heart disease. Some types of saturated fat, such as those found in yogurt and goat and sheep cheese, don't adversely affect cholesterol levels.

>> **Trans fats** were invented by food manufacturers to replace butter, which is more expensive. Unfortunately trans fats, which are currently listed as partially hydrogenated oil on food labels, are worse than saturated fat in causing coronary heart disease. They're found in margarine, cake mixes, dried soup mixes, many fast foods, and many frozen foods, doughnuts, cookies, potato chips, breakfast cereals, candies, and whipped toppings. Food manufacturers have been removing trans fats from numerous foods, but you still may find then in fried foods in restaurants. Keep them out of your diet by reading food labels, which must list them. Some countries, including the United States, have banned trans fats in food processing altogether, and the WHO makes the case for this to be global.

>> **Unsaturated fats** come from vegetable sources such as olive oil and canola oil. There are two forms of unsaturated fats:

- **Monounsaturated fats,** which don't raise cholesterol in the blood. Olive oil, canola oil, and avocado are some examples. The oil in nuts is also monounsaturated.

- **Polyunsaturated fats,** which don't raise cholesterol but can lower good or HDL cholesterol. Corn oil, mayonnaise, and some margarines have this form of fat. Here are the two types of polyunsaturated fats:

- **Omega-3:** Omega-3 polyunsaturated fats are those found in oily fish and some green plants and seeds like flax.

- **Omega-6:** Omega-6 polyunsaturated fats are more often found in vegetable oils and baked processed foods though they're also present in nuts and seeds.

You need both types in your diet, but Western diets have an excess of omega-6 to omega-3 polyunsaturated fats by a ratio of approximately 16:1. This excess is thought to promote unhealthy inflammation. A better ratio from the Mediterranean diet is probably 4:1, which you can achieve by looking out for foods rich in omega-3 fats and reducing the amount of processed foods and vegetable oils you consume, replacing them with EEVO.

REMEMBER

Food is more than its macronutrients, so don't judge an ingredient just by its fat. For example, EVOO and canola oil are different. Both are predominantly monounsaturated fats, but EVOO contains some key antioxidant compounds that are known to have an important health benefit.

Choosing quality fats

The Mediterranean diet, with EVOO, nuts, avocados (introduced from South America), seeds, fish, and fermented dairy is rich in monounsaturated fats, has a good omega-6 to omega-3 ratio, and is relatively low in saturated fat overall. The absence of processed foods, the practice of eating red meat once a fortnight or weekly but only in small amounts, and the presence of these naturally occurring healthy fats make the Mediterranean diet an ideal pattern of eating.

Figuring Out Your Diet

After you know how much to eat of each energy source (carbohydrate, fat, and protein), how do you translate this into actual foods? Foods are usually a mixture of these macronutrients and also contain micronutrients and bioactive compounds (see Chapter 4). Foods interact with each other and have an effect on your gut microbe. The best approach is to consider dietary patterns that contain good quality nutrients and natural, unprocessed foods.

Embracing the Mediterranean diet and other heritage diet patterns

Other dietary guidelines, such as the U.S. Department of Agriculture (USDA)'s MyPlate, focus mostly on macronutrient content of food and ignores micronutrients and lifestyle factors. That's why the Mediterranean diet with so much evidence in its favor is the best option.

We encourage the use of the Oldways Mediterranean Diet Pyramid (see Figure 2-1) with a single caveat. We suggest giving the EVOO portion greater space. The EVOO is the main source of fat in the diet and, as a single ingredient, is unique in its use in the kitchen and its presence in every meal. You can also check out `https://oldwayspt.org/resources/oldways` for more information.

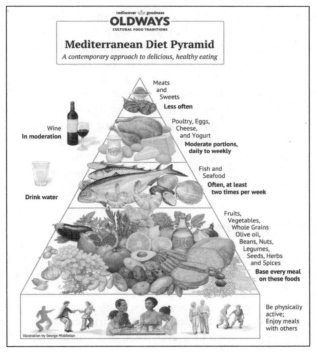

With permission from Oldways

FIGURE 2-1:
The Oldways Mediterranean diet food pyramid.

The Mediterranean diet is considered a *heritage diet* because of its roots in the traditions and culture of the region and because it is composed of local, seasonal, natural, and unprocessed foods. You can look across the world and see other places where people are more likely to enjoy healthy longevity, and you can recognize common themes in their diets, though individual ingredients may vary. Other diets from across the world haven't been studied as much, but it's possible to see common threads in diets from Asia, South America, and Africa, for example. Low glycemic index carbohydrates from a wide variety of colored vegetables and native species of grains, proteins from indigenous beans, peas, lentils, or fish, and healthy unsaturated fats are recognized as well as local types of fermented foods.

The organization that first devised the Mediterranean diet pyramid in consultation with Harvard University recognizes the importance of respecting and celebrating the dietary patterns of other regions and has developed Latin American, Asian, and African Heritage diet pyramids. These pyramids follow the same principles of an excellent diet we describe in Chapter 1. These diets support optimum control of blood glucose for people with prediabetes and diabetes.

REMEMBER

If you have connections with a dietary pattern from another part of the world or you're just passing through, consider which local foods are equivalent to those healthy ingredients of the Mediterranean diet. The one ingredient of the Mediterranean diet that stands out for its unique and powerful health benefits is EVOO. This healthy fat — the fruit juice of the olive — is used in every aspect of the cuisine and is consumed in quantities far greater than any other single food. Fortunately, EVOO is versatile and can be incorporated into other heritage diets to add flavor and health. Many other parts of the world cultivate the olive tree. The journey of the olive tree from its roots in the Middle East through the Mediterranean in the times of the Phoenician traders to North Africa and the United States continues. Olive groves have been planted in Australia, South America, South Africa and even India, China, and Japan.

Counting carbohydrates

People with type 1 diabetes and those with type 2 diabetes who take insulin may find the technique of counting carbohydrates to be the easiest for them. You still need to know how much carbohydrate you should eat in a given day. You divide the total into the meals and snacks that you eat and then, with the help of your healthcare provider, you determine your short-acting insulin needs based upon that amount of carbohydrates and the blood glucose that you measure before that meal.

For example, suppose that a person with diabetes is about to have a breakfast containing 60 grams of carbohydrate. They've found that each unit of lispro insulin controls about 20 grams of carbohydrate intake in their body. Figuring the proper amount of short-acting insulin can be accomplished by a process of trial and error: knowing the amount of carbohydrate intake and determining how many units are needed to keep the blood glucose level about the same after eating the carbohydrate as it was before. (The number of carbohydrate grams that each unit of insulin can control differs for each individual, and another person might control only 15 grams per unit.)

In this example, the person's measured blood glucose is 150 mg/dl (milligrams per deciliter). This result is about 50 mg/dl higher than they want it to be. The person knows that they can lower their blood glucose by 50 mg/dl for every unit of insulin they take. Therefore, they need 3 units of lispro for the carbohydrate intake and 1 unit for the elevated blood glucose for a total of 4 units. For more information on lispro, other types of insulin, and figuring out insulin sensitivity, see our book, the latest edition of *Diabetes For Dummies* (John Wiley & Sons, Inc.).

The person has a morning that is more active than expected. When lunchtime comes, their blood glucose is down to 60 mg/dl. They're about to eat a lunch containing 75 grams of carbohydrate. They take 4 units of lispro for the food but reduce it by 1 unit to a total of 3 units because their blood glucose is low.

At dinner, they're eating 45 grams of carbohydrate. Their blood glucose is 115 mg/dl. They take 2 units of lispro for the food intake and need no change for the blood glucose, so take only 2 units.

TIP

To be a successful carbohydrate counter, you must

>> Have an accurate knowledge of the grams of carbohydrate in the food you're about to eat and how many units of insulin you need for a given number of grams of carbohydrate.

>> Measure your blood glucose and know how your body responds to each unit of insulin.

You can make this calculation a little easier by using *constant carbohydrates*, which means that you try to choose carbohydrates so that you're eating about the same amount at every meal and snack. This approach makes determining proper amounts of insulin less tricky; just add or subtract units based upon your blood glucose level before that meal. A few sessions with your healthcare provider can help you feel more comfortable about counting carbohydrates.

Using a simple calculation

For patients with type 1 diabetes and those with type 2 diabetes who take a shot of rapid-acting insulin before meals and a shot of long-acting insulin once a day, this may be the easiest way to go. And it's just as effective as carbohydrate counting in lowering the hemoglobin A1c.

The method is based on a study published in *Diabetes Care* in July 2008. The authors compared their method with a group that did traditional carbohydrate counting and found no difference. Both techniques lowered the hemoglobin A1c into the normal range.

The targets were a fasting blood glucose of less than 95 mg/dl, blood glucose before lunch and dinner of less than 100 mg/dl, and bedtime glucose of less than 130 mg/dl.

The initial dose of the long-acting insulin (in this case, insulin glargine) was determined by adding all the insulin taken in a day before the study began. The dose was then started at 50 percent of the previous total daily insulin. The dose was adjusted by taking the mean of the previous three-day fasting glucose levels. The adjustment was then made as follows:

If the mean of the last three-day fasting glucose was

- **Greater than 180 mg/dl:** Increase 8 units
- **140 to 180 mg/dl:** Increase 6 units
- **120 to 139 mg/dl:** Increase 4 units
- **95 to 119 mg/dl:** Increase 2 units
- **70 to 94 mg/dl:** No change
- **Less than 70 mg/dl:** Decrease by the same units as the previous increase or up to 10 percent of the previous dose

The dose of the rapid-acting insulin before meals (in this case, insulin glulisine) at first totaled the other 50 percent of the pre-study daily insulin. It was divided into 50 percent for the meal with the most carbohydrate, 33 percent for the middle meal, and 17 percent for the meal with the least carbohydrate. Table 2-3 shows the adjustments made to the rapid-acting insulin based on the pattern of the pre-lunch, pre-dinner, and bedtime glucose patterns of the previous week.

TABLE 2-3

Adjustment of Rapid-Acting Insulin

Mealtime and Bedtime Dose	Pattern of Mealtime Blood Glucose below Target	Pattern of Mealtime Blood Glucose above Target
Less than or equal to 10 units	Decrease by 1 unit	Increase by 1 unit
11 to 19 units	Decrease by 2 units	Increase by 2 units
20 units or greater	Decrease by 3 units	Increase by 3 units

Try this system for yourself under medical supervision. It's easy and it works.

Monitoring Your Micronutrients

Food contains a lot more than just carbohydrate, protein, and fat. Most of the other components are micronutrients (present in tiny or micro quantities), which are essential for maintaining the health of human beings. Examples of micronutrients include vitamins (such as vitamin C and vitamin K) and minerals (such as calcium, magnesium, and iron). Most micronutrients are needed in such small amounts that it's extremely unlikely that you'd ever suffer a deficiency of them. A person who eats a balanced diet by using the pyramid technique or the exchange technique doesn't have to worry about getting sufficient quantities of micronutrients — with a few exceptions, which follow:

>> Adults need to be sure to take in at least 1,000 milligrams of calcium each day. If you're a young person still growing, pregnant, or elderly, you need 1,500 milligrams daily. We suggest you seek advice about supplements, including folic acid, from your healthcare provider. The best food sources of calcium are yogurt, milk, fortified ready-to-eat cereals, and calcium-fortified soy beverages.

>> Some menstruating women lose more iron than their bodies can spare and need to take iron supplements. The best sources of iron are iron-rich plant foods like spinach and lowfat meats.

>> You probably take in much more salt (sodium) than you need and are better off leaving added salt out of your diet.

>> Many people don't get enough vitamin D from gentle exposure to sunlight and from some foods, including dairy and oily fish. If in doubt about your vitamin D status, ask your pharmacist or healthcare provider for advice about supplementation.

>> You should increase your uptake of potassium to help lower blood pressure. The best sources are leafy green vegetables, fruit from vines, and root vegetables. For more information on micronutrients, check out our book, the most recent edition of *Diabetes For Dummies* (John Wiley & Sons, Inc.)

Other compounds in plant foods are very important for maintaining health. They aren't strictly nutrients because they aren't necessary for survival, but they have an important role in protecting you from a multitude of diseases. They're called *bioactive compounds*, and they include polyphenols, carotenoids, and glucosinolates. Chapter 4 discusses them in greater detail.

Recognizing the Importance of Timing of Food and Medication

If you take insulin, the peak of your insulin activity should correspond with the greatest availability of glucose in your blood. To accomplish this, you need to know the time when your insulin is most active, how long it lasts, and when it is no longer active, as the we discuss here:

>> *Regular insulin,* which has been around for decades, takes 30 minutes to start to lower the glucose level, peaks at three hours, and is gone by six to eight hours. This insulin is used before meals to keep glucose low until the next meal. The problem with regular insulin has always been that you have to take it 30 minutes before you eat or run the risk of becoming hypoglycemic at first, and hyperglycemic later when the insulin is no longer around but your food is providing glucose.

>> *Rapid-acting lispro insulin* and *insulin glulisine* are the newest preparations and the shortest acting. They begin to lower the glucose level within five minutes after administration, peak at about one hour, and are no longer active by about three hours. These insulins are a great advance because they free people with diabetes to take a shot only when they eat. Because their activity begins and ends so quickly, these insulins don't cause hypoglycemia as often as the older preparation.

TIP

Given a choice, because of its rapid onset and fall-off in activity, we recommend either lispro or glulisine as the short-acting insulins of choice for people with type 1 diabetes and those with type 2 diabetes who take insulin.

If you're going out to eat, you rarely know when the food will be served. Using rapid-acting insulins, you can measure your blood glucose when the food arrives and take an immediate shot. These preparations really free you to take insulin when you need it. They add a level of flexibility to your schedule that didn't exist before.

If you take regular insulin, keep to a more regular schedule of eating. In addition to short-acting insulin, if you have type 1 diabetes, or in some instances type 2 diabetes, you need to take a longer-acting preparation. The reason is to ensure that some insulin is always circulating to keep your body's metabolism running smoothly. Insulin glargine and insulin detemir are preparations that have no peak of activity but are available for 24 hours. You take one shot daily at bedtime, and they cover your needs for insulin except when large amounts of glucose enter your blood after meals. That is what rapid-acting insulins are for.

Everybody responds in their own way to different preparations of insulin. You need to test your blood glucose to determine your individual response.

Here are a couple other factors that affect the onset of insulin:

» **The location of the injection:** Because your abdominal muscles are usually at rest, injection of insulin into the abdomen results in more consistent blood glucose levels. If you use the arms or legs, the insulin will be taken up faster or slower, depending on whether you exercise or not. Be sure to rotate sites.

» **The depth of the injection:** A deeper injection results in a faster onset of action. If you use the same length needle and insert it to its maximum length each time, you'll ensure more uniform activity.

You can see from the discussion in this section that a great deal of variation is possible in the taking of an insulin shot. It's no wonder that people who must inject insulin tend to have many more ups and downs in their blood glucose. But with proper education, these variations can be reduced.

If you take oral medication, in particular the sulfonylurea drugs like micronase and glucotrol, the timing of food in relation to the taking of your medication must also be considered. For a complete explanation of this balance between food and medication, see the most recent edition of *Diabetes For Dummies*.

In recent years many more people are taking advantage of continuous glucose monitoring systems that are now able to automatically work out how much insulin is required. The technology is advancing at such a pace that it's possible to have *closed-loop* systems, which can administer insulin precisely as necessary in real time to rising and falling blood glucose levels — effectively an artificial pancreas.

Chapter 3

Planning Meals for Your Weight Goal and Glucose Management

You probably have heard of the obesity epidemic where the numbers of people who are classified as being overweight or obese is rapidly increasing across the world. The World Health Organization (WHO) defines overweight and obesity as abnormal or excessive body fat accumulation that may impair health.

A 2021 WHO report observed that worldwide obesity had nearly tripled since 1975. Approximately 39 percent of adults were overweight and 13 percent were obese in 2016, with figures rising each year and countries such as the United States having even higher rates.

You flourish most when you feel comfortable and happy and have optimum mental and physical health. Many people worry about their weight. You like most other people face or have faced social or peer pressure to achieve an ideal body image, and you may experience very real mental or physical illness or disability because of your weight. Your doctor may advise you to lose weight and you may seek support to do so at various times in your life. Many people may feel like trying to be slimmer or to have a different body shape is a lifelong battle.

This billion-dollar industry with it powder shake diets, pills, and even surgery helps some people, but it fails most. Achieving and maintaining a weight that's right for you and that ensures the best possible chances of a long and healthy life may seem an overwhelming challenge. So-called quick fixes and cures that promise immediate and sustained weight loss are almost certainly too good to be true. This chapter explores some of the reasons why losing weight can be difficult, addresses some of the assumptions about being overweight that may not be accurate, and provides some strategies to achieve optimum health through diet and lifestyle changes.

As you read this chapter, consider these few general tips that can help you on your journey:

>> Be compassionate with yourself and others when it comes to weight.

>> Set realistic and achievable weight targets with which you feel comfortable.

>> Be cautious about claims of easy weight loss solutions.

>> Be aware of the risks of excessive rapid weight loss and eating disorders that need medical advice such as anorexia nervosa.

>> Consider any short- or long-term side effects of any medication or surgical option and only consider when offered it by a reputable and registered healthcare professional.

>> Choose a diet and lifestyle approach that's healthy and sustainable in every way.

>> Consider making other lifestyle changes, including exercising more. Being overweight is associated with an increased risk of developing type 2 diabetes, heart disease, stroke, musculoskeletal disorders, and some cancers, but it's just one risk factor of many.

Finding Your Ideal Weight Range

Figuring out an optimum weight isn't necessarily as straightforward as it may first seem. You first need to understand some assumptions more fully. In recent decades there has been a simple approach to weight and weight loss. For many people the advice just doesn't work, which can be frustrating and demoralizing.

Healthcare professionals used to think that being overweight — having a high body mass index (BMI) — was an accurate measure of increased risk of diseases and that being overweight was because people consumed an excess of energy from food and drink (measured in calories) compared to the energy they burnt by activity and exercise. That excess energy would be stored as body fat. If a person could only reduce the calories they take in, or burn them, then they'd be a normal weight. And because fats in a person's diet contain three times as many calories compared to carbohydrates and proteins, the fat was making people fat. To reduce weight, people just needed to have a lowfat/high-carbohydrate diet.

If only things were that simple! Most health professionals now agree that the factors contributing to weight gain are more complicated than this, so it's worthwhile considering in more detail how being overweight is defined and the factors that influence a person's weight.

Measuring your body mass index

The standard measure to establish if a person has excess weight in relation to their height is by calculating BMI.

To calculate your BMI, do the following:

> Divide your weight by the square of your height.

A result above 25 is consistent with being overweight. A result more than 30 falls into the obese category.

For example, a man who is 6 feet tall and who weighs 210 pounds has a BMI of 28.5, which is considered overweight.

BMI is a useful guide that's easy to calculate if you have access to an online calculation tool and you know your weight and height. Seeing where you are on the BMI chart is a good place to start, and your health professional will often begin here.

But BMI isn't necessarily a very accurate measurement of excess body fat associated with poor health because it doesn't distinguish between bone, muscle, and fat mass.

For instance, an American football star or a Welsh rugby player may have a high BMI with additional muscle mass and be phenomenally fit and have a reduced risk of developing type 2 diabetes and other illnesses. Because body mass includes muscle and bone mass, as a person ages having strong bones and muscles to reduce the risk of injury from falls is advantageous.

An older person who has a BMI in an overweight range on a standard chart may have a lower risk of mortality than someone of the same age who is categorized as having a normal weight, and it may not be advisable for certain groups to attempt to lose weight on this basis.

Individuals also store body fat in different places, for reasons not fully understood, and *visceral* — fat surrounding internal abdominal organs — appears to be more harmful than fat stored elsewhere. A person with an *apple body shape* — someone who has increased abdominal girth — is more likely to have increased visceral fat than a person who has a *pear body shape* —where the fat appears visibly to be carried on the hips, thighs, and buttocks.

Counting your calories

Many foods provide information on calorie content. In some countries restaurants also give a calorie count for items on the menu, either voluntarily or through legislation. Like BMI, the number of calories you consume each day can provide you with some useful information but be careful when counting calories.

You may need to reexamine your thinking about the fats you consume. Although fat contains more calories than the other macronutrients, research has confirmed that monounsaturated fats such as olive oil have a much lower tendency to result in a buildup of visceral fat in comparison with saturated fats despite the similarity in calorie count.

In contrast, a diet with high glycemic index carbohydrates such as sodas and added simple sugars such as those you may find in many breakfast cereals or candies, where these sugars are absorbed quickly, can over time increase insulin resistance, fat accumulation, weight gain, and the risk of type 2 diabetes.

Meanwhile, adding fat to a meal of carbohydrates, which also increases calories, actually reduces the speed of absorption of carbohydrates and so may reduce the risk of insulin resistance. Individual foods, including extra-virgin olive oil while adding calories, may increase insulin sensitivity and thereby reduce the risk of long-term weight gain due to the effects of bioactive compounds such as polyphenols. Artificial sweeteners despite zero calories have been found to result in weight gain. One type of calorie may not have the same effect on body weight as another, and the approach of a calorie in versus calorie burned is an oversimplification.

Nurturing your microbiome

Having a healthy and diverse *gut microbiome* — a term that describes the trillions of microbes that live in the human gut — is also important for maintaining optimum weight. Plant foods, such as vegetables, fruits, whole grains, nuts, seeds, beans, peas, lentils and culinary herbs and spices help balance our microbiome. People who are overweight have a less healthy and diverse gut microbiome pattern. Lifestyle factors such as diet, exercise, adequate sleep, and mental health can all affect the trillions of potentially helpful microbes that live in your gastrointestinal tract and that do much of the work of processing the foods you eat before the nutrients are absorbed.

REMEMBER

Everyone has unique gut microbiomes as well as individual genetic profiles that influence how your lifestyle choices result in your body shape and weight. And those choices can influence and even change not only the proportions of good microbes you host but also how your genes are expressed.

If you want to read more about gut microbiome health, check out *Gut Health For Dummies* by Kristina Campbell (John Wiley & Sons, Inc.).

Getting enough exercise

People's sedentary lives have contributed to the statistics that show more and more people have become overweight and obese. However, just as calories intake doesn't necessarily translate directly to becoming fatter, calories burned is an unreliable measure of how much fat people may lose following exercise. Afterall, you can't outrun a bad diet.

However, evidence does support the importance of exercise for everyone, irrespective of weight. Consider the following about the importance of exercise:

>> Exercise can contribute to losing weight and maintaining an optimum BMI.

>> Exercise, like a good diet, promotes good health whether or not you're losing weight.

>> The health gains from exercise can be even more important for people who are overweight or obese.

>> Regular exercise mitigates but can't entirely reverse the increased risks of chronic illnesses associated with being overweight.

Exercise can be fun and even a small amount each week for people who lead otherwise sedentary lives can have profound benefits for cardiovascular health and blood glucose control. We suggest you check out our book, the most recent edition of *Diabetes For Dummies* (John Wiley & Sons, Inc.), for more about how exercise can help you reach and maintain your ideal weight.

Finding foods that satisfy

In recent years researchers have discovered more about appetite and what makes people feel satiated and full. Quite a lot of complicated chemistry goes on and the human body responds to signals from *hormones* — chemical messenger systems such as leptin— that tell your brain that you've eaten enough and give you the sensation of feeling full. Medications have been licensed for use for glucose regulation in diabetes and also to suppress and control appetite in people who are overweight, though the evidence so far suggests that when the drug is stopped, weight is put back on.

No evidence suggests that specific foods can directly affect leptin levels, but some foods score highly on an index of satiety — where people report feeling fuller after eating — although researchers don't entirely understand this mechanism. These foods include vegetables, fatty fish, lean meats such as chicken, eggs, yogurt, olive oil, avocados, and dark chocolate.

The different effects of foods on satiety underlines the need to consider calorie counting with some caution. If foods like olive oil or dark chocolate add some calories to a meal but increase satiety, then encouraging eating them may actually decrease the amount of calories a person consumes over the course of a meal or a day because the person feels fuller and doesn't eat extra calories.

Determining Your Nutritional Needs

As we discuss in these sections, you can figure out how to meet your nutritional needs and achieve your target weight as well as optimize the benefits of a healthy diet. Your diet needs to include the best quality macronutrients and plenty of micronutrients including vitamins and minerals as well as bioactive compounds, which we discuss in Chapter 4.

Focusing on the way people eat

Plenty of evidence shows that the way people eat influences their calorie consumption and how likely they are to gain weight. Consider the following about the way you eat:

- » **Eat slowly and in the company of others.** Eat in company whenever you can. Research shows that sharing and enjoying a meal together at a table rather than in front of the television results in eating a more moderate quantity of food.

- » **Remember portion sizes.** Portion size is perhaps an easier measurement of the food you eat than counting calories. Remember the average plate size has increased by a third in recent decades. You don't need to fill your plate.

- » **Keep leftovers.** You don't need to eat the entire meal. Keep some food in the pan and safely store leftovers for another meal rather than feeling obliged to finish that food that's already in front of you.

- » **Eat slower.** There is a delay in feeling full while eating, so slower eating will allow time for those important messages to get to your brain to tell you that you don't need to eat any more.

TIP

Eat thoughtfully and be conscious of the quantity and quality of foods on your plate. Pause to focus and acknowledge the taste and presentation of your food even if you're in company. Doing so can provide the opportunity to honor the food that you are about to eat, reminding you that it's something to celebrate.

Remembering you're unique

Every person is different in the way that they metabolize food. That's why understanding what works for you as an individual with your own genetic makeup and your different gut microbiome is important.

Some people with diabetes may have access to real-time blood glucose monitoring. It's possible to measure the glycemic index and glycemic load of foods, but each person may respond a little differently to a meal and to individual ingredients. Keeping a food diary that includes changes in your blood glucose gives you feedback that supports what you eat at certain times of the day.

Most people have tried one diet or another at various times in their lives, usually with mixed success. We recommend the Mediterranean diet (as we discuss in Chapter 2), but you may need to tailor it to your own experience and needs. Some people may need to reduce the low glycemic index carbohydrates, thus adopting a lower carbohydrate Mediterranean diet. Others may find that exercise has a more powerful weight-reducing effect, they may need to vary the periods between meals, or they may need to modify the amount they eat daily. Listen to your body and experience and adapt to whatever works best for you, acknowledging your individuality.

Deciding what's most important and making your plan

The science is quite clear: Being overweight is associated with an increased risk of type 2 diabetes and other chronic illnesses, and this triad of excess weight, poor diet, and a sedentary lifestyle influences mortality.

TIP

Ideally aim for healthy weight and BMI, but if you can't quite achieve that goal, remember that you can mitigate much of the risk of being overweight by eating a portion-controlled Mediterranean diet and getting regular exercise. Plan a healthy lifestyle and then focus on the likely outcome, which is to feel happier, healthier, and fitter — while achieving a desirable weight.

Checking Out Other Diets

If you go to the diet section of any large bookstore, the number of choices can overwhelm you. You can find diets that recommend protein and no carbohydrate, carbohydrate and no protein, one type of carbohydrate and not another, all rice, all grapefruit, and on and on. How is it possible for all these diets, many of which are exactly the opposite of others on the same shelf, to actually work for you? The answer is they do and they don't. If you follow any diet closely, you'll lose weight. But will the weight stay off? That's the most difficult part (as we're sure you know).

DOCTOR SAYS

I (Simon) have seen my patients lose weight on diets like the examples described in this section, but I recommend the Mediterranean diet in practice. Sometimes diet plans can achieve quite rapid weight loss in the short term, and as long as they're safe and provide adequate nutrition, then experiencing early success can be a good motivator. But sustaining a healthy weight and enjoying a diet that protects from chronic diseases must surely be the best the long-term goal.

REMEMBER

The Mediterranean diet isn't usually included in lists of diets promoted for weight loss because it's mostly cited for its benefits promoting health and preventing chronic diseases, but perhaps it should be. Studies show that compared with other diets, initial weight loss may be more gradual on the Mediterranean diet, but this diet is much more effective at achieving and sustaining weight reduction and management over a period of years. The Mediterranean diet is one you can live with and enjoy for a lifetime.

WARNING

With the exception of the DASH diet, which the U.S. FDA recommends, none of the diets described in these sections have long-term studies that show, convincingly, that they're better than any other. Each one of them has anecdotal evidence, meaning that one or two or ten people tell you how great they did on this or that diet. But you never hear from those who didn't do so great.

The low carbohydrate group

These diets are based on the claim that carbohydrates promote hunger. By reducing or eliminating them, you lose your hunger as you lose your weight. The first of them, the Atkins Diet, promotes any kind of protein, including protein high in fat. Naturally, other diets were developed promoting very little carbohydrate but less fatty protein. Here are your choices:

>> **Atkins diet:** This plan allows any quantity of meats, shellfish, eggs, and cheese but doesn't permit high-carbohydrate foods like fruits, starchy vegetables, and pasta. Small quantities of the forbidden foods are added in later. The program does recommend exercise but doesn't suggest changes in your eating behavior. Ketogenic diets recommend eating even greater amounts of protein and less carbohydrate in the attempt to use stored fat for energy

>> **South Beach diet:** This diet restricts carbohydrates while the recommended proteins are low in fat, unlike the Atkins diet. Daily exercise is an important component, but the plan doesn't suggest any changes in eating behavior. Over time some carbohydrate is reintroduced into the diet.

>> **Ultimate Weight Solution:** This plan recommends a lot of protein, which naturally results in a reduction in carbohydrate. This program also advises you not to eat foods high in fat. Support groups in which you learn how to modify your eating behaviors are important, and you're supposed to stay in these groups throughout your life. The plan also emphasizes regular exercise, such as walking.

>> **Zone diet:** In this diet, you have to balance your food intake into exact amounts of carbohydrate, protein, and fat. You're not permitted to eat high-carbohydrate and high-fat food. Regular exercise is recommended, but the plan doesn't suggest changes in your eating behavior. You have to continue with this balance throughout life to maintain your weight loss.

The portion control group

These diets recognize that it's not what you eat but how much you eat that determines your weight. They generally follow the recommendations of the government food guidelines. Here are some examples of portion control diets:

>> **DASH diet:** Here, the emphasis is on grains, fruits, and vegetables and restricting the amounts of fat. A further modification for individuals with high blood pressure recommends very little salt. Animal protein, such as meat, fish, and poultry, is limited. An exercise program is suggested but not defined. This diet suggests changes in eating behavior. It's a diet for life (and a very good one).

>> **Nutrisystem:** This diet is comprised of commercially prepared ready-to-eat meals and (shelf-stable or frozen) boxed items, making up 100 percent of the clients' diets, meaning that there's no room for fresh fruits and vegetables, at least in the beginning. Ingredients often contain fillers, vegetable, palm oil, and artificial flavors and coloring that aren't recommended for long-term optimal health. Currently, Nutrisystem offers prepared food meal plans for those desiring to lose weight quickly, are older than 50 years of age, and for those who have diabetes.

>> **Weight Watchers, now known as WW:** This plan uses a point system in which foods are given points according to the amount of fat, fiber, and calories in them. To get to and maintain a certain weight, you're given a daily number of points. As long as you stay within these points, you'll be successful. Therefore, foods that have large amounts of calories will use up your daily points quickly, so relying on low glycemic index vegetables and lean protein as the basis of your diet are key. The program suggests exercise and changes in your lifestyle.

>> **Noom:** One of the more recent diet plan companies, Noom is an app-based fitness and weight loss program that you can access 24/7. It includes psychological strategies to create sustainable weight loss. It's more flexible in that you don't have to cut out all carbs and count calories, and it teaches tips and tricks to lose weight. Some American insurance companies, such as Blue Cross

Blue Shield, offer free Noom memberships at the time of writing this book. Noom considers physical activity levels and other lifestyle factors to help people lose weight and keep it off. They offer 16-week custom plans and focus on redefining daily habits so that you're not dependent on meal delivery and can enjoy fresh, homemade food. For those who don't have a personal health coach or nutrition professional at their disposal, the app can help them to incorporate some of the strategies that we discuss in this book.

A diet that emphasizes weight training

The Abs diet is similar to the diets that recommend a balanced approach to eating, with carbohydrates that aren't refined and dairy and meat that are low in fat as the most suggested foods. However, the major emphasis in this diet is on a program called "Total Body Strength Training Workout" to build muscles. Changes in eating behavior aren't a large part of the program. To maintain weight loss, you must eat and exercise as the diet prescribes for your entire life.

More extreme diets

These diets require a level of participation that may be difficult for people who have a life. You really need to give your time and energy to staying on the diet. If you go away for a few weeks and stay within their program, you'll have some short-term success. But after you return home, sticking to the program gets difficult. Here are the two major programs currently available:

>> **Dean Ornish Program:** This plan allows fruits, vegetables, and whole grains along with the leanest of meats and poultry. You can't eat processed foods or drink caffeine or alcohol, and you must avoid sugar, salt, and oil. Exercise is recommended as is help with eating behaviors. Meetings are an important part of this program, which you're supposed to follow for life.

>> **Pritikin Eating Plan:** Whole grains, vegetables, and fruits are essential foods, and the diet allows almost no protein or fat. Exercise is a part of the program as is changing your lifestyle to promote better eating behaviors. You're expected to follow this program for life. Only Pritikin and a few others have been able to do this.

>> **Paleo diet:** This diet is supposedly based on the diet that ancient ancestors ate — plenty of meat, nuts and vegetables but little of modern agricultural foods like dairy, wheat, and legumes. But anyone who thinks that modern meat is anything like the meat that hunter-gatherers ate is sadly mistaken.

Ancient people didn't suffer from today's modern diseases of old age because they died young. This diet placed last among experts for *U.S. News & World Report* for many years with respect to health, weight loss, and ease of following.

A more recent and extreme development from the paleo diet is the carnivore diet that recommends only eating meat or meat-based products, which is the exact opposite of most public health advice.

» **Biggest Loser:** Based on a television show by the same name, this diet features small frequent meals consisting of lean protein, lowfat dairy, fruits, vegetables, whole grains, beans, and nuts. There is a huge amount of exercise associated with the diet. This program is very hard to sustain in real life.

Chapter **4**

Bioactive Compounds — Nutrition Is More than Nutrients

The discovery of bioactive compounds, produced by plants to protect them from their challenging environment, is probably the most exciting development in nutrition of recent years. *Polyphenols, carotenoids,* and *glucosinolates* — the three classes of bioactive compounds — are likely to be the most important things you eat that you've never even heard of! This chapter takes a much closer look at what they are, how they work, and where we can find them. Many thousands of distinct biochemicals are in food, and research is beginning to uncover fascinating and important effects on human health.

Part 2 has recipes that have been specifically crafted to include a wide variety of bioactive compounds, which we refer to as bioactives, to help you, your family, and friends, who have or don't have prediabetes or diabetes, to benefit from a bioactive-rich diet.

More than half of all of today's modern medicines are derived from plants, not from macronutrients or micronutrients, but from the chemistry of bioactives. The ancient Greek father of medicine Hippocrates was aware of these powers when he said, "Let food be thy medicine and medicine be thy food."

Staying Healthy with Bioactive Compounds

More than likely you've heard of the macronutrients carbohydrates, fats, and proteins. Chances are most of you also know a little bit about many of the micronutrient vitamins and minerals that are needed in smaller quantities to survive. Chapter 2 of this book and our books, the most recent editions of *Diabetes For Dummies* and *Diabetes Meal Planning and Nutrition For Dummies* (John Wiley & Sons, Inc.), look in more detail at these nutrients including how to get enough in your diet.

What you probably aren't as familiar with are plant *bioactive compounds.* The many thousands of plant-produced bioactive compounds are different from macronutrients and micronutrients; they aren't strictly nutrients because the definition of a *nutrient* is a chemical that you need to find in your foods to sustain life. The compounds we discuss in this chapter aren't necessary for surviving but are important for thriving. As the name suggests, they have biological activity — they impact your body in many ways, and their many effects are important for maintaining health and preventing a multitude of diseases. That means, if you want to live your best life, you need to understand more about them and to spend more time finding out about them and talking about them as much as carbohydrates and calcium, proteins and potassium, or saturated fat and sodium.

Here we investigate the effects of bioactive compounds and identify the characteristics of the foods that contain them.

Recognizing where to find bioactives

When nutrition professionals talk about individual foods that are particularly healthy, they may be thinking about their macro or micronutrient content. For example, ancient whole grains contain low glycemic index, complex carbohydrates that support good blood glucose balance, beans are a fantastic source of protein and fiber, olive oil is a fat that helps keep cholesterol levels down, and oranges contain vitamin C and potassium. All these plant foods contain nutrients as well as those individual ones highlighted, but what these and many other so-called superfoods also have in common is the abundance of bioactive compounds.

REMEMBER

Vegetables, fruits, nuts, extra-virgin olive oil (EVOO), seeds, dark chocolate, red wine, herbs, spices, teas, and coffee are all rich sources of a variety of polyphenols and other bioactives. The Mediterranean diet, which we discuss in Chapter 2, promotes health because of its balance of natural foods with high quality macronutrients and micronutrients combined together, but it may be the presence of a wide range of bioactives that supercharge its beneficial effects.

We're passionate about healthy and tasty food and enjoy studying and teaching nutrition and cuisine. The story of bioactives and the benefits they can provide to everyone, especially those living with prediabetes or diabetes, is one of the most fascinating, inspiring, and exciting subjects that will continue to develop over the next few years. For the first time, we dedicate entire chapters to bioactive compounds in our other *Diabetes For Dummies* books. Remember, you read it here first.

REMEMBER

There is no definition of the word "superfood" and so we use the term with caution. The trouble comes when the food industry uses, or abuses, that term to market particular products. For example, kale is a green leafy vegetable that has many bioactive compounds, but the processed food industry has added kale to chips and advertised it as a "superfood chip" with implied health benefits, despite the numerous additives and unhealthy processing methods.

Identifying some benefits

Researchers aren't always entirely sure how bioactive compounds work to promote health, but the effects are broad. However, they are closely studying the bioactive effects of polyphenols to get a clearer picture. Here are some of the main benefits to polyphenols:

>> **They help regulate blood sugar levels.** That's why they're particularly beneficial for people with prediabetes or diabetes. They can improve insulin sensitivity and reduce the risk of insulin resistance.

>> **They support brain health.** Some polyphenols have been found to be *neuroprotective*, meaning they protect nerve cells from damage and may reduce the risk of neurodegenerative diseases like Alzheimer's and Parkinson's disease. They can also improve memory and cognitive function.

>> **They enhance gut health.** Polyphenols can act as prebiotics, nourishing beneficial gut bacteria. A healthy gut microbiome is essential for digestion, nutrient absorption, and overall immune function.

>> **They work as antioxidants (see Figure 4-1).** They neutralize harmful chemicals called *free radicals* in the body. Free radicals can damage cells and contribute to aging and various diseases. By neutralizing these free radicals, polyphenols can reduce oxidative stress and lower the risk of chronic diseases such as cardiovascular diseases, cancer, and neurodegenerative diseases.

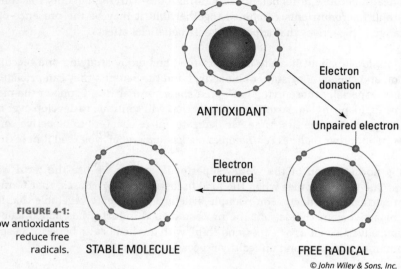

Electron donation

ANTIOXIDANT

Unpaired electron

Electron returned

FIGURE 4-1: How antioxidants reduce free radicals.

STABLE MOLECULE

FREE RADICAL

© John Wiley & Sons, Inc.

>> **They reduce inflammation.** Polyphenols have *anti-inflammatory properties,* which means they can reduce inflammation in the body. Chronic inflammation (which we discuss in the section "Reversing Inflammation" later in this chapter) is linked to numerous health problems including diabetes, heart disease (the most common complication of diabetes), and *autoimmune diseases* (chronic inflammation because of a misdirected immune response to the body's own cells). Polyphenols help inhibit inflammatory pathways, thereby reducing the risk of inflammation-related diseases.

>> **They improve cardiovascular health.** Polyphenols can improve cardiovascular health by promoting healthy blood circulation, reducing blood pressure, and preventing the oxidation of LDL cholesterol, which damages blood vessel walls and causes inflammation and blood clot formation. These effects contribute to a lower risk of heart disease.

>> **They prevent cancer.** Research is ongoing, but some polyphenols have shown the potential to prevent certain types of cancer. Their antioxidant properties help protect cells from DNA damage that can lead to cancer.

TECHNICAL STUFF

Bioactives have a lot of unknowns. Researchers are intrigued by their ability to apparently disappear at times — they can often be found in the gut and urine but may be impossible to identify elsewhere in the body. Many seem to be broken down in the gut, or changed by gut microbes, and perhaps these new compounds or metabolites called *postbiotics* are most active. Researchers are also challenged by measuring their antioxidant effects and understanding how such tiny concentrations can have such powerful effects at a cell level. Some researchers have theorized that they recharge each other, enhance the body's own antioxidant pathways, or act on our genes in other ways.

Reversing Inflammation

Many chronic diseases including diabetes, heart disease, stroke, neurodegenerative diseases, and many cancers are associated with chronic inflammation. To comprehend the potential harm of chronic inflammation, you need to understand how the protective processes of *acute,* or short-term inflammation, become damaging when they aren't resolved and instead become long term.

Understanding what inflammation is

Inflammation is a natural response of a person's immune systems to injury or infection. It plays a crucial role in defending the body, eradicating harmful bacteria and viruses and promoting tissue repair. *Acute inflammation* occurs rapidly and involves many features of a person's immune response including the release of chemicals that can target and kill bacteria or viruses and cells that capture and ingest the localized damaged tissues as well as promote healing and a return to normal cell functions.

As part of this process, the human immune system releases a controlled burst of highly reactive oxidizing molecules — internally produced free radicals that chemically destroy any invaders or compromised cells before a healing and restructuring takes place. Your immune system mostly does a brilliant job and keeps you safe and well despite the hazards of life. A good diet supports this normal and beneficial functioning of your immune cells.

REMEMBER

On the other hand, *chronic inflammation* is when the processes of inflammation persist over a longer period. It happens in response to a persisting infection, autoimmune disorders, or exposure to damage from tobacco smoke, pollution, radiation, or unhealthy chemicals directly in your diet or those formed during metabolism that your body fails to use or excrete. Chronic inflammation leads to continuous tissue and organ damage, impaired healing processes, and the development of conditions like rheumatoid arthritis, inflammatory bowel disease, diabetes, cardiovascular disease, and stroke, which are known to involve chronic inflammation of cholesterol deposits in blood vessel walls. Chronic inflammation, by damaging DNA, can also lead to an increased risk of many types of cancer.

TECHNICAL
STUFF

The chemical triggers of chronic inflammation can occur when there's an excess of free radicals — highly reactive molecules often containing oxygen atoms, called reactive oxygen species, which are charged and that seek vulnerable molecules from which they can "steal" electrons to neutralize their reactive needs, rebalancing the charge like a magnet that attracts a metal.

Such forces can damage molecules from which the electrons are taken. This is an *oxidation reaction*, and your body tries to manage excessive oxidation with internal balancing antioxidant processes called *redox systems* as well as utilizing antioxidants in your diet. Compounds like polyphenols in foods may act as generous donors of electrons to satisfy the free radicals' need for chemical balance. When the human body doesn't have sufficient capacity to control the level of reactive oxygen species with antioxidants then, they may go on to cause oxidative damage to important structures in the body. This may include the protective fats of cell membranes, potentially harmful LDL cholesterol, and cell structures including proteins and DNA. This state is called *oxidative stress*, and the chain reaction of damage without healing can result in a proinflammatory immune response and chronic inflammation.

Identifying what increases inflammation

Certain times during the day you are most at risk of oxidative stress. In addition to external environmental triggers of oxidative stress, such as pollution, smoking, ultraviolet light, and radiation, one of the greatest challenges is much closer to home — the food you eat. With numerous by-products, including free radicals being formed, you need all the antioxidant support you can get.

These foods increase oxidative stress and are proinflammatory:

>> **Processed foods:** Those high in refined sugars and other additives can promote inflammation. These include many fast foods, sugary snacks, and processed baked goods.

>> **Sugary drinks:** Beverages like soda, energy drinks, and sugary fruit juices can cause spikes in blood sugar, which results in a proinflammatory state

>> **Processed meat:** Processed meat, possibly due to the additives, have been associated with inflammation. Red meat without the protection of co-ingredients in a bioactive-rich marinade may also result in a chronic inflammatory state.

>> **Refined carbohydrates:** Foods made with white flour such as white bread and many baked goods cause rapid increases in blood sugar, contributing to inflammation.

>> **Some fats:** Trans fats and some forms of saturated fats may promote inflammation.

>> **Alcohol:** Excessive alcohol consumption may cause inflammation, including, but not limited to, inflammation of the liver.

>> **Artificial additives:** Certain additives have been shown to be proinflammatory, including some artificial sweeteners, the preservative sodium nitrite, and high-fructose corn syrup. Many others are suspected of having these effects.

>> **Vegetable oils:** Certain vegetable oils such as corn, soybean, and sunflower are high in omega-6 polyunsaturated fats. Although these fats are essential in moderation, excess intake, especially when the balance with omega-3 polyunsaturated fats is disrupted, they can promote inflammation. Under heat, these oils may be less stable, producing trans fats and other breakdown products that make foods fried in these oils proinflammatory.

REMEMBER

In recent years, health professionals and public health organizations have advised people to increase consumption of unsaturated fats because of the association between saturated fats, LDL cholesterol, and heart disease. This may have paradoxically resulted in a harmful increase in inflammatory foods especially where high omega-6 vegetable or seed oils are concerned. Researchers are beginning to understand the importance of inflammation in chronic diseases, but for many people exposed to unhealthy vegetable oils and spreads, this may be rather too late.

TIP

Spikes in blood glucose result are proinflammatory. Prediabetes and diabetes are proinflammatory conditions and result in a state of oxidative stress. People with diabetes need to focus on a diet that not only maintains glucose balance but also is rich in anti-inflammatory bioactive compounds.

Researchers are discovering more about foods and their ability to promote or reduce inflammation. Some chemicals in the blood — including C-reactive protein (CRP), interleukin-6 (IL-6), and tumor necrosis factor alpha (TNF-alpha) — are referred to as *biomarkers of inflammation*. Researchers can analyze them to measure inflammation and are compiling lists of foods with their effects on inflammation. Although researchers are in the early stages of understanding the effects fully, they've created a Dietary Inflammatory Index (DII) where diets with processed foods score very poorly in comparison with anti-inflammatory dietary patterns rich in bioactive compounds like the Mediterranean diet.

Reversing inflammation — Plant power

The way to reverse inflammation is where plants come to the rescue. Although many people take them for granted, plants are extraordinary. Eating plant nutrients can reverse harmful chronic inflammation in the body, which may contribute to the prevention of many chronic diseases.

Imagine yourself to be a small apple seed. First, you must survive in the soil. When the time is right, you must appear and spread small leaves to capture the light and warmth of the spring. Your photosynthesis combines the energy from sunlight with carbon dioxide in the air and water from the earth to produce glucose for growth and you release the by-product oxygen.

Your environment can be difficult as you mature — you can't uproot yourself to move to a safer place. You may be destined to live and flourish for many years, even after the animals that eat your fruit and disperse your seeds have seen many generations come and go. You need to protect yourself from the UV light and heat of summers, from the harsh winters, and from reactive oxygen in the air that surrounds you and will threaten your blossom and fruit, browning any exposed flesh and degrading it before it's ready. You also have the challenge of pests, infections, and creatures that may be tempted to take your fruit before your seeds are mature and strong.

The evolutionary response to these pressures is the formation of protective compounds. Although perhaps less necessary for a life in a low-risk environment, in nature these secondary metabolites are essential for health and survival.

REMEMBER

Bioactive compounds can protect and support the plant in several ways. They can

>> Prevent the potentially damaging chemical reactions of oxidation, which is increased with heat and light exposure.

>> Have antimicrobial activity and repel insects, increasing if for imminent danger or the plant is injured.

>> Taste bitter or pungent to deter animals from eating the plant or its fruit, which may lessen as a fruit ripens to maturity if it's designed to be eaten. Alternatively, some plants protect themselves by producing harmful or toxic compounds throughout their life cycle as a long-term survival strategy.

>> Provide color changes to signal to animals when a fruit is ripening and ready for eating, using the animal to spread its seed.

Plants can increase levels of these compounds at times of stress and change the proportions when there's a need to adjust color or taste. Plants can even communicate with each other, often through root and soil ecosystems and neighbors may adapt to warnings from others that a rise in protective compounds may be necessary.

You can see all this in practice in an apple. Polyphenols are concentrated in the exposed outer layers as protection. If you cut open an apple, you can see the processes of oxidation occurring rapidly. An apple changes taste and color through the season as the seed matures and becomes ready for dispersal.

Plants or (plant products such as honey) containing bioactive compounds can support human health with antioxidant, anti-inflammatory, and even antimicrobial effects. Knowing how to recognize the ways to get the best from plant bioactives is a fun and tasty experience!

TIP

Children learn from their parents and social groups at an early age about which plants can be good for their health, including some that are bitter or pungent. Children notice how bioactive compounds like polyphenols can sometimes be bitter, spicy, or pungent. As they learn from their parents and social groups about what's safe to eat, they develop a taste for herbs, spices, and other plants that have interesting flavors and that can provide a variety of bioactive compounds. That's why, especially for most children, broccoli is an acquired taste.

Some evidence suggests people get to like familiarity in what they eat, and that perhaps they're getting used to the dulled-down tastes of processed foods, with added sugars, fats, and salts. The key may be to have as much variety as you can in the plants in your food and drink and to enjoy and explore flavors and tastes you haven't necessarily been used to.

Understanding Bioactives

The following sections discuss the three types of bioactive compounds: carotenoids, glucosinolates, and polyphenols.

Colorful carotenoids

Carotenoids (see Table 4-1) are a group of organic pigments found in plants, algae, and some bacteria. They're responsible for the red, orange, and yellow colors in various fruits and vegetables, such as carrots, tomatoes, and kale. Carotenoids, such as beta-carotene, are important because the human body can convert them into vitamin A, which is essential for vision, immune function, and overall health. Additionally, carotenoids possess antioxidant properties, helping to neutralize harmful free radicals in the body.

TABLE 4-1 **Carotenoids in Foods and Possible Bioactivity**

Carotenoid Type	Food Sources	Potential Health Benefits
Alpha-carotene	Carrots, sweet potatoes, pumpkins, winter squash	Antioxidant, eye health, immune system support
Beta-carotene	Carrots, sweet potatoes, spinach, kale, apricots	Antioxidant, vision health, immune system support, skin health
Beta-cryptoxanthin	Oranges, papayas, peaches, mangoes	Antioxidant, immune system support, joint health
Lutein	Spinach, kale, collard greens, broccoli, avocado	Antioxidant, eye health, brain health, heart health
Lycopene	Tomatoes, watermelon, pink grapefruit, papaya	Antioxidant, heart health, prostate health, skin health
Zeaxanthin	Spinach, kale, collard greens, broccoli, eggs	Antioxidant, eye health, skin health, cognitive function, heart health

Glorious glucosinolates

Glucosinolates (refer to Table 4-2) are sulfur-containing compounds predominantly found in cruciferous vegetables like garlic, broccoli, cabbage, and mustard greens. When these vegetables are chopped or chewed, glucosinolates are broken down into bioactive compounds, including isothiocyanates and indoles. These compounds have been studied for their potential cancer-fighting properties. They may help the body detoxify and eliminate carcinogens, and they also have anti-inflammatory and antioxidant effects.

TABLE 4-2 **Glucosinolates in Foods and Possible Bioactivity**

Glucosinolate	Food Sources	Potential Health Benefits
Gluconasturtiin	Watercress, garden cress, nasturtium flowers	Antioxidant, anticancer properties, respiratory health
Glucoraphanin	Broccoli, cauliflower, brussels sprouts, cabbage	Anticancer properties, detoxification, anti-inflammatory
Glucotropaeolin	Radishes, cabbage, watercress, mustard greens	Antioxidant, anti-inflammatory, anticancer properties
Progoitrin	Brussels sprouts, mustard greens, kale	Anticancer properties, thyroid health, anti-inflammatory
Sinapine	Broccoli, brussels sprouts, mustard seeds	Antioxidant, anti-inflammatory, cardiovascular health
Sinigrin	Mustard seeds, horseradish, wasabi, arugula	Anticancer properties, anti-inflammatory, digestive health

Plentiful polyphenols

Polyphenols (see Table 4-3) are a large group of naturally occurring compounds found in plants. They have antioxidant properties, which means they can help protect the body's cells from oxidative stress and damage caused by free radicals. Polyphenols are abundant in foods such as fruits, vegetables, tea, coffee, red wine, and dark chocolate. Different types of polyphenols include flavonoids, phenolic acids, and lignans. Research suggests that polyphenols may have various health benefits, including reducing the risk of chronic diseases, improving heart health, and supporting brain function.

TABLE 4-3   **Polyphenols in Foods and Possible Bioactivity**

Polyphenol Type	Example	Food Sources	Potential Health Benefits
Flavonols	Quercetin	Onions, apples, berries, broccoli, green tea, capers, citrus fruits	Antioxidant, anti-inflammatory, cardiovascular health, allergy relief
Flavonols	Kaempferol	Kale, spinach, broccoli, green tea, strawberries, fennel	Antioxidant, anti-inflammatory, cardiovascular health, anticancer properties
Flavonols	Myricetin	Berries, grapes, red wine, pomegranate, walnuts, red onions	Antioxidant, anti-inflammatory, brain health, anticancer properties
Flavanols (Catechins)	Epicatechin	Green tea, cocoa, red wine, apples, berries, cherries, pears	Antioxidant, cardiovascular health, blood sugar regulation
Flavanols (Catechins)	Epigallocatechin gallate (EGCG)	Green tea, matcha, apples, berries, cocoa, dark chocolate	Antioxidant, metabolic health, brain health, weight management
Flavanones	Hesperetin	Citrus fruits (oranges, lemons, grapefruits), tomatoes, parsley	Antioxidant, cardiovascular health, anti-inflammatory
Flavanones	Naringenin	Grapefruit, tomatoes, oranges, lemons, grapefruit juice, hops	Antioxidant, cardiovascular health, metabolic health
Flavones	Luteolin	Parsley, celery, chamomile tea, thyme, sage, peppermint	Antioxidant, anti-inflammatory, brain health, anticancer properties
Flavones	Apigenin	Parsley, celery, chamomile tea, artichokes, basil, celery seed	Antioxidant, anti-inflammatory, brain health, anticancer properties

(continued)

TABLE 4-3 *(continued)*

Polyphenol Type	Example	Food Sources	Potential Health Benefits
Anthocyanins	Cyanidin	Blueberries, blackberries, cherries, grapes, cranberries, eggplant	Antioxidant, cardiovascular health, brain health, anti-aging
Anthocyanins	Delphinidin	Blueberries, cranberries, raspberries, blackcurrants, red radishes	Antioxidant, cardiovascular health, brain health, anti-inflammatory
Hydroxybenzoic acids	Gallic acid	Coffee, tea, blueberries, blackberries, strawberries, red wine	Antioxidant, anti-inflammatory, cardiovascular health, anticancer properties
Hydroxybenzoic acids	Protocatechuic acid	Green tea, apples, pears, cinnamon, cocoa, cherry, vanilla	Antioxidant, anti-inflammatory, metabolic health, brain health
Hydroxycinnamic acids	Caffeic acid	Coffee, whole grains, apples, pears, artichokes, lettuce, parsnips	Antioxidant, anti-inflammatory, cardiovascular health, anticancer properties
Resveratrol	Resveratrol	Red grapes, red wine, peanuts, mulberries, dark chocolate, pistachios	Antioxidant, anti-inflammatory, cardiovascular health, brain health
Secoiridoides	Oleuropein, oleocanthal, Tyrosols	Extra-virgin olive oil	Anti-inflammatory, cardiovascular health including oxidation of LDL cholesterol, antioxidant properties
Lignans	Secoisolariciresinol	Flaxseeds, sesame seeds, whole grains, berries, cruciferous vegetables	Antioxidant, hormonal balance, cardiovascular health, anticancer properties
Lignans	Enterolactone	Flaxseeds, sesame seeds, whole grains, berries, cruciferous vegetables	Hormonal balance, anticancer properties, cardiovascular health

Raising Bioactives and Bacteria in the Gut

Bioactive compounds don't simply get eaten, absorbed, and immediately go to work. It's more complicated than that. Researchers are just starting to understand the gut microbiome's role. The *gut microbiome*, a complex community of trillions of microorganisms living in your digestive tract, plays a crucial role in your health. Understanding how the microbiome works and how to keep it in good shape is important.

DOCTOR SAYS

You may see advertisements for supplements that contain extracts of various polyphenols. Unfortunately little evidence supports taking them. There's a big difference between getting bioactive compounds from the natural foods in your diet and taking a concentrated extract in a pill. My advice is to enjoy the tastes, colors, and combinations of polyphenols and other bioactive compounds in healthy, nutritious foods.

Looking at what the gut microbiome does

Polyphenols and other bioactives influence the gut microbiome and vice versa. Scientists are only just beginning to see how crucial this relationship is. Here's an overview of the microbiome's importance:

» **Digestion and nutrient absorption:** Gut bacteria help break down complex carbohydrates and fiber that human digestive enzymes can't process. This breakdown aids in digestion and allows the body to absorb essential nutrients.

» **Immune system support:** A significant portion of the immune system is located in the gut. Beneficial gut bacteria contribute to the development and function of the immune system, protecting against harmful infections and supporting overall immune health.

» **Metabolism and energy regulation:** The gut microbiome influences metabolism, including how the body stores and extracts energy from food. Imbalances in the gut microbiota have been linked to obesity and other illnesses.

» **Production of vitamins and enzymes:** Certain bacteria in the gut produce essential vitamins (like B vitamins and vitamin K) and enzymes that the body can't produce on its own. These substances are critical for various bodily functions.

» **Mental health and brain function:** Emerging research suggests a strong connection between the gut and the brain, often referred to as the *gut-brain axis.* Imbalances in the gut microbiome have been associated with mental health conditions such as depression, anxiety, and even neurological disorders.

» **Protection against infections:** Beneficial bacteria in the gut can prevent harmful foreign microbes from colonizing the intestines. They do this by competing for resources and producing substances that inhibit the growth of harmful microbes.

>> **Influence on chronic diseases:** An unhealthy microbiome has been linked to several chronic diseases, including inflammatory bowel diseases, diabetes, autoimmune disorders, and even certain types of cancer. Research in this area is ongoing, but it suggests a significant role for the gut microbiota in these conditions. A healthy gut microbiome is associated with lower rates of these illnesses.

>> **Response to medications:** Gut bacteria can influence how medications are metabolized in the body, potentially affecting the efficacy and side effects of various drugs.

For more detailed information about your gut health, check out *Gut Health For Dummies* by Kristina Campbell (John Wiley & Sons, Inc.).

Seeing how polyphenols affect the gut microbiome

Maintaining a diverse and balanced gut microbiome through eating a healthy diet, regularly exercising, and avoiding unnecessary antibiotics is crucial for overall health. Research on how polyphenols interact with the gut microbiome is a relatively new and rapidly evolving field, but here are several ways in which polyphenols can influence the gut microbiota:

>> **Prebiotic effects:** Some polyphenols act as *prebiotics,* which means they provide a source of nutrition for beneficial gut bacteria (refer to the next section for more details). These compounds can stimulate the growth and activity of specific beneficial bacteria, such as *Bifidobacteria* and *Lactobacilli*.

>> **Antimicrobial effects:** Polyphenols can also have antimicrobial properties, which means they can inhibit the growth of harmful bacteria in the gut. This selective antimicrobial activity can help maintain a healthy balance of gut bacteria.

>> **Composition changes:** Polyphenols can influence the overall pattern of the gut microbiota. Different polyphenols can favor the growth of specific bacterial species, leading to changes in the diversity and abundance of gut microbes.

>> **Production of short-chain fatty acids (SCFAs):** Gut bacteria ferment dietary fibers and polyphenols to produce SCFAs, which have various health benefits. Polyphenols can influence the production of SCFAs, which play a role in gut health and immune function.

>> **Anti-inflammatory effects:** Polyphenols can change inflammatory pathways in the gut. Chronic inflammation in the gut can disrupt the balance of the microbiota, and polyphenols' anti-inflammatory properties can help maintain this balance.

>> **Improvement to gut barrier function:** Polyphenols have been shown to improve the lining of the gut, which forms a barrier between the gut and the rest of the body. A healthy gut barrier is essential for preventing the passing of harmful substances from the gut into the bloodstream.

REMEMBER

The effects of polyphenols on the gut microbiome can vary depending on the specific type of polyphenol, the dose, and individual differences in gut microbiota composition. The interaction between polyphenols and the gut microbiome is complex and the subject of much ongoing research.

Examining probiotics and prebiotics

Many foods you eat are prebiotics or probiotics. Such foods can support a healthy and diverse gut microbiome. Understanding their effects and where you can find them is important:

>> **Probiotics:** They're live beneficial bacteria that, when consumed in adequate amounts, add to the diversity and health of the microbiome. They can often be found in fermented foods. Examples of probiotic-containing foods include yogurt, some cheeses, kefir, pickles, kimchi, sauerkraut, kombucha, and tempeh.

>> **Prebiotics:** They're nondigestible fibers and polyphenols and other plant compounds that promote the growth and activity of beneficial gut bacteria. They essentially act as food for probiotics, the beneficial bacteria in the gut. Examples of prebiotics are green leafy vegetables, onions, garlic, oats and many other whole grains, fruits, and vegetables.

Combining prebiotics and probiotics from a variety of foods that also contain interacting bioactive compounds is a way to ensure you get the most from your helpful gut microbes that support your health. That's why we talk of the quality of foods rather than just their macronutrient constituents. For example, high quality protein sources include beans and nuts because they're also rich in prebiotic fiber and many type of polyphenols.

EATING THE RAINBOW

You have probably heard the expression "eat the rainbow," which is good advice. Eating these plant polyphenols and other plant compounds gives you the rainbows of colors in your food unless of course it includes ultraprocessed foods like blue bubble gum–flavored ice cream. You need to include a variety of colored vegetables and fruits in your diet. The pigments are often bioactive compounds like carotenoids and polyphenols that can produce yellow, orange, red, purple, and green hues. Often a greater concentration of color means higher concentrations of the antioxidant compounds.

The relationship between color and antioxidant effects was known long before scientists had the science to explain it. A real-world example comes from the United States during the Prohibition Era. A grape variety called *Alicante Bouschet* was known for its thick, heavily pigmented purple skin and the presence of the colors in the grape's flesh. This hardy grape could be transported from California vineyards to the East Coast where it would arrive still in good condition and able to be made into contraband alcoholic drinks. With its high levels of protective polyphenols, the variety had evolved to become particularly hardy and was resistant to oxidation and deterioration. It had thrived in France due to it ability to overcome a common insect blight that had ravaged vineyards. As with many polyphenol-rich fruits, the grape has quite a tannic, robust and pungent flavor as a young wine, and it's likely to be a good source of antioxidant and anti-inflammatory polyphenols if enjoyed in moderation with food, Mediterranean style.

Choosing Bioactive Quality

Knowing something about plant bioactive compounds — the best sources, the colors, taste, and how the plant responds to its environment — means you can choose foods that are likely to have the most beneficial effects.

Here are a few examples of plant bioactive compounds at work:

» Tomatoes grown in sunshine, exposed to natural UV sunlight and warmth, contain higher levels of the carotenoid lycopene than those heavily irrigated and raised in greenhouses for an increased yield.

» Many nuts, cereals, vegetables, and fruits concentrate their protective polyphenols in the outer skin or husks. Oftentimes these skins or husks are edible and can provide an added dose of fiber as well.

Most people don't think about how they can increase the polyphenols in their diets, but it can be very easy to figure out how to recognize polyphenol-rich foods and to incorporate them into your meal planning.

Making polyphenols part of your diet

Foods that are rich in polyphenols are often delicious and add beneficial nutrients, color and flavor to meals.

Here are a few ways you can increase your intake of polyphenols:

» If you enjoy red wine, drink a glass with food (the polyphenols mix and are better) and choose a pungent grape variety like Tannat, Alicante, Malbec, or Durif with plenty of tannins.

» Drink a variety of teas, including herbal teas, and coffee during the day.

» Add herbs and spices, garlic, and chilis to meals to add interesting tasting polyphenols.

» When eating chocolate, eat bitter. Dark, 80 percent or higher cacao, is highest in polyphenols and one you'll come to love the taste!

Getting behind extra-virgin olive oil

The Mediterranean diet has one particularly polyphenol-rich ingredient – extra-virgin olive oil (EVOO). In fact, EVOO is consumed in a quantity matched by no other single food and is a great way to get some unique and very special polyphenols.

People in the region use it not only to cook with, but also to add flavor and texture. EVOO contains many types of polyphenols including the secoiridoids, tyrosols, oleuropein, and oleocanthal. These polyphenols have powerful anti-inflammatory and antioxidant effects and contribute to the many proven health benefits associated with regular consumption of the oil.

Here are some benefits to using EVOO:

» It has substances that reduce inflammation, an important contributor to both cancer and diabetes.

» It prevents heart disease and stroke by lowering bad cholesterol and raising good cholesterol and reducing inflammation.

>> It reduces blood pressure.

>> People who consume higher levels of EVOO have less rheumatoid arthritis and lower rates of dementia.

>> It improves bone mineralization and calcification.

>> It coaxes more nutrients out of the food.

>> It reduces the negative effects of toxins in food.

The olive is a fruit, though botanists would formally class it as a *drupe.* The olive tree produces olives in harsh and challenging environments and responds to stress with fewer, but higher polyphenol olives. The best EVOOs for health are those where the olives are harvested early, where they're exposed to some environmental pressures such as growing in a dry climate with only minimal necessary irrigation, higher altitude, and perhaps without the spraying of pesticides and excess fertilizer use. These oils may be a little more expensive to produce because of decreased yield, but they have the sought-after flavors of fruitiness, bitterness, and pungency, softened by food, and are likely to be high in healthful polyphenols.

Some of the polyphenols in EEVO have been studied to establish how they affect its flavor (see Table 4-4). Some bitterness and pungency is considered a positive taste attribute for a high-quality extra-virgin olive oil and indicates that it is healthy, too, because of these polyphenols.

TABLE 4-4   ## Phenolic Compounds in EEVO

Phenolic Compound	Taste Profile
Hydroxytyrosol	Bitter, pungent, slightly sweet
Tyrosol	Mildly bitter, slightly sweet
Oleuropein	Bitter, pungent, robust, herbal
Ligstroside	Bitter, pungent, slightly sweet
Oleocanthal	Peppery, slightly spicy, tingling sensation
Oleacein	Bitter, pungent, complex, slightly fruity
Verbascoside	Bitter, astringent, slightly sweet
Lignans (such as pinoresinol)	Woody, herbal, slightly bitter
Flavonoids (such as luteolin)	Bitter, astringent, slightly citrusy, herbal

Chapter 5

Choosing Delicious and Healthful Foods

Every trip to the supermarket is an adventure. This chapter is about coping with the challenge of going grocery shopping without being lured into buying items that aren't good for your diabetes nutritional plan. But it's also about overcoming your natural desire to take home what you know isn't good for you.

The good news is that research shows that as soon as you're established on a healthy and nutritious diet and lifestyle, you'll come to prefer it. You'll gradually lose the taste for unhealthy, artificially sweetened, high-salt, and saturated fat processed foods. You'll begin to look forward to nourishing yourself with healthier, homecooked favorite foods, and you'll actively look for great ingredients that help you look and feel your best.

Going to the Supermarket with a Plan

If you have a hobby, you've probably developed a series of steps by which you can accomplish your hobby in the most efficient manner, whether it's painting pictures or raising tomatoes. If you paint pictures, you certainly wouldn't start painting without deciding on a subject and buying the right paints, brushes, and canvas. If you raise tomatoes, you prepare the soil, add amendments such as manure, and buy the seeds or, more likely, the plants. You use a watering system as well as tomato cages to hold up your crop.

Plan your excursion to the market in the same careful manner (the following sections help you do just that). Decide in advance what you need that complies with your nutritional plan. Chapters 2 and 3 look at the nutrients and types of foods that provide excellent nutrition and are best for optimum control of blood glucose. You can use those suggestions to make a shopping list to make sure that you purchase what you need. To that list, add the perishables that you'll use immediately, such as meat and poultry or fish, milk and other dairy products, and, of course, fruits and vegetables.

TIP

Eat something before you go to the market so that you aren't hungry as you walk down the aisles.

Understanding a supermarket's layout

A supermarket is like a huge menu set up to entice you. Most markets are set up in the same way (see Figure 5-1), and this setup isn't by accident. It's arranged to encourage you to buy. What people buy on the impulse of the moment is often the most calorie-concentrated, processed, and expensive food that is least appropriate for their health yet most profitable for the store.

All the perishable food in many supermarkets is arranged around the store's perimeter. The high-calorie foods are in the aisles in the middle of the store. Unless you want to take the long way around, you must go through those aisles to get to the meat, milk, fruit, and vegetables. You pass the loose candies, the cookies, the high-sugar cereals, and all the other no-nos. If you prepare a list and buy only from the list, you won't purchase any of those foods. Walking into the market hungry and without a list is dangerous for your health.

TIP

Sometimes the supermarket employs someone who's trained to help people with medical conditions make the best selections. Check with your grocery store to find out whether such a person is on staff and spend some time touring the aisles with them. You can get some valuable insights that make handling a shopping trip easier.

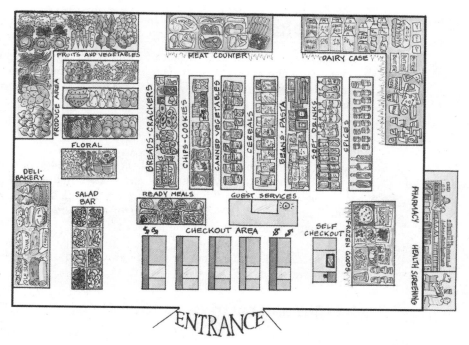

FIGURE 5-1:
A typical
supermarket
layout.

Illustration by Liz Kurtzman

Here are some additional keys to shopping the market most effectively:

>> Shop at the same supermarket each time.

>> Go to the supermarket when it isn't crowded.

>> Don't walk every aisle.

>> Head straight to the areas with the fresh foods — produce, dairy, seafood, poultry, and so on, and skip the processed food aisles as much as possible.

>> Don't be tempted by free samples. They're usually high in calories to appeal to your taste buds.

>> If you bring your kids (we advise that you leave them at home with someone) to the store, make sure that they aren't hungry. If they are, then buy some apples at the express counter before continuing your shopping.

>> Stock up on whole foods, such as fruits and vegetables that are on sale as well as bulk grains, beans, lentils, and good quality extra-virgin olive oil (EVOO) to keep in the pantry.

>> Be especially careful in the checkout lane, where stores force you to run through a gauntlet of goodies — none of which are good for you.

The bakery

Use the bakery section of your store to your advantage. Seek out fresh, whole-grain breads and ask for them to be thinly sliced for you. It's a great idea to purchase whole-wheat pita bread (which you can freeze to use later) as a go-to staple. Some bakeries have fresh multigrain breads, sourdough breads, and whole-wheat bagels and wraps. Skip the other shelved, packaged varieties that are usually highly processed.

TIP

Choose to make your own desserts, such as those in Chapter 12, and skip desserts in the store. They usually contain too much saturated fat and simple carbohydrates; however, you don't have to give up everything. If you enjoy it on occasion, a small portion of a rich dessert as part of an otherwise healthful meal won't derail your overall health goals.

These sections identify some of the items you may encounter when walking through the bakery.

Muffins and pastries

Muffins and pastries are usually high in fat, but in deference to the popular belief that fat makes people fat, stores now sell lowfat muffins and pastries. The problem is that these still contain many calories, high glycemic carbohydrates, and added artificial ingredients, so don't overdo it.

TIP

If you must indulge, try a smaller portion, share your muffin with a friend, or choose something else altogether. A popular choice is angel food cake, but watch out because, even though it's totally fat-free, it's filled with calories.

Breads

A common theme in this chapter is to help you look for indicators of processed foods. Regulating authorities may consider these preservatives safe, but researchers are continuing to discover new and hidden effects — for example, on the human gut microbiome or on the glycemic index. Although the absence of preservatives may reduce the shelf life of a loaf of bread, you can always freeze good quality bread and take out a slice at a time when you need it.

Sourdough techniques and breads made from traditional ancient grains are naturally lower glycemic index so explore rye, spelt, barley, or khorasan breads. Select breads that have at least 2 grams of fiber per slice and whole-grain breads. Bagels and English muffins should be whole-grain as well. Don't forget that they're usually too large, so plan on eating a serving of half or less. (That goes for any bread.)

Breads that are brown in color aren't necessarily whole-grain. They may just have additives like caustic sulfite caramel (E150b) to make them look healthier (this is one of the first tricks of the food industry you may see on your shopping trip). Why not play a game and see if you can spot the next (and the next) trick in the food aisle. Because bread is such a basic item that has been a staple for humankind since the beginning of agriculture, it shouldn't be a heavily processed food but in modern times it usually is. On the same shelf you may find a bread packed with artificial preservatives, sweeteners, stabilizers, thickeners, and gelling agents to change its shelf life or consistency with another bread that's much more simply and naturally produced. This is why we suggest you make your own bread when possible.

Produce

Fruits and vegetables are in the produce section. Vegetables in particular are the foundation of your excellent diet. Stores continue to offer the usual apples, pears, and bananas, but today they stock more fruits and vegetables that you may never have seen before. Here is where you can add some real variety and those all-important natural colors to your diet. Try some of these new items, and you may discover that you can substitute them for the cakes, pies, chips, and other concentrated calorie foods that you now eat. For example, you may find that you like some of the new varieties of melons, which are sweet and have a great texture yet a low glycemic load.

The other benefit to trying new fruits and vegetables is that you get a variety of vitamins and minerals from the different sources. Each differently colored vegetable provides different vitamins, so pick out a variety of colors.

Keep the following in mind as you peruse the produce:

>> Seek good value and interesting and diverse vegetables for every meal, every day of the week. And you don't need to worry about nutritional value in the produce department. For example, you may notice that a carrot doesn't have any nutritional label. It doesn't need one because it's a carrot. There are no tricks here.

>> To prolong their season, you can freeze some of the fruits, especially the berries, and use them as you need them.

>> Remember that dried fruits have very concentrated carbohydrate and can be used sparingly.

>> Choose in-season fruits and vegetables. Seasonal produce is cheaper and contains more of the nutrients that your body needs at that time.

>> Decide when you're going to consume your produce. The ripeness of the fruits and vegetables that you buy depends on your needs. If you're going to eat them immediately, or within a day, buy the ripest you can find. (Each vegetable has a specific ripened period; look up ripeness of each item online.) If you choose to buy produce that you'll be eating the next week, choose items that aren't completely ripe.

>> Save a trip to the store by planning wisely. Some produce naturally stays fresh longer when refrigerated. Apples, oranges, onions, Brussels sprouts, broccoli, cabbage, cauliflower, carrots, celery, radishes, pears, fennel, and beets generally last longer than a week when refrigerated. We like to keep them on hand in case we can't get to the supermarket.

>> Enjoy fruits and veggies in as many ways as possible. Whether or not you buy packaged veggies compared to nonpackaged, such as spinach or carrots, is up to your personal preference. The important thing is to eat fresh produce. Local and organic are the best options.

>> Keep root vegetables, such as potatoes, turnips, onions, and rutabaga separately in a cool, dry place. They don't need refrigeration.

The dairy case

At the dairy case, you can make some very positive diet modifications. Go for the best fermented dairy products such as yogurt, cheeses, or kefir. Remember these important pointers when choosing dairy food:

>> Choose full-fat yogurt (which you can have with a cut-up piece of fruit for breakfast), which is better than a lowfat version that may be flavored with fruit syrup and added sugars.

Although the saturated fat in full-fat yogurt (and cheese) may be flagged as red on the nutritional label, a moderate serving of yogurt each day has been shown to improve blood glucose control and to have no added risk of heart disease.

>> Artisan sheep and goat milk cheese can be very beneficial to your diet, especially the aged varieties. Cheese has beneficial effects on the gut microbiome and is a great source of calcium. Processed cheeses, however, can contain added ingredients like salt, dyes, preservatives, and emulsifiers, so purchase a local, traditional cheese.

The deli counter

We always recommend fresh seafood, poultry, and meat instead of what can be purchased at a deli counter. A simple boiled egg can be a much better choice than the processed luncheon meats, sausages, bacon, frankfurters, meat spreads, and prepared foods offered at deli counters.

WARNING

Recent studies show that these processed meats are dangerous to your health. The World Health Organization (WHO) has classified many preserved meats as carrying a possible risk of cancer, especially bowel cancer, which may be due to the preservatives in combination with the meat proteins. Nitrates occur naturally in vegetables and may well have beneficial effects on your health, but nitrites in preservatives, most commonly in the form of sodium nitrite (E250), may be carcinogenic when the proteins in cooked meats combine to form compounds called *nitrosamines*. Some traditional ham producers only use salt to preserve, which may be healthier than using artificial preservatives as long as people are aware of the levels of salt in their diet overall.

If you choose prepared salads from this area, pick out those that contain EVOO instead of cream. Don't be afraid to ask a deli employee about the exact ingredients in these prepared foods. Typically these prepared foods come in multigallon tubs and are filled with preservatives. Part 2 presents simple recipes that you can make that taste better than deli options.

REMEMBER

A better and healthier option to these deli prepared salads: Buy fresh salad ingredients in the produce department and make your own salad with lettuce, tomatoes, cucumber, peppers, feta cheese, nuts and seeds.

The fresh meat and fish counter

The fresh meat and fish counter provides some good choices for your protein needs. When at the meat counter, consider the following:

>> Buy no more than a normal serving for each family member. Just because the meat attendant has cut a 12-ounce piece of swordfish doesn't mean that you have to buy the whole thing. Some stores give you just the piece you want. If not, wrap and freeze what you don't need to cook that day for another day. Or cook the excess portion and eat it for lunch or dinner the following day.

>> For convenience, you can get two servings at one time if you know you have the willpower to save the second serving for another meal. Ask the attendant to cut the fish in half so you aren't tempted to eat the whole thing. Enjoying plenty of vegetables and EVOO with your meal will ensure that you're satisfied.

>> Buy skinless poultry to eliminate a major source of the fat in chicken. Slow cooking is a great way to preserve juices and maximize flavor with other ingredients.

>> Eat fish at least twice a week because of the positive effect it has on blood fats. Remember that a fish such as tuna or salmon is good for you and contains *Omega-3 polyunsaturated fats,* which are good for heart and brain health as well as for losing weight.

>> If you're a vegetarian or vegan or don't feel like eating meat, you can buy lentils, beans, and other legumes that provide protein and are a powerhouse of other nutrients and fiber.

REMEMBER

The fresh meat and fish counter usually offers breaded or battered fish to make your life easier — you only have to put it in the oven. The problem is that the breading or batter often contains too much butter, fat, artificial ingredients, and salt. Ask the person serving you for a list of the ingredients in the breading or batter. Or better yet, skip the prepared fish and head for the fresh. If you notice a very fishy smell, then the fish isn't very fresh.

Frozen foods and diet meals

When the season for your favorite fresh fruits and vegetables is over, the frozen food section may stock these items. However, because markets now often bring in more varieties of fresh food from all over the world year-round, you may not need to turn to frozen products as much.

WARNING

Food manufacturers are producing a variety of frozen foods, which you can heat in the microwave oven. These meals are often high in unhealthy fat and salt, however. Be sure to read the food label, which we explain in the section "Deciphering the Mysterious Food Label" later in this chapter. Avoid frozen foods mixed with cream or cheese sauces.

Are frozen diet foods a good choice for you? Many patients complain that they lack time to prepare the right foods. For those people, prepared diet meals work very well. For people who like to involve themselves in food preparation — for example, people who bought this book for the wonderful recipes — this isn't the way to go.

Low-carbohydrate foods are also being made by many of the food manufacturers. See our discussion of the various types of diets in Chapter 3 for ways that these foods can fit in your nutrition plan.

Canned and bottled foods

Canned and bottled foods can be healthful and can help you quickly make recipes calling for ingredients such as tomato sauce. Check the Nutrition Facts label (refer to the section "Deciphering the Mysterious Food Label" later in this chapter) to determine what kind of liquid a food is canned in. Unhealthy oil adds a lot of fat calories, so look for the same food canned in water or EVOO. Make sure the list of ingredients is as easy to understand as possible — with natural and recognizable contents.

REMEMBER

The case against sugar and high–fructose corn syrup keeps getting stronger. Not only does it lead to weight gain, but it also increases blood pressure, raises the risk of gout, causes liver damage, and accelerates the aging process. It's not the sugar in fruits and vegetables but also the *added sugar* that the manufacturer inserts during processing and that you add to your diet in the form of sugar, syrup, high–fructose corn syrup, and molasses. Don't buy canned and bottled foods with added sugar and keep your additions to a minimum.

When purchasing canned and bottled foods, consider the following:

TIP

>> Look for low-salt varieties because canned vegetables often contain too much salt. Canned fruits often contain too much sweetener, so you're better off with fresh if possible.

>> Watch for this marketing trick: Stores often display higher-priced canned foods at eye level and lower priced products on lower shelves. Also, store brands are often less expensive and just as good as name brands.

>> Avoid bottled foods that include fruit juice drinks, which are high in sugar and low in nutrition. You're better off drinking pure fruit juice rather than a juice drink diluted with other ingredients.

>> The same principle is true for bottled and canned soda, which has no nutritional value and lots of calories. Substitute water for this expensive and basically worthless food that really doesn't quench your thirst (soft drinks often leave an aftertaste, especially the diet drinks). Try adding lemon or lime to your water.

Snack aisle

You probably frequently feel like eating a little something between meals. Your choice of foods may make the difference between weight gain and weight control, between high blood glucose levels and normal levels. We prefer that you skip the processed snacks in favor of some of these fresh options as well as the recipes in Chapter 7.

Here are the best selections to choose as you make your way around the supermarket:

>> **Fresh fruit:** A typical serving is 60 to 80 calories.

>> **Fresh vegetables:** Carrots, celery, and so forth.

>> **Nuts and seeds:** Unsalted, unroasted almonds, walnuts, pistachios, cashews, sesame seeds, chia seeds, and flaxseeds

>> **Flavored rice cakes:** These items are filling without adding too many calories. But watch out for added preservatives or stabilizers.

>> **Fruit and fig bars:** These items can satisfy hunger without many calories. A couple of fig cookies, for example, will set you back only 120 calories.

>> **Lowfat and low sugar granola:** Watch out for regular granola, which is high in calories. Depending on the brand, ½ cup of lowfat granola contains 220 to 250 calories.

>> **Plain popcorn:** If you prepare it in an air-popping machine or a microwave oven, it contains only 30 calories per cup and is free of salt and fat.

>> **Raisins and other dried fruit or nuts and trail mix:** Stick to small portions. A quarter of a cup of raisins is only 130 calories. A handful of unsalted nuts are a fantastic superfood snack. Add Greek yogurt if desired.

This list should give you enough choices to satisfy your hunger without wrecking your diabetic control.

Herbs and spices

When shopping for herbs and spices, keep these herbs and spices in your kitchen. You can forget you ever needed a saltshaker (remove it from your table while you're at it):

>> **Parsley:** You can add parsley to many dishes to give them a fresher taste, add nutrients, and increase the flavor of other herbs and spices, like the ones in tomato sauce. A salad of lentils, beans, and parsley is a perfect Mediterranean dish. Parsley contains high amounts of vitamins A, C, and K and has anti-inflammatory effects. People in the Mediterranean use it to combat high blood pressure, allergies, and other conditions.

>> **Sage:** Sage has a persistent smell and a lemony, woody flavor, which lends great taste to chicken, eggs, onions, and apples. Sage also goes great in bean dishes. Add it to poultry dishes and roasts. Sage adds delicious taste to fish or

chicken when wrapped together in parchment paper. Some researchers suggest that sage may contribute to improved memory, lower cholesterol, prevent cancer, and improve blood sugar control.

>> **Cilantro:** Cilantro comes from the leaves of the plant *Coriandrum sativum*. The seeds of the same plant make up coriander. Cilantro is said to help balance blood sugar and has aphrodisiac properties. It brings out the flavor of other foods and can be sprinkled on cooked dishes and added to soups. If you don't like cilantro, substitute parsley.

>> **Basil:** Basil is one of our favorite herbs. It's one of the oldest herbs used in Mediterranean cooking and is also said to elevate the mood and regulate blood sugar. Needless to say, basil is also considered an aphrodisiac. Basil has a million uses. You can add it to tomatoes with a little olive oil; use it in pesto sauce; add it to other herbs and spices; include it in soups and stews; and use it with fish, chicken, teas, and on and on.

>> **Pepper:** Pepper is the king of spices. It was the major ingredient in the Mediterranean spice trade for hundreds of years, and in the first century CE one of the main gates to Alexandria, Egypt, was known as the Pepper Gate. There are several colors of pepper from different stages of the same plant, but we're talking about black pepper here.

Black pepper differs from place to place and depending upon where it's grown can have a very different taste. Because it can be added to almost every type of recipe, it's fun to experiment with different types of pepper to add different flavors to your food. We recommend freshly ground pepper because it has a lot of volatile oils, so if it's pre-ground, it loses its aroma quickly. Black pepper boosts the absorption of other spices, such as turmeric, so use them together. Black pepper is anti-inflammatory and has antibacterial and antioxidant properties.

>> **Unrefined sea salt:** The human body actually requires sodium chloride to live. Because processed foods contain too much processed salt, as does a lot of modern cooking, salt has gotten a bad rap. When salt is required in recipes, we recommend small amounts of unrefined sea salt that you can find in most organic and regular supermarkets labelled as unprocessed sea salt. These salts still contain their original mineral content and don't have added chemicals that table salt does. The human body needs these nutrients to properly process sodium, so a little bit can be beneficial unless your doctor specifically suggests avoiding all salt.

REMEMBER

Besides the wonderful tastes that herbs and spices add to your food, they are some of the most concentrated sources of bioactive antioxidant and anti-inflammatory polyphenols. Herbs and spices have been valued for possible medicinal effects for millennia.

TAKING ADVANTAGE OF FARMERS' MARKETS

Modern farmers' markets bring together produce from local farmers with extremely fresh fish and poultry. Take it from us: There is nothing tastier than an heirloom tomato just picked by the farmer and sold to you that day. Many of the farmers have made their farms organic, which means their produce is free from harmful pesticides. Although farmers' markets often include bakeries, you can easily walk past those stands. If you do stop there, opt for delicious, freshly baked whole-wheat breads — they're wonderful on your Mediterranean diet.

The vegetables at farmers' markets have just been picked and are at the peak of their taste — unlike those in the supermarkets, which are grown more for their lasting qualities than their taste. The same is true of the fruits. Compare farmers' market strawberries with supermarket strawberries, and you'll never buy supermarket strawberries again.

The produce you find there can cost a bit more than produce in the supermarkets (but often they cost less!). If the produce does cost more, the difference is worth every penny. Plus, you're supporting local growers and getting the best that money can buy. The produce may be very seasonal, but who says that melons should be enjoyed in January?

The other noteworthy thing about the farmers' markets is the general air of festivity to be found there. Everyone is smiling! Farmers are happy to explain how they grow the produce and which ones they most recommend. If by chance you buy something and it isn't up to your standard, the farmer will likely replace it the next week or give you your money back. And you can taste everything! It's okay to go to the farmers' market hungry — the fruits and vegetables you taste won't hurt you!

As we discuss in Chapter 4, growing foods less intensively means they're more likely to be rich in polyphenols and other bioactive compounds. A tomato grown in full sunlight is exposed to more UV light than a tomato grown in a large glasshouse and tastes much more interesting. Research shows that the concentrations of bioactive compounds such as lycopene may be as much as a third higher.

Identifying the Must-Have Staples

You can set yourself up for success by having the following items in your pantry. Pantries aren't just storage space for things that you purchase in bulk. Up until a century ago, kitchens all over the world required pantries in order to be able to provide balanced meals on a daily basis. Nowadays, a good pantry can set you up for cooking flavorful and nutritious meals in less time than it takes to order takeout.

Stocking your pantry

Most people have been there before — an unexpected guest comes over, something is preventing you from getting to the grocery store to buy fresh ingredients, or maybe you just don't feel like going out or paying delivery fees. An easy, fun, and inexpensive way to stay on top of your health goals is to cook from your pantry. Challenge yourself to come up with the most flavorful meals you can using what you've got on hand.

Here's what we recommend keeping on hand to make last-minute meals a cinch.

» **Cereals, pastas, and grains**

- Barley
- Brown rice — short, medium, and basmati
- Farro
- Millet
- Pearl couscous and smaller grain couscous
- Quinoa
- Stone-cut oatmeal
- Wheat berries
- Whole-wheat pasta (various shapes), preferably slow-dried

» **Beans and legumes**

- Dried and/or no-sodium-added canned chickpeas, black beans, cannellini beans, and your favorites
- Lentils of all varieties: red, green, brown, and black

» **Nuts, dried fruit, and seeds**

- Unsalted almonds, walnuts, pistachios, cashews, pine nuts
- Sesame seeds, chia seeds, flaxseeds
- Dried dates, raisins, unsweetened dried apricots, cherries, and cranberries

>> **Condiments and flavor enhancers**

- EVOO — the freshest and best quality you can find

- Low-sodium tamari

- No-sugar-added mustards

- Spices: allspice, anise seeds, black pepper, caraway seeds, pure Ceylon cinnamon, cilantro, cloves, coriander, cumin, fennel seeds, ground ginger, green cardamom pods, herbes de Provence, marjoram, mint, nutmeg, oregano, paprika, peppercorns, red pepper, saffron, sage, sumac, tarragon, thyme, turmeric, unrefined sea salt, za'atar

- Unrefined coconut oil, if desired

>> **Drinks**

- Coffee

- Teas

- Tisanes (herbal teas)

>> **Canned and jarred goods**

- Artichokes

- Canned or jarred tuna in water

- No-sodium-added jarred vegetables of your choice

- Olives

- Roasted red peppers

- Sardines

REMEMBER

We always prefer fresh, seasonal vegetables when possible. Frozen vegetables are also good to keep on hand. That said, we still advise stocking up on shelf-stable items to carry you through times that shopping isn't possible. Rinse and drain these well before eating and add additional EEVO, herbs, and spices to your taste.

>> **Baking ingredients**

- Almond, soy, or rice milk

- Flours: Almond, whole-wheat, barley, cornmeal

- Leaveners: Baking powder, baking soda, dried yeast

- Raw cane sugar

- Raw honey

- Vanilla extract

AMY'S ANTI-INFLAMMATORY SPICE MIX

This mix tastes great in bean, poultry, meat, and seafood dishes. Use fresh, organic spices for best results. Yield is approximately 1 to 1½ cups and it serves approximately 20.

Follow these easy steps:

1. **Add ½ cup turmeric, ½ cup dried ginger, ¼ cup ground cinnamon, and 1 teaspoon freshly ground black pepper.**

2. **Store in an airtight container in a cool, dark pantry for up to a month.**

Recognizing essentials for the fridge and freezer

You can stock your refrigerator to help keep you on track with nutritional goals and have the ingredients on hand to prepare the recipes in this book.

Here's what we recommend:

>> **Dairy**

- Aged sheep cheese, such as Manchego or pecorino
- Fresh goat cheese
- Plain, full-fat Greek yogurt
- Whole milk or unsweetened almond or rice milk

>> **Produce**

- Aromatics, such as onions, garlic, shallots, celery, carrots
- Cruciferous vegetables, such as cauliflower, broccoli, brussels sprouts
- Fruit, such as apples, berries, clementines, kiwifruit, mandarins, lemons, limes, oranges, pears, pomegranates
- Hearty vegetables, such as cabbage and peppers (they usually last at least a week)
- Leafy greens, such as arugula, collard and dandelion greens, kale, and spinach
- Root vegetables, such as potatoes, rutabaga, turnips

Deciphering the Mysterious Food Label

Most packaged foods have a food label known as the Nutrition Facts label, which isn't really mysterious if you know how to interpret it. It was designed to be understood. Figure 5-2 shows a typical food label. The Food and Drug Administration regulates the contents of the Nutrition Facts label in the United States, and other countries with the equivalent regulating or trading standards organization regulate theirs. The following sections walk you through what the label means and discuss some drawbacks when using this label.

Examining the label

Updates to the U.S. Nutrition Facts label were introduced in 2016 to show the product's percentage of an average maximum recommended saturated fat intake. For example, naturally occurring sugars in the matrix of fiber in fruit have a different effect than added sugars. Presentation of serving sizes and numbers of servings has been improved and references to vitamins and minerals are now included.

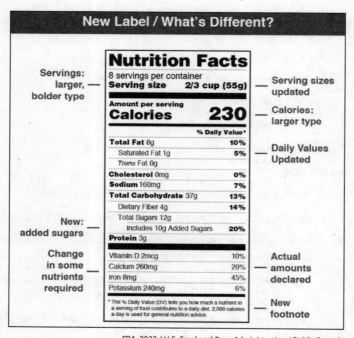

FIGURE 5-2:
A Nutrition Facts food label.

FDA, 2023 / U.S. Food and Drug Administration / Public Domain

Here are a few things that are important when deciphering labels:

>> Remember that ingredients are listed in the order of the amount of the ingredient from highest to lowest.

>> Read the ingredient list first. If the food has high-fructose corn syrup, artificial colors, hydrogenated fats, and artificial sweeteners, or if it isn't made the way you'd make it at home, leave it behind. You can use other products nearby that meet your higher standards.

>> Manufacturers can say many things on the front of food packets within the labeling laws of their country: gluten-free, cholesterol-free, low-sodium, and so forth. Just because it says any of these doesn't mean that the food is healthy.

>> After reading the ingredients list, you need to read the nutrient label to see if you're getting great nutrient density from this food.

You can find similar labels in Europe and elsewhere. Many of them sometimes have voluntary or compulsory traffic light–labeling systems where the amounts of fat, saturated fat, salt, and sugar are highlighted in red, yellow, or green to denote the government view on the healthiness of the product.

For example, the European Union (EU) recommends its member countries adopt the new Nutri–Score system, which grades and colors products from A (green) to E (red) based on an algorithm that computes negative scores for high energy, sugar, salt, and saturated fat along with positive attributes such as fruit, vegetable, fiber, nuts and legume content, and the amount of protein and fiber. This system isn't clear of controversy because the energy content or number of calories in a food may not be the best measurement of how healthy the food is, additives in processed foods including artificial sweeteners don't contribute to the score, and bioactive compounds that may be very beneficial for health aren't included.

Governments must do more to inform consumers of the nutritional value (or hazards) of products in a highly processed food environment which has been described as *obesogenic* — one that tends to result in weight gain in the population, but it's important that the information is accurate and comprehensive.

Considering drawbacks to these labels

Current government regulated ways of labelling nutrition including FDA and European guidelines may have the following flaws and limitations, though it can be argued that they are better than no system at all:

» Total fat levels aren't as important as the types of fats people eat, and perhaps healthy unsaturated fats should be emphasized more.

» Not all saturated fat is created equal, and the saturated fat in dairy products may well have health benefits, yet it may result in a red traffic light warning.

» Artificial sweeteners give a reassuring green to the sugar column of a traffic light–labelling system, but the WHO described them as potential cancer-causing chemicals.

» The EU Nutri-Score may indirectly measure important micronutrient and bioactive compounds like polyphenols by the vegetable content. Most other nutritional labels don't specifically recognize them.

» The list of added ingredients may be extensive in processed foods. Some evidence may suggest that they might potentially harm, but that's often not represented on food labels. For example, if a food contains toxic substances created from the way in which it's manufactured, the label doesn't reveal that information.

A high consumption of ultraprocessed foods is associated with an increased risk of chronic illnesses including diabetes, but many of the artificial ingredients aren't included in nutrition labels. Researchers don't yet know whether that's because of a combination of high saturated fat, added sugars, and salt or whether it also relates to the addition of artificial preservatives and stabilizers and a lack of bioactive compounds.

Some countries allow specific and regulated health claims on some foods that fulfill the often-demanding requirements of health claims legislation. For example, it includes foods high in unsaturated fat or fiber in the United States and Europe. The EU has an authorized health claim for EVOO, which contains a specified minimum level of certain polyphenols that have beneficial health effects on LDL cholesterol.

Making Sense of Ingredients Lists

Although nutrition labels can be useful, probably more revealing is the list of ingredients. Most countries require this list be published in smaller print with items listed in the order of quantity that they appear in the product.

TIP

Even if you're in a hurry in the supermarket, pay special attention to the ingredients list. Nutrition labels list the macronutrients and some micronutrients in the product, whereas the ingredient list must provide details about everything that goes into the product. This list can be revealing about the product.

For example, a margarine spread advertises that it contains olive oil, but on closer scrutiny you notice that the olive oil is refined with a tiny percentage of EVOO. Furthermore, the product contains numerous artificial additives to provide color, emulsifiers and stabilizing agents to give the product consistency, and preservatives to prolong shelf life.

Every food ingredient in countries like the United States must be considered safe for human consumption, but as history shows, researchers and consumers may not yet know some of the effects of new additives and preservatives on health. Eating only what you recognize as a natural ingredient is common sense. Keep to the unprocessed foods familiar in the Mediterranean and other heritage diets.

2

Healthy Recipes That Taste Great

Chapter **6**

Breakfast Dishes

An Italian adage says, "Good morning! Today's a new day. Try your best and make it a masterpiece." It's their belief that the right mindset and an appealing breakfast is a great way to ignite your inspiration and balance your blood sugar while enjoying yourself in the process. A big part of keeping your blood sugar steady is eating regularly. Typically, the longest break without food during a day comes at night. While your body rests and revitalizes itself, your blood glucose level takes a nosedive. Starting each day the right way with a healthy balanced breakfast is one of the greatest ways to improve your health.

Breakfast is a subject of love, intrigue, misunderstanding, and debate to many. In this chapter, we explain what a delicious and nutritious breakfast can look like while giving you ideas for quick breakfasts and offering other options for when you have a bit more time to linger over breakfast.

DOCTOR SAYS

Research has shown that eating a substantial breakfast in the morning can reduce your appetite throughout the day and help you lose weight. One study showed that overweight women with metabolic syndrome (a cluster of conditions including high blood pressure, high blood sugar, high cholesterol, and too much body fat around the waist) were able to lose weight and belly fat better by eating a big breakfast than by following a conventional 1,400-calorie diet. The larger breakfast was also shown to prevent diabetes and heart disease. Additional research has shown that those individuals who eat a big breakfast burn twice as many calories as those individuals who eat a larger dinner. Eating a big breakfast has also been linked to improved mood and metabolism, as well as making better food choices throughout the day. Starting the day with 30 grams of protein is actually recommended by neuro-therapists for optimal brain function.

Be sure to read the Note in each recipe to find out about its nutritional values. Also refer to the book's Introduction for some recipe conventions we use.

Understanding Diabetes-Friendly Breakfasts

Breakfast is a critical meal, particularly for people with diabetes. Getting your day off to a steady, balanced start sets you up for success the rest of the day. Check out Part 1 if you need help planning your meals for the day based on your individual needs. The following sections can help you make the right breakfast choices.

Breakfast recipes are always the most challenging for me (Amy) to write. It's not that they're difficult per se, but people have very different issues of what constitutes a proper breakfast. People's personal breakfast preferences also vary greatly, even within the same cultures. Many people like sweet breakfasts, some like to enjoy big breakfasts leisurely, others like savory breakfast items, and others only eat breakfast if it can be prepared quickly and consumed on the go.

Breakfast foods and styles also vary from culture to culture. Americans and Northern Europeans enjoy Italian egg dishes at breakfast time that are eaten for lunch and dinner in Italy. Similarly, they often enjoy the hearty Middle Eastern bean-based dishes such as fuul and falafel for lunch and dinner, normally eaten in their native cultures at breakfast time. For this reason, in this chapter I include recipes that fit each of those needs and can also be enjoyed at snack time in smaller quantities or with a salad and some lean protein for lunch or dinner.

You may want to choose a combination of quick yogurt, almond, and fresh fruit if you're in a hurry, or you can try a scrambled egg and whole-wheat toast with some vegetables. Even leftovers from a nutritious lunch or dinner can make a satisfying and savory breakfast option. Brush up on the recipes in this chapter for inspiration to fit each and every type of morning. Whether you're eating on the go, can enjoy alone, or have the time to savor a truly leisurely breakfast with others, there's something to suit your style and please your palate.

By planning ahead, you can utilize these recipes to make a delicious breakfast that fits well into your diabetes-friendly meal plan and busy schedule. The recipes come with a warning, though! Some are so tasty that you may want to enjoy them at other times of the day as well!

Getting the most out of your breakfasts

Regardless of what type of foods that you eat or when, keep these guidelines in mind:

>> Choose healthful fats, good quality carbohydrates, and proteins that are low in fat. Not all nutrients are created equal.

>> Make sure that good sources of all three macronutrients (protein, fat, and carbohydrate) are present in each of the meals that you consume.

>> Choose organic, clean ingredients as much as possible.

>> Aim for 9 to 12 servings of fresh produce per day. The majority of your meals should be based on fresh vegetables and some fruit.

>> Try to eat larger meals earlier in the day, such as at breakfast or lunch, and keep your evening meal a bit lighter.

One of the reasons why people often skip breakfast is because their day is already harried enough and they can't find the time to cook or eat something that's already prepared. If the thought of making breakfast while you're trying to get the kids off to school is too much or you have a long commute and have to be out the door bright and early, you're not alone. Maybe you're just not a breakfast person or you'd rather spend the time sleeping 15 more minutes, exercising, or meditating.

Whatever your reason for not wanting a long, drawn-out breakfast, the following list is for you. Here are some grab-and-go breakfasts to have on hand:

>> A serving of Greek yogurt with fruit or crudites

>> A handful of almonds and an orange

- A serving of *labneh* (strained Middle Eastern yogurt cheese) and a piece of whole-wheat pita bread with dates

- A hardboiled egg, a handful of walnuts, and a piece of aged cheese

- A serving of whole-milk ricotta with a drizzle of local honey

- A serving of overnight or rolled oats with fresh fruit

- A serving of fresh fruit salad with a few tablespoons of Greek yogurt

- A smoothie made out of ½ cup Greek yogurt, 1 ripe banana, ½ cup strawberry slices, and a few ice cubes

Instead of turning to fast food or sugary cereals on a busy morning or skipping breakfast even though you're really hungry, keep these formulas and foods on hand to carry you to lunchtime. Enjoy them with a sense of gratitude and look forward to whatever part of your day brings you the most joy.

Figuring out which fruit is right for you

We are amazed at the number of people who omit fruit from their diets after they're diagnosed with diabetes. Even those patients who continue to eat foods that aren't healthful believe that fruit will be especially harmful to them. The truth is that even though you shouldn't eat fruit in copious amounts, a serving of fresh fruit (especially if it's from the list in this section) along with a handful of plain nuts and/or a serving of plain Greek yogurt is always a better meal or snack option than processed, fast, and junk foods.

Although fruit is full of natural sugars and your body processes them quickly, you don't have to (and shouldn't) mark them off your list completely. Fresh and dried fruits (with no sugars added) offer a wide spectrum of vitamins, minerals, and antioxidants that are beneficial to the body as a whole. Choose these fruits that you most enjoy and rotate them so that you're consistently eating the rainbow, that is, enjoying fresh fruits and vegetables with a wide variety of colors.

Whole fruit, rather than juice, is a better choice for everyone, and especially those with diabetes. The fiber and skin in whole fruit slow down the digestion of the fruit, resulting in a more gradual rise in your blood sugar level.

TIP

Don't overlook nutritious fruit, especially those with a low glycemic index (GI) for dessert instead of sugar coated alternatives. Remember to buy organic fruits and vegetables when possible and to clean them properly with a produce–cleaning agent (such as a mixture of water and distilled vinegar or a nontoxic version from a health food store) so that you can enjoy their skins when appropriate.

Here's a list of fruits with a lower GI (which we discuss in more detail in Chapter 2):

- » Apples
- » Apricots
- » Blueberries
- » Cherries
- » Grapefruit
- » Grapes

- » Kiwifruits
- » Oranges
- » Peaches
- » Pears
- » Plums
- » Strawberries

And just for balance, here are a few fruits with a higher GI:

- » Bananas
- » Cantaloupes
- » Dates
- » Mangoes

- » Pineapples
- » Raisins
- » Watermelons

REMEMBER

Just because a certain fruit has a higher GI doesn't mean you can't eat it. Just take it into consideration when you plan when you eat it and what you eat with it. Plan to eat smaller amounts of high GI foods.

Kiwifruit, Mandarin, and Pomegranate Salad with Yogurt

PREP TIME: 5 MIN	YIELD: 2 SERVINGS

INGREDIENTS

½ cup (112g) Greek yogurt (organic and sheep or goat milk if possible)

1 ripe kiwifruit, halved, peeled and sliced into thin rounds

1 mandarin, peeled and segmented

¼ cup (44g) pomegranate seeds

1 tablespoon (7g) ground flaxseeds

1 teaspoon (7g) raw honey

DIRECTIONS

1 Dollop ¼ cup of the yogurt over each plate. Arrange ½ of the kiwifruit around the border of 1 side of yogurt on each plate. Arrange ½ of the mandarin around the border of the other side of each plate.

2 Sprinkle ½ of the pomegranate seeds and top the yogurt with ½ of the flaxseeds. Drizzle ½ teaspoon of honey over each plate and serve.

TIP: Blend the salad for a quick and nutritious breakfast smoothie on the go. This dish is fun to make with kids and can be prepared the night before, if necessary. Just hold off on adding honey until serving.

NOTE: The addition of yogurt to fruit reduces the glycemic load and increases satiety. Pomegranate seeds, also called arils, have polyphenols called ellagitannins and flaxseeds have omega-3 fats.

NOTE: Figure 6-1 shows how to seed a pomegranate.

PER SERVING: *Calories 147 (From Fat 43); Fat 5g (Saturated 2g); Cholesterol 0mg; Sodium 24mg; Carbohydrate 22g (Dietary Fiber 4g); Protein 7g. Sugars 16g.*

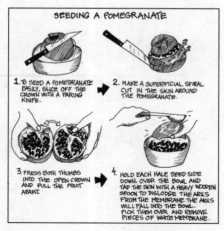

SEEDING A POMEGRANATE

1. To seed a pomegranate easily, slice off the crown with a paring knife.

2. Make a superficial spiral cut in the skin around the pomegranate.

3. Press both thumbs into the open crown and pull the fruit apart.

4. Hold each half, seed side down, over the bowl and tap the skin with a heavy wooden spoon to dislodge the arils from the membrane. The arils will fall into the bowl. Pick them over and remove pieces of white membrane.

FIGURE 6-1: Seeding a pomegranate.

Illustration by Liz Kurtzman

Summer Berry and Seed Yogurt Parfaits

INGREDIENTS

1 cup (148g) blueberries, blackberries, and strawberries

½ cup (72g) plain, unsalted, whole almonds

1 cup (224g) Greek yogurt

2 tablespoons (28g) chia seeds

1 tablespoon (9g) sesame seeds

2 teaspoons (14g) raw honey

1 teaspoon (2g) ground cardamom

DIRECTIONS

1 Place ½ of the berries and almonds in 2 bowls. Pour the yogurt over the top.

2 Scatter 1 tablespoon chia seeds and ½ teaspoon of sesame seeds and ½ of the honey over each bowl's contents.

3 Sprinkle the cardamom over the top of each bowl and serve.

TIP: This parfait can do double duty as a healthful dessert. To serve it after a meal, whisk an additional tablespoon of honey, a teaspoon of pure vanilla, and a dash of cinnamon into the yogurt before using it. Serve in pretty dessert bowls, custard cups, or martini glasses.

NOTE: For the berries, you can use one kind of berry at a time, two types, or a combination of all three — blueberries, blackberries, and strawberries.

NOTE: When in season, fresh peaches, plums, and cherries also taste great in this recipe. Raw (unprocessed) honey contains antibacterial compounds, and sesame seeds are a great source of fiber and contain the lignan compound pinoresinol that may help regulate blood glucose as well as other antioxidant and anti-inflammatory polyphenols.

VARY IT! Blend the ingredients together the night before for a nutritious breakfast or snack on the go!

PER SERVING: *Calories 471 (From Fat 276); Fat 31g (Saturated 6g); Cholesterol 0mg; Sodium 46mg; Carbohydrate 35g (Dietary Fiber 12g); Protein 21g. Sugars 18g.*

Banana Beauty Smoothie

PREP TIME: 5 MIN	YIELD: 2 SERVINGS

INGREDIENTS

2 cups (480ml) unsweetened, plain, full-fat kefir

1 tablespoon (10g) flaxseeds

½ cup (72g) fresh strawberries

1 overripe banana

1 cup (250ml) ice

DIRECTIONS

1 Place all the ingredients into a blender and blend on high until smooth and creamy.

2 Pour into 2 glasses and serve cold.

NOTE: This is called a beauty smoothie because it contains ingredients that are said to be particularly beneficial to the hair and skin. Strawberries are a great way to get more fiber, vitamin C, and healthy cancer-preventing polyphenols into your diet. Bananas are rich in vitamin A, B, and E, making them powerful agents that are often applied directly on the skin as masks. The presence of live cultures along with lactic acid, zinc, and other minerals and enzymes in yogurt make it a great choice for improving skin condition as well as improving your gut microbiome. Flaxseed was cultivated in Babylon as early as 3000 BCE and contains a high amount of omega-3 fatty acids.

VARY IT! Plain Greek yogurt can be used in place of kefir in this recipe if desired.

VARY IT! Any fresh fruit — pomegranate arils, berries, apples, oranges, or a combination — can be used. Be sure to choose fruits like cherries, grapefruit, and apples that have a lower GI for best results.

PER SERVING: *Calories 242 (From Fat 94); Fat 10g (Saturated 5g); Cholesterol 30mg; Sodium 127mg; Carbohydrate 30g (Dietary Fiber 4g); Protein 10g. Sugars 21g.*

Morning Fruit, Nut, and Cheese Platter

PREP TIME: 5 MIN	YIELD: 2 SERVINGS

INGREDIENTS

1 apple or pear, sliced into quarters

¼ cup (36g) whole plain, unsalted almonds

¼ cup (36g) unsalted walnut halves

2 ounces (55g) whole-milk ricotta or goat cheese

2 soft Medjool dates, or your favorite dates

1 teaspoon (7g) raw honey

DIRECTIONS

1 Arrange the apple or pear, almonds, walnuts, cheese, and dates in separate sections on a serving platter.

2 Drizzle the cheese with honey and serve.

TIP: Substitute your favorite fresh fruit from the list of low GI fruits earlier in this section when they're in season.

TIP: Choose plain, unsalted nuts. You can make this platter to enjoy the next morning or as an on-the-go snack. Just be sure to slice the apple or pear at the last minute to avoid browning or drizzle them with lemon juice and turn to coat. Nuts are an integral part of the Mediterranean diet with unsaturated fats, fiber, and many antioxidant and anti-inflammatory polyphenols. They're an important source of essential micronutrients like iron, potassium, selenium, zinc, magnesium, and copper.

VARY IT! In addition to creamy ricotta and soft goat cheese, you can also use 2 ounces of aged Parmigiano-Reggiano or Manchego cheeses, which also offer a good source of calcium, protein, and vitamins.

PER SERVING: *Calories 358 (From Fat 190); Fat 21g (Saturated 4g); Cholesterol 14mg; Sodium 26mg; Carbohydrate 39g (Dietary Fiber 7g); Protein 10g. Sugars 30g.*

Moroccan-Style Avocado and Citrus Smoothie

PREP TIME: 5 MIN   YIELD: 2 SERVINGS

INGREDIENTS

1 ripe avocado, peeled and pitted

1 cup (240ml) cold water

½ (120ml) cup ice

½ cup (48g) ground almonds

2 mandarins, peeled and seeds removed

DIRECTIONS

1 Place all the ingredients into a blender and blend on high until smooth and creamy.

2 Pour into 2 glasses and serve cold.

NOTE: Traditionally, fresh, homemade almond milk is used in this recipe instead of the water, ice, and ground almonds. Because it can be difficult to find natural almond milks without a lot of sweeteners and additives, I (Amy) altered this recipe. However, if you have a clean source of almond milk, you can use 1 cup instead of the water and ground almonds.

NOTE: Morocco is full of fresh juice stands. Each seasonal fruit is pressed into delicious, added sugar-free drinks on demand. Some people like to mix orange juice with the avocado as well, but I enjoy it in its pure form. Avocados are an all-round healthy fruit containing monounsaturated fats, rich in vitamins B, C, E, and K along with minerals and bioactive carotenoid compounds.

VARY IT! You can use any fresh fruit — bananas, pomegranate seeds, berries, apples, oranges, or a combination — in this recipe. Be sure to choose those like cherries, grapefruit, and apples that have a lower GI for best results.

PER SERVING: *Calories 304 (From Fat 211); Fat 23g (Saturated 3g); Cholesterol 0mg; Sodium 10mg; Carbohydrate 24g (Dietary Fiber 8g); Protein 6g. Sugars 10g.*

Putting together protein-packed punches

In the United States and many countries around the world, eggs are an important breakfast staple. Remember, however, that even though eggs offer a multitude of health benefits, they aren't the only breakfast protein. In fact, many people with diabetes and other health complications must limit their intake of cholesterol, and eggs are an easy target for removal. We recommend eating a serving of eggs or egg whites on a regular basis unless a nutritional professional has instructed you otherwise. (Check out the section "Enjoying Egg-ceptional Dishes" later in this chapter for smart ways to include eggs at breakfast.) Consider the many other protein choices when you're deciding which breakfast items you'd most like to enjoy.

Here's a list of protein-rich foods that might make a good addition to your breakfast table if you like sweet breakfasts:

>> Plain Greek yogurt with a serving of low GI fresh fruit from the list in the previous section

>> 2 tablespoons of peanut butter on whole-wheat toast

>> Handful of plain almonds or walnuts with a serving of warm quinoa and fresh berries

>> Steel cut oats with protein powder, topped with berries

>> A smoothie with 8 ounces milk (regular or unsweetened almond, oat, or rice), 2 tablespoons nut butter, and berries or other low GI fruit

If you like savory breakfasts, here are some options:

>> A serving of homemade hummus or other beans with whole-wheat pita

>> One 4-ounce grilled chicken breast or fish fillet with vegetables

>> ½ cup lentils with fresh or steamed broccoli, EVOO, and lemon juice

>> ¼ cup cottage cheese with diced grape tomatoes

Starting with Whole-Grain Goodness

Whole grains can and should be a part of each of your diabetes-friendly meals. Steel cut oats, quinoa, barley, bran, bulgur, millet, organic whole wheat berries, and brown rice should be your grains of choice on a regular basis.

When you received your diagnosis of diabetes, maybe you thought your days of eating waffles and pancakes were over. Although starting the morning off with pancakes dripping with butter and maple syrup probably isn't in your current eating plan, you can still enjoy equally mouthwatering treats in the morning on occasion, especially if you use whole grains and the recipes in this book.

When purchasing bread, choose those that are truly 100 percent whole, unprocessed grain. Baking your own bread, when time permits, is a wonderful way to spend time engaging in an ancient ritual, save money, and enjoy healthful grains more often. Refined grains are processed to remove the bran and the hull, and along with them, up to 90 percent of the nutrients, including vitamins E and B. Whole grains have a lower GI than refined grains, so whole grains are less likely to send your blood glucose soaring and then dipping. The protein, fat, and fiber in whole grains slow their absorption into the bloodstream. In addition, whole grains make you feel fuller and stay fuller longer.

TIP

When buying processed foods, read labels carefully to ensure that the food you're getting is made from whole grains. Don't just look for "wheat" bread; make sure it says "whole wheat." By law, bread can be called "whole wheat" in some places, and only actually contain a percentage of whole-wheat flour mixed with all-purpose or refined flour. In addition, some manufacturers add caramel color or molasses to refined flour and sell the bread as "wheat bread," potentially confusing hopeful healthy eaters. Choose the food with more fiber.

Pink Beet Hummus and Avocado Toast

| PREP TIME: 10 MIN | COOK TIME: 2 MIN | YIELD: 4 SERVINGS |

INGREDIENTS

4 slices good quality whole-wheat, barley, or oat bread

4 teaspoons (20ml) Amy Riolo Selections or extra-virgin olive oil, divided

1 cup (168g) cooked beets

¼ cup (60g) tahini

¼ cup (56g) Greek yogurt

⅛ teaspoon (.6g) salt or fleur de sel

2 ripe avocadoes, halved and pitted

DIRECTIONS

1 Toast the bread in a toaster or under the broiler to desired doneness.

2 Drizzle ½ teaspoon of olive oil over each piece of toast.

3 Place the beets in a food processor. Add the tahini, Greek yogurt, and salt to the food processor. Pulse the food processor on and off. Add water, tablespoon by tablespoon, to get an extra-creamy consistency (you should need less than ¼ cup in total). Scrape down the sides of the food processor and puree for 1 to 2 additional minutes, or until extremely creamy. Taste and adjust seasoning if necessary.

4 Slather ¼ of the beet dip across each piece of toast. Scoop the avocado out of the shell and place the flesh from each half of the avocado on each piece of toast. Drizzle the remaining olive oil, approximately ½ teaspoon, on each piece of toast. Sprinkle with salt and serve warm.

NOTE: Refer to the color insert for a photo of this dish.

PER SERVING: *Calories 449 (From Fat 275); Fat 31g (Saturated 5g); Cholesterol 0mg; Sodium 367mg; Carbohydrate 40g (Dietary Fiber 12g); Protein 10g. Sugars 6g.*

COOKING BEETS AHEAD OF TIME

To prepare the beets for this recipe, preheat your oven to 425 degrees F. Scrub the beets well with a vegetable brush and prick them. Place them on a baking sheet or in a roasting pan and cook until tender (approximately 30 to 45 minutes depending on size). Allow to cool, then peel, and use. Cooked beets last up to a week in the refrigerator, so cook more than you need and use them at a later date.

I also cook potatoes, sweet potatoes, and pumpkin at the same time to make the most of the energy, space in the oven, and my time. That way I have cooked recipes ready to go throughout the week when I need them.

🍅 Warm Quinoa with Raspberries and Cocoa Almond Cream

PREP TIME: 10 MIN	COOK TIME: 15 MIN	YIELD: 2 SERVINGS

INGREDIENTS

½ cup (85g) dry quinoa, rinsed

2 teaspoons (4g) plain, powdered cocoa (unsweetened), fair trade certified, if possible

1 teaspoon (5ml) pure vanilla

½ cup (120ml) unsweetened almond milk

2 teaspoons (7g) pure raw honey

1 cup (148g) fresh raspberries or blueberries

2 tablespoons (18g) raw sesame seeds

DIRECTIONS

1 Bring 1 cup of water to a boil in a medium saucepan over high heat. Add the quinoa, cocoa, and vanilla, stir, reduce the heat to low, and cover. Allow to simmer until all the liquid is absorbed, about 10 to 15 minutes. Remove from the stove and allow to cool completely.

2 Stir in the almond milk and honey to sweeten, if desired.

3 Place the quinoa in 2 bowls, top with the raspberries and sesame seeds and serve warm.

TIP: Quinoa (see Figure 6-2) is considered a complete plant protein, so it's a great alternative to meat, fish, and dairy for lunch. Prepare it in advance to toss into salads like this recipe, or eat it with a few berries, nuts, and a drizzle of cinnamon and honey with almond milk for breakfast.

NOTE: Warm quinoa puts a surprising spin on breakfast, and the addition of cocoa adds rich, chocolaty taste and antioxidants. Raspberries contain anthocyanin and ellagitannin polyphenols with blueberries rich in flavonoid and stilbene polyphenols. Cocoa is rich in polyphenols including catechins and procyanidins. Cocoa beans contain as much as 8 percent polyphenols by dry weight.

PER SERVING: Calories 282 (From Fat 73); Fat 8g (Saturated 1g); Cholesterol 0mg; Sodium 4mg; Carbohydrate 47g (Dietary Fiber 7g); Protein 9g. Sugars 13g.

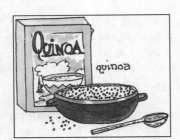

FIGURE 6-2: Quinoa.

Illustration by Liz Kurtzman

Whole-Grain Waffles with Warm Apple Spice Compote

PREP TIME: 5 MIN | COOK TIME: 10 MIN | YIELD: 2 SERVINGS

INGREDIENTS

1 egg

2 teaspoons (10ml) pure vanilla extract, divided

¼ cup (60ml) organic milk or almond milk

1 tablespoon (7g) milled or ground flaxseeds

1 cup (120g) barley or whole-wheat flour

Pinch salt

½ teaspoon (2.3g) baking soda

2 teaspoons (9.4g) unsalted butter, melted, or extra-virgin olive oil, for waffle maker and compote

2 fresh apples, diced

1 teaspoon (2g) ground pure cinnamon

¼ teaspoon (.5g) ground cloves

1 teaspoon (5ml) pure vanilla extract

2 tablespoons (42g) raw honey

DIRECTIONS

1 In a medium bowl, whisk together the egg, vanilla, and milk. Stir in the flaxseeds, flour, salt, and baking soda, mixing well to combine. If the batter seems too thick, add water, a tablespoon at a time (it may take up to ½ cup), to make the batter a consistency of a slightly thicker than normal pancake batter.

2 Heat 1 teaspoon butter in a large wide skillet over medium-high heat. Add the apples and toss to coat with butter. Cook, stirring often, for 5 to 10 minutes, uncovered, until they begin to soften. Sprinkle the cinnamon and cloves over the apples and stir in vanilla and honey.

3 Brush the waffle maker with the melted butter or oil. Pour approximately ⅓ cup of batter onto the hot maker. Using a spoon, spread the batter to the corners before shutting the lid.

4 Cook until the waffles are puffy and golden, about 3 to 5 minutes. Spoon apple compote over the warm waffles and serve immediately.

NOTE: Waffle makers vary from manufacturer to manufacturer, so test yours out — both to find out exactly how much batter you need to make the proper-sized waffle on your iron and to check the amount of time it takes to accurately cook the waffles. Some waffle makers have lights to tell you when the iron is preheated and when the waffles have finished cooking.

NOTE: Refer to the color insert for a photo of this recipe.

TIP: Make extra waffles and freeze them in airtight plastic bags to use at another time.

PER SERVING: *Calories 474 (From Fat 98); Fat 11g (Saturated 2g); Cholesterol 109mg; Sodium 132mg; Carbohydrate 89g (Dietary Fiber 13g); Protein 14g. Sugars 38g.*

Creamy Bulgur, Peach, and Almond Bowls

PREP TIME: 10 MIN	COOK TIME: 5 MIN	YIELD: 2 SERVINGS

INGREDIENTS

½ cup (70g) fine bulgur (cracked wheat)

1 cup (240ml) water

1 teaspoon (5ml) pure vanilla

2 teaspoons (14g) pure raw honey, if desired

½ cup (120ml) unsweetened almond milk

2 ripe peaches, pitted and cut into bite-sized pieces

2 tablespoons (19g) raw almonds, finely chopped

½ teaspoon (1g) pure ground cinnamon

DIRECTIONS

1 Place the bulgur in a large glass bowl and bring 1 cup of water to a boil in a medium saucepan over high heat.

2 Pour the boiling water over the bulgur and cover with a plate.

3 Allow to sit for 8 to 10 minutes, or until the water is absorbed and the bulgur is tender. Add the vanilla, honey, and almond milk and stir.

4 Stir in the peaches and almonds. Sprinkle with cinnamon and serve.

TIP: Keep bulgur in the cupboard for quick meals. Because it doesn't require actual cooking, it's great to make and enjoy in the warmer months — in fact, it's my (Amy) go-to summer cereal.

NOTE: Bulgur is a whole grain rich in fiber, known to be associated with a healthy gut microbiome that reduces the risks of colon cancer and heart disease and helps to regulate blood glucose levels. Bulgur also has plenty of minerals and vitamins. In fact, bulgur is the same form of wheat that's used to make traditional tabbouli salad with lots of parsley, diced tomatoes, and cucumbers.

VARY IT! If you have more time or want to enjoy a warm cereal with the same flavors, cook barley, rice, or whole wheat berries and prepare them the same way. Swap the peach for other low GI fruits.

PER SERVING: *Calories 237 (From Fat 54); Fat 6g (Saturated 0g); Cholesterol 0mg; Sodium 6mg; Carbohydrate 43g (Dietary Fiber 10g); Protein 8g. Sugars 13g.*

🍅 Blueberry and Almond Pancakes

INGREDIENTS

½ cup (56g) almond flour

¾ cup (90g) whole-wheat flour

¼ cup (56g) Greek yogurt

2 teaspoons (9g) baking powder

½ cup (120ml) whole milk or almond milk

1 teaspoon (5ml) vanilla extract

3 egg whites

1 teaspoon (4.7g) butter

DIRECTIONS

1 In a medium bowl, combine the almond flour, whole-wheat flour, Greek yogurt, baking powder, milk, vanilla, and egg whites and mix well to combine.

2 Whisk until smooth. If the batter is very thick, add in more milk, a tablespoon at a time, until it's the consistency of a slightly thin cake batter.

3 Coat a large, wide skillet with the butter; place over medium heat until hot. Spoon ¼ cup batter for each pancake. Sprinkle a few of the remaining ½ cup of blueberries on top.

4 When bubbles form on top of the pancakes, turn them over. Cook until the bottom of each pancake is golden brown. Serve with blueberry syrup.

Syrup

INGREDIENTS

2 cups (296g) fresh blueberries, or frozen berries, thawed, divided

1 teaspoon (2g) cinnamon

1 tablespoon (21g) honey

1 teaspoon (5ml) almond extract

½ cup (120ml) water

DIRECTIONS

1 Place 1½ cups blueberries, cinnamon, honey, almond extract and ½ cup water in a medium saucepan over medium-high heat. Stir with a wooden spoon and bring to a boil.

2 Reduce the heat to low, and simmer, uncovered, for 5 to 10 minutes until the blueberries burst and a thick syrup is formed. Remove from the heat and set aside.

PER SERVING: *Calories 267 (From Fat 93); Fat 10g (Saturated 2g); Cholesterol 6mg; Sodium 61mg; Carbohydrate 37g (Dietary Fiber 6g); Protein 12g. Sugars 15g.*

☺ Oatmeal with Berries, Cocoa, and Almonds

PREP TIME: 10 MIN	COOK TIME: 15 MIN	YIELD: 2 SERVINGS

INGREDIENTS

1 cup (240ml) water

½ cup (88g) steel cut oatmeal

1 teaspoon (5ml) pure vanilla

2 teaspoons (4g) plain, powdered cocoa (unsweetened), fair trade certified, if possible

2 teaspoons (14g) pure raw honey

½ cup (120ml) unsweetened almond milk

1 cup (148g) fresh raspberries or blueberries

2 tablespoons (19g) raw sesame seeds

DIRECTIONS

1 Bring 1 cup of water to a boil in a medium saucepan over high heat. Add the oatmeal and vanilla, stir, reduce heat to low, and cover. Allow to simmer until all the liquid is absorbed, about 10 to 15 minutes. Stir in the cocoa.

2 Remove from the stove. Stir in the almond milk and honey to sweeten, if desired.

3 Place the oatmeal in 2 bowls and top with raspberries and sesame seeds. Serve warm.

TIP: Steel cut oats are the best option for people with diabetes because they're the least processed version of oat groats available. They also have a lower GI than quick- or slow-cooked rolled oats.

NOTE: Cocoa adds a decadent flavor profile to standard oats, but you can leave it out of the recipe. Cocoa not only contains important poly-phenol antioxidants, but it also provides a sense of fullness, which helps to regulate appetite though the day. Oatmeal, in addition to being low GI, low in saturated fat, and high in fiber, contains beta glu-can, which can help lower cholesterol and blood glucose. Some almond milks contain preservatives, but many are available with just almond and water. Try to choose a clean almond milk.

VARY IT! Make the oats in advance and then store them overnight. In the morning, add almond milk, fruit, and seeds, if desired.

PER SERVING: *Calories 295 (From Fat 71); Fat 8g (Saturated 1g); Cholesterol 0mg; Sodium 5mg; Carbohydrate 51g (Dietary Fiber 9g); Protein 3g. Sugars 14g.*

Stocking Up on Baked Goods

Baking can be one of the greatest pleasures of life. Unfortunately many people associate the ancient ritual of baking with many people's modern addiction to sugar and unhealthful foods. Actually, though, the more that you indulge in baking wholesome items instead of buying ones whose ingredients can't be traced, the better off you'll be. Baking from scratch allows you to choose the quality of ingredients that you use, prevents the need for chemicals and additives, and provides a great creative outlet. Recent studies even show how baking can be a mood elevator. If you've ever wanted to bake, now is a great time to start.

Having diabetes doesn't mean you have to deprive yourself of the ease (and deliciousness!) of grabbing a muffin, biscuit, or slice of quick bread. Plan ahead and keep some of these heart-healthy handfuls on hand for breakfast on the go.

TIP

We help you ease into using whole grains in this section by using a blend of almond, barley, and whole-wheat flour. You can find whole-wheat flour in the baking aisle in just about any grocery store, and you can order specialty flour online.

Chocolate Zucchini Nut Bread

PREP TIME: 12 MIN	COOK TIME: 45 TO 60 MIN	YIELD: 20 PIECES

INGREDIENTS

1 teaspoon (5 ml) Amy Riolo Selections or extra-virgin olive oil

½ cups (180g) whole-wheat flour

1 cup (112g) almond flour

¼ cup (24g) cocoa powder

½ cup (158g) pure maple syrup

½ cup (46g) chopped, unsalted almonds

1 teaspoon (2g) cinnamon

1 teaspoon (5ml) pure vanilla extract

2 teaspoons (9g) baking powder

2 egg whites

1 cup (244g) unsweetened applesauce

½ cup (112g) Greek yogurt

2½ cups (310g) grated zucchini

DIRECTIONS

1 Preheat the oven to 350 degrees F. Oil 2 loaf pans, 9 x 5 inches or 8 x 5 inches.

2 In a large bowl, combine the whole-wheat flour, almond flour, cocoa powder, maple syrup, almonds, cinnamon, and baking powder.

3 In another medium bowl, combine the egg whites, applesauce, and yogurt. Mix in the zucchini. Then combine with the flour mixture.

4 Pour the mixture into the loaf pans. Bake 45 minutes to 1 hour. Insert a toothpick in the center of the loaf. When it comes out clean, the bread is done. Cool in the pan for 5 minutes and then cool completely on a wire rack.

NOTE: Zucchini is a versatile and healthy vegetable with plenty of fiber, minerals, and vitamins, especially B6, which may help to regulate blood glucose. It also contains polyphenols such as zeaxanthin and lutein, which reduce oxidative stress and may have anticancer effects.

NOTE: You can also make muffins with this same batter; just line 2 (12 whole) muffin tins with paper liners and fill each well ¾ full. Bake at 350 degrees F for 20 to 25 minutes, or until a toothpick inserted into the center comes out clean.

TIP: Don't bother peeling the zucchini before grating it. Just wash it and grate away.

VARY IT! If you aren't concerned with high cholesterol, use 3 whole eggs instead of 6 egg whites in this recipe.

PER SERVING: Calories 118 (From Fat 45); Fat 5g (Saturated 1g); Cholesterol 0mg; Sodium 10mg; Carbohydrate 16g (Dietary Fiber 3g); Protein 4g. Sugars 7g.

🍅 Homemade Whole-Grain Bread

PREP TIME: 20 MIN PLUS 1 HR FOR RISING	COOK TIME: 30 MIN	YIELD: 18 PIECES

INGREDIENTS

2½ cups (600ml) warm water

1 tablespoon (12g) active, dry yeast

2 teaspoons (14g) honey

1 teaspoon (5g) salt

6 cups (720g) barley flour, or whole-wheat flour, or a combination of the two, plus extra for kneading

4 teaspoons (20ml) Amy Riolo Selections or extra-virgin olive oil, divided

3 teaspoons (9g) sesame seeds

DIRECTIONS

1 In a large bowl, add the warm water. Sprinkle the yeast over the water and mix until dissolved. Allow to sit for 5 minutes to make sure that the yeast is actively working. When bubbles appear on the top, add the honey and salt.

2 Gradually mix in 6 cups of flour, with a wooden spoon, adding up to 2 more cups, 1 cup at a time, if needed, until the dough pulls away from the side of the bowl.

3 When the dough becomes a ball, place it on a flour-dusted surface and knead until smooth, about 5 to 10 minutes (refer to Figure 6-3). Roll the dough into a 12-inch log; then divide into three equal pieces.

4 Shape each piece into a 4-inch dome-shaped loaf. Grease a baking sheet with 1 teaspoon of the oil. Place the loaves on the baking sheet. Cover with a kitchen towel and place in a draft-free area to rise until doubled, about 1 hour.

5 Preheat the oven to 350 degrees F. Uncover the loaves and brush each loaf with 1 teaspoon olive oil, and sprinkle with 1 teaspoon sesame seeds.

6 Bake until lightly golden, about 20 to 30 minutes. Let cool slightly and serve warm.

NOTE: The ingredients list calls for 6 cups of flour, but the amount that you need depends on how finely milled the flour is, as well as the temperature and humidity level of the room that you're baking in. I've used up to 8 cups of flour when baking it on humid days.

NOTE: This bread is great for any meal, breakfast or not. It also makes a good accompaniment to most main dishes and small plates in this book.

(continued)

NOTE: Preparing your own bread gives you mastery over its ingredients, and you can always ensure that it's low GI and rich in vitamins and minerals with healthy flour including flours from ancient grains. You can avoid the unnecessary and unwanted added ingredients sometimes found in processed breads.

VARY IT! If you happen to be able to find millet flour, you can always make it in this recipe. Millet bread was a daily staple of the ancient Greek philosopher Pythagoras, who in addition to mathematics, taught nutrition, music, and philosophy at the school he founded in Crotone, Italy in the sixth century BCE.

PER SERVING: *Calories 152 (From Fat 18); Fat 2g (Saturated 0g); Cholesterol 0mg; Sodium 107mg; Carbohydrate 30g (Dietary Fiber 5g); Protein 6g. Sugars 1g.*

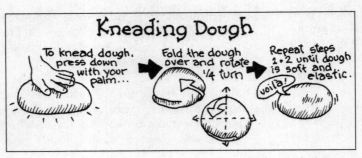

FIGURE 6-3:
Knead dough by pressing, folding, and rotating it.

Illustration by Liz Kurtzman

THE BOUNTY OF WHOLE-GRAIN BREADS

In the United States, more and more people are eliminating bread from their diets for fear that it isn't nutritious and healthful. Like all other foods, however, it's important to decipher the good from the bad. Ultraprocessed bread made with unpronounceable ingredients, poor quality processed bleached wheat, artificial sweeteners, and preservatives isn't good for anyone, let alone individuals who have been diagnosed with diabetes or are trying to avoid it.

We are fans of wholesome, homemade, and artisan breads that allow you to enjoy its flavors and textures without any unwanted ingredients. Baking bread is therapeutic and allows you to control the ingredients that you put into the bread that you eat. If you're not a baker, choose the most wholesome versions of bread that you can find, and be sure to enjoy it in small quantities along with protein and healthful fats in order for it to not cause a spike in blood sugar.

Here are some types of breads to seek out:

- 100 percent whole grains (whole wheat, barley, teff, rye, millet, oat)

- Those with sourdough or natural starters

- Varieties that are free of additional sweeteners and other additives

- Breads that are sold fresh in a bakery and not those that are packaged for long shelf lives

Enjoying Egg-ceptional Dishes

"Better to have an egg today than a chicken tomorrow!" This Italian proverb is the equivalent to the English "A bird in the hand is better than two in the bush" saying. In addition to their ease of use, eggs are an inexpensive, versatile, and nutritious ingredient.

REMEMBER

Choosing eggs gives you a protein power punch to start your day. In fact, one egg contains 7 grams of high-quality protein, only 75 calories, and 1.6 grams of saturated fat and many nutrients such as minerals, vitamins, iron, lutein, and carotenoids.

This simple food also contains all essential amino acids. Eggs are also a source of B complex vitamins, vitamins A, D, and E, selenium, and zinc. However, egg yolk (the yellow center) also contains a significant amount of cholesterol. Consequently, low-cholesterol diets restrict the number of eggs allowed each week. People with diabetes should limit their eggs to a couple per week for the same reason.

Eggs are a staple in the Mediterranean diet. People in the southern European portion of the region eat them strictly for dinner, and sometimes lunch, whereas the North African and Middle Eastern countries also eat them for breakfast. Although they were traditionally viewed as a meat substitute in many countries because of their lower cost, many Mediterranean egg dishes are so savory that they're often preferred over meat. For best results, use organic eggs from pasture-raised chickens. Regardless of when you choose to serve them, these egg-based dishes will quickly become family favorites.

TIP

One great way to enjoy eggs but limit your cholesterol is to enjoy egg whites, use a combination of whole eggs and egg whites, or enjoy them on occasion. Because the egg yolk contains the dreaded cholesterol, limiting your intake of yolks may be enough to keep egg whites on your list.

Baking egg pies and quiches

These baked breakfast egg dishes are a great way to make delicious, healthy meals for a group. They're a great choice for elegant brunch entertaining or a weekday when you have a little extra time. Alternately, you can make a pie or quiche, cool it completely, and then cut it into individual servings and freeze them for later.

Portobello Mushrooms with Poached Egg Florentine

PREP TIME: 10 MIN	COOK TIME: 25 MIN	YIELD: 4 SERVINGS

INGREDIENTS

4 fresh Portobello mushrooms, cleaned and trimmed

1 tablespoon (15ml) Amy Riolo Selections or extra-virgin olive oil

2 ounces (55g) goat cheese

4 eggs

¼ cup (56g) Greek yogurt

⅛ teaspoon (.6g) salt

1 tablespoon (15ml) fresh lemon juice

⅛ teaspoon (.6g) pepper, to taste

Handful of fresh baby dill, or your favorite combination of herbs, reserving a few pieces for garnish

3¼ cups (100g) fresh baby spinach

DIRECTIONS

1 Heat the oven to 425 degrees F. Place the mushrooms, gill-side up, on a baking tray. Drizzle with olive oil and bake for 10 minutes, or until eggs are cooked through.

2 Remove from the oven and top each with ¼ of the goat cheese (about ½ ounce), using a knife to slather it across the top.

3 To poach the eggs, bring a pot of water to a gentle boil, then salt the water. With a spoon, begin stirring the boiling water in a large, circular motion. When the water is swirling like a tornado, add the eggs. Cook for about 2½ to 3 minutes. Using a slotted spoon, remove the eggs and place them on a dish lined with a paper towel.

4 Combine the yogurt, salt, lemon juice, pepper, and dill in a blender, or whisk by hand until smooth and creamy and set aside.

5 Wilt the spinach by heating a large wide skillet over medium heat. Add the spinach and stir quickly for 1 to 2 minutes until it releases water and cooks down. Divide the spinach among each of the 4 mushroom caps. Place a poached egg on top of each.

6 Spoon a ¼ of the sauce on top of each mushroom and garnish with extra dill or other herbs and serve.

NOTE: This recipe combines the classic "Florentine" notions of a poached egg with spinach and a sauce and adds powerful nutritional benefits by using a Portobello mushroom for "toast" and a yogurt, citrus, and herb-based sauce instead of the classic Hollandaise made with butter and egg yolks. Mushrooms are an excellent nutritional source of vitamin D, which is otherwise made through your skin's exposure to light — and people often don't get quite enough especially in temperate climates.

PER SERVING: *Calories 191 (From Fat 121); Fat 13g (Saturated 5g); Cholesterol 222mg; Sodium 219mg; Carbohydrate 6g (Dietary Fiber 2g); Protein 13g. Sugars 3g.*

Baked Italian Eggs with Tomatoes, Garlic, and Herbs

PREP TIME: 15 MIN	COOK TIME: 15 MIN	YIELD: 4 SERVINGS

INGREDIENTS

2 tablespoons (30 ml) Amy Riolo Selections or extra-virgin olive oil, divided

1 pint (298g) cherry tomatoes (yellow, orange, and red if possible, halved)

1 clove garlic, minced

Handful fresh basil

2 cups (40g) baby arugula or kale

4 eggs

⅛ teaspoon (.6 g) salt

1 teaspoon (.6 g) pepper or to taste

DIRECTIONS

1 Preheat the oven to 425 degrees F. Heat 1 tablespoon olive oil in a large skillet over medium-high heat. Add the cherry tomatoes and stir to coat and cook, about five minutes, or until slightly tender. Add the basil and arugula and cook for an additional 5 minutes until greens are tender.

2 Line an 8-inch square glass baking dish or 4 ovenproof rame-kins with the remaining tablespoon of olive oil. Pour the tomato mixture into the bottom of the dish or divide evenly among the ramekins.

3 Make 4 wells in the mixture and break the eggs into each (or place one in each ramekin). Season with salt and pepper.

4 Bake, uncovered for 5 to 10 minutes, or until eggs are set. Remove from the oven and serve warm.

TIP: The flavor of the cherry tomatoes really enhances this dish; if they aren't in season, use diced, no-salt-added, boxed, or jarred tomatoes, or leftover tomato sauce.

TIP: When you're short on time, but want a delicious and nutritious dish, do like the people in Italy do — they serve this dish as part of a light dinner with salad or greens and cheese.

NOTE: Tomatoes are a fantastic source of the carotenoid lycopene, which has been studied for its possible anticancer effects particularly prostate cancer. Green herbs including basil (arugula is classified as a lettuce but is similar) are rich in antioxidant polyphenols; garlic and onions contain anti-inflammatory glucosinolates and polyphenols like quercetin. For the benefits of EVOO, see Chapter 4.

NOTE: You can find a photo of this recipe in the color insert.

VARY IT! You can use any leftover vegetables or tomato sauce instead of the cherry tomatoes in this dish. If you're watching your cholesterol, use 2 or 3 egg whites instead of whole eggs per serving.

PER SERVING: *Calories 147 (From Fat 108); Fat 12g (Saturated 3g); Cholesterol 212mg; Sodium 135mg; Carbohydrate 4g (Dietary Fiber 3g); Protein 7g. Sugars 1g.*

Smoked Salmon and Eggs Toast

PREP TIME: 5 MIN	COOK TIME: 12 MIN	YIELD: 4 SERVINGS

INGREDIENTS

4 slices good quality whole-wheat, barley, or oat bread

4 teaspoons (20 ml) Amy Riolo Selections or extra-virgin olive oil, divided

8 ounces (224 g) smoked salmon

4 eggs, or 8 egg whites

½ cup (75g) cherry tomatoes, halved

⅛ teaspoon (.6 ml) salt or fleur de sel, plus extra for water

⅛ teaspoon (.6 ml) pepper, to taste

DIRECTIONS

1 Toast the bread in a toaster or under the broiler to desired doneness. Drizzle ½ teaspoon of olive oil over each piece of bread. Place 2 ounces of smoked salmon on top of each piece of toast.

2 To poach the eggs, bring a pot of water to a gentle boil and then salt the water. With a spoon, begin stirring the boiling water in a large, circular motion. When the water is swirling like a tornado, add the eggs and cook for about 2½ to 3 minutes.

3 Using a slotted spoon, remove the eggs and place one on top of each piece of toast.

4 Heat a small skillet over medium–high heat, add remaining 2 teaspoons of olive oil. Add the cherry tomatoes and stir to coat. Cook for 2 to 3 minutes until warm and the tomatoes release their juices.

5 Plate the toasts on a platter and transfer the tomato mixture to a bowl on the same platter. Sprinkle with salt and pepper and serve warm.

TIP: Serve this simple toast as lunch or dinner paired with a green leafy salad.

NOTE: Smoked salmon is an easy and nutritious option alternative to processed lunch meats. Salmon contains healthy omega-3 polyunsaturated fats, and the black pepper not only enhances flavor but also adds health benefits.

VARY IT! Use hardboiled egg slices or scrambled eggs, or Greek yogurt to make this dish even easier. If avocados aren't ripe or are too pricy, substitute sautéed fresh spinach, collards, or kale.

PER SERVING: *Calories 309 (From Fat 130); Fat 14g (Saturated 3g); Cholesterol 225mg; Sodium 733mg; Carbohydrate 25g (Dietary Fiber 3g); Protein 21g. Sugars 3g.*

Mediterranean Egg, Vegetable, and Pita Plate

PREP TIME: 5 MIN	YIELD: 2 SERVINGS

INGREDIENTS

2 Persian cucumbers or 1 English cucumber, sliced

2 Roma tomatoes, sliced

1 handful fresh mint or parsley, or a combination of both, cleaned

½ cup (112g) Greek yogurt

2 hardboiled eggs

2 tablespoons (30 ml) Amy Riolo Selections or extra-virgin olive oil

⅛ teaspoon (.6 ml) salt

1 whole-wheat pita, cut into quarters

DIRECTIONS

1 On two separate plates or a large platter, arrange the cucumber slices and tomatoes in a decorative pattern on half of the plate. Add the fresh mint and/or parsley to the center of the plate.

2 Dollop the Greek yogurt on one quadrant of the plate.

3 Slice the hardboiled eggs into quarters and place next to the yogurt.

4 Drizzle the egg and labneh with olive oil and sprinkle with sea salt. Serve with warm pita triangles (2 per person).

TIP: Serve this quick and nutritious Middle Eastern power plate as a great portable lunch or dinner. Assemble it in plastic containers the night before and store in the fridge to make it easier to transport.

NOTE: Tomatoes and cucumbers are a fantastic combination. The plentiful polyphenols and carotenoids in tomatoes are complemented by the lignan class of polyphenols found in cucumbers, which have potential anticancer effects and may add protection against cardiovascular disease.

VARY IT! Use a combination of your own favorite vegetables and cook the egg in a different way if you choose.

PER SERVING: *Calories 374 (From Fat 204); Fat 23g (Saturated 5g); Cholesterol 212mg; Sodium 384mg; Carbohydrate 30g (Dietary Fiber 4g); Protein 16g. Sugars 7g.*

Trying your hand at omelets

Omelets are among the best and easiest ways to get a burst of protein to start your day. In this section, we give you one flavorful recipe to keep your taste buds hopping.

FACING FACTS ABOUT FETA CHEESE

If you haven't tried this terrific Greek cheese, here's your chance. It's a soft, salty cheese that has a tangy bite. It crumbles very easily and is an easy addition to salads, eggs, or stuffed in olives. The commercially available variety is made from cow's milk and sold in small squares, usually in plastic tubs covered in plastic wrap. You can find it in the gourmet or specialty cheese section of your local grocery. If you're up for a little more searching, you can purchase traditional Greek feta, or a similar product made with a combination of sheep and goat milk cheese in many places. Cheeses made with sheep and goat milk contain more calcium and phosphorous than cow's milk cheeses.

Feta is lower in fat and calories than many aged cheeses yet contains more calcium than many other cheeses, which is great for bones and teeth. As a fermented food, it also contains powerful probiotics that are good for bones and gut health. Conjugated linoleic acid found in feta is also believed to help promote weight loss. Sheep and goat milk contains shorter chain saturated fats — those that are less likely to cause a rise in harmful LDL cholesterol.

One of the best things about feta is its tangy flavor profile that enhances simple, vegetable-based recipes. A little can go a long way. So if you're looking for flavor but don't want to weigh down your food with lots of cheese and fat, feta's a good choice. Look for flavored feta cheese for a change of pace. You can find it blended with sun-dried tomatoes and basil, and peppercorns.

Spinach, Kale, and Feta Cheese–Filled Omelets

PREP TIME: 5 MIN	COOK TIME: 10 MIN	YIELD: 2 SERVINGS

INGREDIENTS

1 tablespoon (15 ml) Amy Riolo Selections or extra-virgin olive oil

1 small yellow onion, diced

1 cup (30g) chopped spinach

1 cup (40 g) chopped kale

¼ cup (15g) finely chopped fresh herbs (parsley, basil, oregano, dill, mint, or your choice)

2 whole eggs

4 egg whites

½ cup (75g) crumbled plain Greek feta cheese

1 small plum tomato, chopped

DIRECTIONS

1 Add the olive oil to a large, wide skillet and place over medium heat. Sauté the onion until tender, stirring occasionally, about 6 minutes.

2 Add the spinach and kale and cook until wilted, about 4 minutes. Stir in the herbs.

3 In a medium bowl mix the eggs and egg whites. Pour the egg mixture over the spinach and kale mixture in the skillet. Cook over low heat, stirring occasionally until the eggs are almost cooked.

4 Top with the feta cheese and tomatoes and cover until the eggs are puffy, about 5 minutes. Fold the omelet in half and serve.

NOTE: Leafy green vegetables like spinach and kale are a fabulous source of nutrients — fiber for cardiovascular disease prevention and a healthy microbiome, potassium to normalize blood pressure, and folate that has been shown to protect against heart attacks and strokes. Vitamins, including A, C, and E, as well as minerals and many polyphenols add to the well-known benefits.

TIP: Leftover omelets make great sandwiches when layered between slices of whole-grain bread. Use whichever greens or leftover vegetables that you have to make this quick meal any time.

VARY IT! If feta cheese isn't your favorite, substitute whole-milk ricotta or a bit of goat cheese instead.

PER SERVING: *Calories 341 (From Fat 183); Fat 20g (Saturated 8g); Cholesterol 245mg; Sodium 640mg; Carbohydrate 20g (Dietary Fiber 3g); Protein 22g. Sugars 12g.*

» **Preparing snacks in advance**

» **Adding dips and sauces to snacks**

» **Preparing mini meals**

» **Including base recipes to save calories and money**

Chapter **7**

Successful Snacking

Healthful snacking is the best way to get you started in balancing your blood glucose throughout the day. By eating a snack that contains the three macronutrients — carbohydrates, protein, and fat — along with powerful antioxidants, you can avoid the dips and surges in blood sugar levels that are caused by going for long periods without eating. Many people, however, have difficulty prioritizing the preparation of snacks, and they often skip them.

In this chapter, we give you many great choices for healthful snacking, whether you're traveling, working outside the home, or spending the day inside. Look here for enticing new ways to enjoy simple snacks throughout the day, sensational salsa recipes with tips for creating your own varieties, and a great selection of dips and dippers — no need to skimp on taste. Just remember to choose appropriate portion sizes and pace yourself. You have a whole lot to enjoy.

Be sure to read the Note in each recipe to find out about its nutritional values. Also refer to the book's Introduction for some recipe conventions we use.

Enjoying Snacks

People with diabetes have a common misconception that they need to eat less. Those individuals trying to watch their weight, especially if not following a plan prepared by a nutrition professional, often attempt to go longer periods without meals, skip snacks, and in general try to avoid even thinking about food. This approach can be harmful.

In addition to walking and physical exercise, eating the proper snacks in between meals can give you the energy that you need to keep your body performing at optimal levels. Begin thinking about food as your friend, which can help you achieve your health goals and provide pleasure. These snack ideas are high in healthier unsaturated fats and include a variety of nuts, whole grains, fruits, and vegetables. The focus on using good-quality extra-virgin olive oil (EVOO) and eating high-fiber foods is especially important for people with diabetes.

REMEMBER

All people get energy from the food they eat. Food is made up of fat, protein, carbohydrate, and vitamins and minerals. It's up to you to choose the most nutritious forms of those components. When you eat, your body converts the carbohydrate to glucose, which then enters your bloodstream. The cells in your body use this glucose for energy to fuel your bodily functions. Even though all nutrients have an impact on blood glucose, carbohydrates have the biggest impact, so people with diabetes need to eat the proper amounts of carbohydrates and to balance them with other healthful ingredients.

Consuming three large meals a day can lead to spikes in blood glucose with dips several hours afterwards. More frequent, small meals and snacks create a healthier blood glucose profile avoiding the highs and lows (see Figure 7-1).

FIGURE 7-1: Blood glucose levels with intermittent large meals and more frequent smaller meals or snacks.

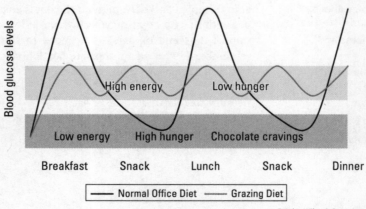

© John Wiley & Sons, Inc.

Keeping healthy snacks at the ready

Creating a plan to keep snacks on hand is an easy way to feel full longer, enrich your diet with additional nutrients, and take charge of your health.

TIP

Here are a few tips to remember:

>> Never leave home without water and a simple snack — even if it's just a handful of raw nuts and a few raw veggies or a piece of fresh fruit.

>> Wash fruit and vegetables upon purchase and store in the refrigerator for ease of use.

>> Keep your refrigerator, cupboards, and freezer stocked with snackable items such as those that are used in the recipes in this chapter (see the nearby sidebar about shopping).

>> Make salads in advance and store them without dressing in the refrigerator for a quick snack.

>> Prepare hummus, lentil dip, kale chips, and spiced edamame and chickpeas in advance and store in individual size portions to grab and go.

>> Keep plain, full-fat Greek yogurt in single servings on hand as a great snack because it contains all three macronutrients.

>> Set aside a few minutes before bed each night to either prepare or make a note of which snacks to take with you or enjoy at home the next day.

SNACK SHOPPING LIST

Keep these items on hand to whip up snacks in minutes:

- **Dairy:** Plain Greek yogurt, cottage cheese, plain yogurt
- **Fresh fruit:** Apples, bananas, kiwifruit, oranges
- **Fresh vegetables:** The more the merrier, especially if you're talking about the green leafy kinds: celery, carrots, cherry tomatoes, broccoli and cauliflower heads, edamame, cucumbers, fresh kale, spinach, corn, arugula, lettuces
- **Pantry:** Almond butter, black beans, roasted red peppers, flaxseeds, red lentils, sesame seeds, dried dates, chickpeas, good-quality EVOO, tahini sauce, unsalted raw almonds, walnuts

Mixing it up with vegetables and fruits

Whether you have diabetes or not, basing your diet on mostly plant-based foods is always a good idea. Remember to search for fresh, seasonal produce and eat a wide variety of colors (remember the rainbow) daily. When planning snacks, always start with fresh vegetables and fruit because they help you get additional servings in each day.

DOCTOR SAYS

I (Simon) met one of the most respected researchers of the Mediterranean diet, Professor Antonia Trichopoulou. She said, "In Greece we eat three times the quantity of vegetables in comparison with the UK and United States. It is not necessarily that we Greeks like vegetables any more than you, but we enjoy them with delicious and abundant extra-virgin olive oil."

REMEMBER

We're not talking about the starchy vegetables — such as beans, peas, lentils, corn, and potatoes — that really belong in the starch list of exchanges, but rather the vegetables that contain much less carbohydrate. These vegetables include asparagus, bok choy, green beans, cabbage, carrots, cauliflower, chard, collards, kale, arugula, spinach, Brussels sprouts, broccoli, peppers, carrots, cucumbers, onions, summer squash, turnips, and water chestnuts.

Use these vegetables for snacks and in meals. They fill you up but add very few calories. Some are just as good when frozen and defrosted as they are when fresh (because they're flash frozen immediately after picking). Especially good snack vegetables include baby carrots, cucumbers, and pieces of sweet pepper. Your cart at the market should reflect the Mediterranean diet pyramid with an emphasis on fresh vegetables and fruits.

Here we share a simple yet tasty toast, fruit salad, and regular salad that diners of all ages will enjoy. Chapter 9 is dedicated to salads, so flip there for additional ideas for snacking.

🍎 Apple and Almond Butter Toast

PREP TIME: 2 MIN	COOK TIME: 2 MIN	YIELD: 2 SERVINGS

INGREDIENTS

2 slices whole-grain bread (consider Homemade Whole-Grain Bread in Chapter 6)

2 tablespoons (32g) organic, unsweetened almond butter

1 medium apple, cut into thin slices

DIRECTIONS

1 Toast the bread until desired doneness.

2 Slather with almond butter.

3 Top with apple slices.

NOTE: Almond butter is very healthy, containing healthy fat, proteins, minerals, and antioxidants, as long as it's simply made from almonds. Choose 100 percent almond butter and avoid additives, salt, and especially palm oil.

TIP: This snack is quick to prepare but best not prepared in advance because the apple might discolor. Gala and Red Delicious apples work best in this recipe, but feel free to swap out your favorite.

VARY IT! Skip the toasting step or use gluten-free rice cakes as a base for the almond butter and fruit. Swap the apple for pear or kiwifruits as desired. Top with ground flaxseed if desired.

PER SERVING: *Calories 240 (From Fat 103); Fat 11g (Saturated 1g); Cholesterol 0mg; Sodium 187mg; Carbohydrate 33g (Dietary Fiber 5g); Protein 5g; Sugars 12g.*

Kiwifruit, Banana, and Orange Fruit Salad with Almond Butter

PREP TIME: 5 MIN   **YIELD: 2 SERVINGS**

INGREDIENTS

2 kiwifruits

1 banana

1 orange or 2 mandarins

2 tablespoons (32g) organic, unsweetened almond butter

DIRECTIONS

1 Peel kiwifruits and slice into thin rounds. Slice each round in half to create a half moon.

2 Slice the banana into rounds.

3 Peel the orange or mandarins and break into segments.

4 Arrange half of the banana slices to look like palm tree trunks (refer to Figure 7-2).

5 Use the kiwifruit segments to create the foliage on the tops of the trees.

6 Spread almond butter at the base of trees and arrange orange segments on top.

NOTE: Kiwifruit is the star of this snack and contains numerous vitamins and bioactive compounds as well as a compound called actinidin that aids in the breakdown and absorption of protein. The skin is edible if you want to increase your fiber intake even more.

NOTE: This dish is popular with the little hands in the family and does double duty as an easy dessert.

VARY IT! If you prefer to use another source of protein, you can spread ½ cup plain, full-fat Greek yogurt on the bottom of the plate before assembling the trees and skip the almond butter. Alternately, you could scatter whole almonds around the plate.

PER SERVING: *Calories 231 (From Fat 91); Fat 10g (Saturated 1g); Cholesterol 0mg; Sodium 75mg; Carbohydrate 36g (Dietary Fiber 6g); Protein 5g; Sugars 21g.*

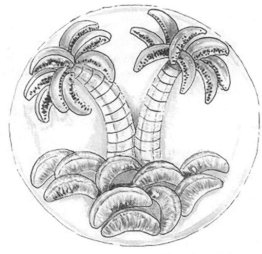

FIGURE 7-2:
Kiwifruit, Banana, and Orange Fruit Salad with Almond Butter.

Illustration by Liz Kurtzman

☝ Black Bean, Corn, and Red Pepper Sunshine Salad

PREP TIME: 5 MIN   YIELD: 2 SERVINGS

INGREDIENTS

½ cup (86g)cooked black beans (see the recipe in this chapter)

¼ cup (39g) frozen corn, thawed, or fresh

2 roasted red peppers, rinsed and diced (see the recipe in this chapter)

2 cups (60g) fresh baby spinach

2 tablespoons (30ml) Amy Riolo Selections or extra-virgin olive oil

Pinch of salt

⅛ teaspoon (.27g) pepper

Juice, 1 lime

DIRECTIONS

1 Combine the beans, corn, roasted red peppers, and spinach in a large bowl.

2 If eating immediately, toss with the olive oil, sea salt, black pepper, and lime.

3 If storing, divide into 2 airtight containers and place in the fridge and dress with the olive oil, salt, pepper, and lime before serving.

NOTE: This snack combines the polyphenols of EVOO with bioactive compounds due to the colors of corn and peppers. Black beans are a powerhouse of fiber, vitamins and minerals and a great source of protein. They have been shown to increase insulin sensitivity so are a great choice for regulating blood sugar.

VARY IT! Use no-sodium added canned beans of your choice instead of dried black beans; be sure to rinse them well and omit the added salt in this recipe if using them.

NOTE: Check out a photo of this recipe in the color insert.

PER SERVING: *Calories 242 (From Fat 130); Fat 14g (Saturated 2g); Cholesterol 0mg; Sodium 110mg; Carbohydrate 24g (Dietary Fiber 8g); Protein 7g; Sugars 6g.*

SOAK AND COOK YOUR OWN BEANS

To cook and soak beans for this recipe, follow these steps:

1. **Place dry beans in a large heat.**

2. **Proof bowl and cover with water overnight.**

   The next day, place in a pot and cover with water.

3. **Bring to a boil over high heat, reduce the heat to low and cook, 45 mins to 1 hour, or until tender.**

I like to prepare dried beans once a week to have them on hand. If you forget to soak the beans the night before, you can follow the same process but cover them with boiling water for 1 hour and then drain and cook the same way.

☁ Baked Kale Chips

PREP TIME: 10 MIN | COOK TIME: 15 TO 20 MIN | YIELD: 4 SERVINGS

INGREDIENTS

3 teaspoons (15ml) Amy Riolo Selections or extra-virgin olive oil

½ cup (48g) ground unsalted almonds

¼ cup (28g) ground flaxseed

½ teaspoon (1g) smoked paprika

Pinch of salt

2 egg whites

One 10-ounce (284g) bunch fresh kale, rinsed, dried, and stems removed, torn into bite-sized pieces

DIRECTIONS

1 Preheat the oven to 300 degrees F. Coat 2 baking sheets with 1 teaspoon olive oil. Place the almonds on a sheet of wax paper or small plates.

2 As soon as the almonds are cool, transfer them to a small bowl and stir in the flaxseed and paprika mixture.

3 In a small, deep bowl, whisk together the egg whites until foamy. Dip the edges of kale leaves into the egg whitewash. Then dip the kale leaves into the almond mixture to coat the egg whites.

4 Place the dipped kale leaves on the baking sheet. Repeat with the remaining kale, leaving a ¼-inch space between them.

5 Drizzle 1 teaspoon olive oil over the kale on each of the baking sheets. Bake for 15 to 20 minutes, or until crispy.

NOTE: Kale and EVOO with seeds, nuts, and a dash of paprika deliver a small dose of a variety of polyphenol compounds and beta-carotene, vitamin C, and the micronutrient selenium. You don't need the additives so often found in processed chips.

TIP: Clean and prepare the kale and ground almonds the day before so that they take less time to come together. I like to make large batches and store in airtight containers in individual serving sizes in the refrigerator. Be sure to dry the kale very well.

PER SERVING: Calories 180 (From Fat 115); Fat 13g (Saturated 1g); Cholesterol 0mg; Sodium 99mg; Carbohydrate 12g (Dietary Fiber 5g); Protein 8g; Sugars 1g.

Filling your fridge with dairy

You can enjoy delicious dairy on a diabetes-friendly diet. As with all other ingredients, it's important to keep in mind that not all types of dairy are created equal. We're interested in dairy that will provide the most protein and nutrients. These recipes focus on yogurt and cottage cheese, but goat cheese, traditional feta, and ricotta as well as small amounts of aged sheep milk cheeses can also be a great choice.

CONSUMING SMALL DOSES OF DAIRY

Goat, sheep, cow, and buffalo milk all provide excellent dairy products. Nutrient contents vary in different types of milk and also depending upon how the cheeses are made. Milk and its products contain a healthful dose of animal protein (about 9 grams per 6-ounce serving), plus other nutrients such as calcium, vitamin B2, B12, potassium, and magnesium. Calcium has been shown to have beneficial effects on bone mass in people of all ages, but check nutritional labels to choose brands of milk and yogurt that contain at least 20 percent of the daily recommended value of both calcium and vitamin D. (Because vitamin D boosts calcium absorption, but isn't naturally present in dairy, most Western companies add it.)

Aged cheese contains a good amount of probiotic and microbial content that are good for a healthy gut. It's also a great source of hunger-curbing protein and calcium. Researchers believe it slows down the absorption rate of carbohydrates eaten at the same meal, balances blood sugar levels, and improves mood. It also contains the same calcium benefits as milk and yogurt. The zinc content in cheese is believed to protect skin, hair, and nails, as well as help tissue growth and repair.

Yogurt with live active cultures (probiotics) helps to maintain the natural balance of organisms, known as microflora, in the intestines. Digestive concerns such as lactose intolerance, constipation, diarrhea, and irritable bowel syndrome (IBS) have been shown to improve with probiotic consumption. Plain, full-fat Greek and regular yogurt are great choices for vegetarians and for athletes looking for a post-workout snack. The protein helps muscle recovery and water absorption, which can improve hydration. One 8-ounce serving contains approximately 60 percent of the recommended daily B12 intake for adult women along with good amounts of phosphorous, potassium, riboflavin, iodine, zinc, and vitamin B5.

Spice-Infused Yogurt with Berries and Flaxseeds

INGREDIENTS

1½ cups (340g) Greek yogurt

½ cup (72g) strawberries fresh or frozen

½ cup (74g) blueberries, fresh or frozen

1 tablespoon (7g) ground flaxseeds

1 teaspoon (7g) raw honey

½ teaspoon (1.3g) cinnamon

DIRECTIONS

1 Place ¾ cup yogurt into each of 2 clear glasses or dessert bowls.

2 Top with half of the berries and flaxseeds.

3 Drizzle each with ½ teaspoon honey and sprinkle ½ of cinnamon over each one.

NOTE: The combination of cinnamon in yogurt is an amazing way to nurture your gut microbiome, especially with the richness of the varieties of polyphenols found in red, blue, and purple berries. Flaxseeds are a great source of omega-3 fats and natural, raw unprocessed honey is a sugar with anti-inflammatory, antioxidant, and antimicrobial effects.

TIP: Make this recipe the night before left covered in the refrigerator to enjoy anytime.

VARY IT! Combine ingredients in the blender for a fast smoothie.

PER SERVING: *Calories 223 (From Fat 87); Fat 10g (Saturated 5g); Cholesterol 0mg; Sodium 62mg; Carbohydrate 21g (Dietary Fiber 3g); Protein 16g; Sugars 13g.*

Herbed Cottage Cheese with Pears and Pistachios

PREP TIME: 3 MIN	YIELD: 2 SERVINGS

INGREDIENTS

1 cup (110g) cottage cheese

¼ cup (23g) finely chopped fresh mint or parsley

2 pears, washed and cut into quarters, skin on

1 tablespoon (15ml) Amy Riolo Selections or extra-virgin olive oil

2 tablespoons (16g) shelled unsalted pistachios, roughly chopped

DIRECTIONS

1 Place the cottage cheese into a bowl and stir in the mint or parsley. Divide half of the cottage cheese onto 2 small plates.

2 Arrange the pear quarters around the cottage cheese (4 per plate). Drizzle each plate with ½ tablespoon olive oil.

3 Sprinkle with 1 tablespoon pistachios per plate and serve.

NOTE: Another combination of fruit with EVOO is a delightful way to mix great nutrition with delicious flavor. Pears are rich in vitamin C and have a good glycemic profile, with the EVOO improving the insulin response. Pistachios are great unsaturated fats with fiber, minerals, and polyphenols.

TIP: If making this dish ahead of time, cut the pears at the last minute so that they don't brown or coat them with lemon juice.

VARY IT! Swap the cottage cheese for plain, full-fat Greek yogurt or ricotta or 2 ounces of plain feta cheese.

PER SERVING: *Calories 322 (From Fat 139); Fat 15g (Saturated 4g); Cholesterol 0mg; Sodium 431mg; Carbohydrate 34g (Dietary Fiber 7g); Protein 16g; Sugars 18g.*

Spiced Edamame and Chickpeas

PREP TIME: 5 MIN | COOK TIME: 25 MIN | YIELD: 4 SERVINGS

INGREDIENTS

3 quarts (2.8L) water plus
¼ cup (60 ml)

1 teaspoon (5g) salt

8 ounces (227g) fresh
edamame, or frozen, shelled

½ teaspoon (1.3g) arrowroot
starch

1 tablespoon (15ml) Amy Riolo
Selections or extra-virgin
olive oil

2 cloves garlic, finely minced

¼ teaspoon (.66g) red chili
flakes

1 teaspoon (2g) fresh ginger,
grated or ¼ teaspoon (.45g)
dried and ground

1 tablespoon (18g) tamari

1 tablespoon (21g) raw honey

8 ounces (227g) cooked
chickpeas

DIRECTIONS

1 Bring 3 quarts of salted water to boil in a large pot over high heat. Turn the heat down to medium. Add the edamame and cook for 5 minutes, or until barely fork–tender. Drain well.

2 In a small bowl, whisk together ¼ cup water and arrowroot starch until smooth.

3 In a large, wide skillet heat the olive oil over medium heat. Add the garlic, chili flakes, and ginger. Sauté for 1 to 2 minutes or just until garlic releases its aroma.

4 Add the tamari and honey and stir well. Stir in the arrowroot mixture, whisking quickly. Reduce to a simmer and allow to cook for only 1 to 2 minutes to avoid sauce being too thick.

5 Remove from the heat and stir in the edamame and chickpeas. Allow to cool and serve.

NOTE: Edamame and chickpeas are great for nicely balanced carbs and proteins. The spiciness of chili comes from capsaicin — an anti-inflammatory polyphenol with possible anticancer and heart-protecting qualities.

TIP: If you want to make a meal out of this snack, serve this dish atop a serving of brown rice, quinoa, barley, or millet.

VARY IT! You can omit the chickpeas and use 1 pound edamame, if desired.

PER SERVING: *Calories 222 (From Fat 72); Fat 8g (Saturated 1g); Cholesterol 0mg; Sodium 863mg; Carbohydrate 28g (Dietary Fiber 8g); Protein 12g; Sugars 9g.*

Sweet Sesame-Studded Energy Bites

PREP TIME: 10 MIN   YIELD: 6 SERVINGS

INGREDIENTS

½ pound (227g) soft dates, pitted

2 tablespoons (30 ml) water

¼ pound (113g) whole unsalted almonds

1 teaspoon (5 ml) pure vanilla

1 teaspoon (2g) ground cardamom

½ teaspoon (1.3g) Ceylon cinnamon

½ cup (75g) sesame seeds, toasted

DIRECTIONS

1 Place the dates, 2 tablespoons water, almonds, vanilla, cardamom, and cinnamon into a food processor. Pulse to form a smooth paste.

2 Shape the dough into date-sized balls. Spread the sesame sheets onto wax paper or a plate.

3 Roll the date balls in the sesame seeds to coat. Arrange on a platter and serve.

NOTE: Dates are a powerhouse of polyphenols and have been studied for reducing the risk of bowel cancer. Sesame seeds, the paste of which has been used as tahini for thousands of years, are a great source of fiber, B vitamins, healthy fats, proteins, polyphenols, and minerals. Sesame has been studied for its potential effects to reduce blood pressure.

TIP: Use Medjool dates for best results. You can make this recipe in advance and store in the refrigerator. In the Arabian Peninsula, these date bites are usually served as accompaniments to cardamom-infused Arabic coffee. Store in an airtight container for up to a week.

VARY IT! You can transform these energy bites into dessert by stuffing each with a whole almond, rerolling it, and dipping it in melted dark (85 percent or more) chocolate for an occasional indulgence.

PER SERVING: *Calories 292 (From Fat 145); Fat 16g (Saturated 2g); Cholesterol 0mg; Sodium 6mg; Carbohydrate 36g (Dietary Fiber 7g); Protein 7g; Sugars 26g.*

Preparing Mini Meals

You may be wondering what a mini meal is and why it matters. Some studies show that eating four smaller meals, instead of three larger ones can prevent the onset of diabetes in the first place. After a person receives a diabetes diagnosis, however, many medical professionals assert that eating smaller meals throughout the day is the best approach for people with type 2 diabetes. Eating more yet smaller meals at regular intervals throughout the day, up to 6 times a day, can be particularly beneficial.

As with snacks and regular meals, the mini meals should be balanced and contain good-quality carbs, protein, and healthful fats such as olives and EVOO, avocados, and nuts. You can consider many of the recipes in the section "Enjoying Snacks" earlier in this chapter and in Chapter 8 as great mini meal options.

TIP

In addition to discussing what to eat with your nutrition professional, discuss when and how many meals a day are appropriate for you. Everyone has a different structure, metabolism, and lifestyle, so find the eating strategies that suit your particular needs the most.

Savoring Salsas

The word "salsa" means *sauce* in both Spanish and Italian. The world has fallen in love with the Mexican condiment, which is commonly served at restaurants. Most store-bought versions, however, have too much sugar and vinegar, so they aren't nearly as good as the homemade variety. Plus, the homemade varieties are full of antioxidants and other nutritious ingredients. Why bother with those versions when it's so easy to create your own? We think you'll agree that these salsa recipes taste anything but simple.

Stocking essentials for scrumptious salsas

Add the standard salsa seasonings to any grain or legume for a tasty and nutritious treat anytime. You can flavor cooked brown rice, quinoa, or any cooked beans with any of these tasty additions:

- » Cilantro
- » Garlic
- » Lime juice or lemon juice
- » Onions
- » Peppers (such as serranos and jalapeños)
- » Tomatoes

WARNING

Use caution when slicing and dicing hot peppers such as jalapeños. Use your knife, not your fingers or fingernails, to remove the super-spicy ribs and seeds, and consider wearing gloves if you have sensitive skin. The pepper oil can get stuck under your nails, making it painful if you touch your eyes, nose, or any other moist parts later. And if your skin is exposed to sunlight with residual pepper oil, you can get a nasty burn.

SALSA 101

The word "salsa" originates from the word "to salt" because salt was a highly taxed and coveted ingredient. Salt was also used to preserve ingredients, so adding it to recipes provided additional flavor, much in the way that modern sauces do. In the English language, salsa often refers to Mexican-style salsas, but you can enjoy scores of versions as long as they're made with healthful ingredients.

Be aware of purchased sauces or salsas from any type of cuisine and stick to those that you make yourself or only include healthful ingredients such as those listed in the "Stocking essentials for scrumptious salsas" section. Fresh herbs, garlic, citrus juice, onions and shallots, peppers, tomatoes, along with extra-virgin olive oil provide you with the flavor that your palate craves and the nutrients that your body needs in no time.

Mexican Salsa

INGREDIENTS

Juice of 2 limes

½ teaspoon (2.4g) salt

1 pound (454g) fresh tomatoes, cored and chopped

½ medium onion, diced

1 tablespoon (5g) fresh chopped jalapeño pepper

1 small garlic clove, chopped fine

½ cup (8g) fresh chopped cilantro

1 cup (172g) cooked white or black beans

4 carrots, peeled and cut into sticks

4 celery stalks, peeled and cut into sticks

2 cucumbers, cut into rounds

DIRECTIONS

1 In a mixing bowl, combine the lime juice and salt. Stir to dissolve the salt.

2 Add the tomatoes and coat them with the juice. Add the onion, jalapeño, garlic, and cilantro and stir.

3 Stir in the beans and serve with the vegetables to dip.

NOTE: Salsa is a fantastic way to boost your health with the lycopene and polyphenol in tomatoes, the glucosinolates from garlic and onion, and the plentiful vegetables and the lime juice that reduce the glycemic load of carbohydrate foods that accompany it.

TIP: If you prefer a smooth rather than chunky salsa, toss all the ingredients in a food processor and process the mixture in pulses until it reaches the consistency you desire.

VARY IT! If you're serving this salsa as an appetizer to precede a larger meal and not as a stand-alone snack, omit the beans.

PER SERVING: *Calories 159 (From Fat 9); Fat 1g (Saturated 0g); Cholesterol 0mg; Sodium 349mg; Carbohydrate 34g (Dietary Fiber 9g); Protein 7g; Sugars 13g.*

Adding citrus and other fruits to salsas

To give your salsa a fruity twist, don't bother with bottled lemon or lime juice. Fresh is definitely the way to go. Squeezing the juice out is easy to do, and the flavor is far superior.

Here's how to get the most out of your citrus fruit (check out Figure 7-3 for details):

1. **Roll the fruit on a hard, flat surface, pressing down fairly hard to break up the juice sacs.**

2. **Cut the citrus fruit in half width-wise.**

3. **Holding one half in one hand, stick the tines of a fork into the fruit pulp and squeeze the fruit.**

Twist the fork as needed to release as much juice as possible.

TIP

Juice your fruit over a separate bowl, not into other ingredients. Doing so helps you catch any errant seeds that may try to sneak their way into your delectable dishes.

Lemon and lime aren't the only fruity flavors you can add to your salsas. Check out the following yummy salsas featuring mango and pineapple.

FIGURE 7-3:
A fork is a handy tool in juicing a citrus fruit.

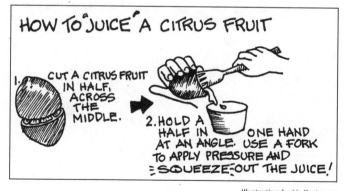

Illustration by Liz Kurtzman

🍅 Mango Salsa Spread

PREP TIME: 15 MIN | **YIELD: 4 SERVINGS**

INGREDIENTS

1 large ripe mango, peeled, pitted, and chopped

½ small red bell pepper, seeded and chopped

1 cup (227g) Greek yogurt

1 green onion, green and white parts, chopped

2 tablespoons (12g) minced fresh ginger

Juice of 1 lime

3 tablespoons (3g) fresh chopped cilantro

4 brown rice cakes (36g)

DIRECTIONS

1 In a medium mixing bowl, combine all the ingredients and mix well. Cover and refrigerate until ready to serve.

2 Divide the mango salsa onto rice cakes and serve.

NOTE: Figure 7-4 shows how to core and seed a red pepper.

PER SERVING: *Calories 130 (From Fat 28); Fat 3g (Saturated 2g); Cholesterol 0mg; Sodium 52mg; Carbohydrate 21g (Dietary Fiber 2g); Protein 6g; Sugars 10g.*

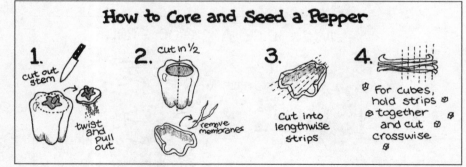

How to Core and Seed a Pepper

1. cut out stem — twist and pull out

2. cut in ½ — remove membranes

3. Cut into lengthwise strips

4. For cubes, hold strips together and cut crosswise

FIGURE 7-4: Coring and seeding a pepper.

Illustration by Liz Kurtzman

🍅 Warm Pineapple Salsa

PREP TIME: 20 MIN	COOK TIME: 15 MIN	YIELD: 4 SERVINGS

INGREDIENTS

1 tablespoon (15ml) Amy Riolo Selections or extra-virgin olive oil

½ cup (46g) slivered almonds, chopped

1 small onion, thinly sliced

2 teaspoons (4g) curry powder

2 cups (330g) fresh pineapple, diced

1 tablespoon (15 ml) cider vinegar

¼ teaspoon (1.2g) salt

1 tablespoon (21g) raw honey

4 slices Ezekiel bread, cut into quarters

DIRECTIONS

1 In a small saucepan, heat the olive oil over medium heat. Add the almonds and gently toss in the oil. Add the onion and cook until tender and until the almonds are golden brown.

2 Add the curry powder, pineapple, vinegar, salt, and honey. Bring the mixture to a boil, reduce the heat, and simmer for 5 to 10 minutes. Remove the salsa from the heat and set aside.

3 Heat your broiler on low and toast the bread quarters until crispy, flipping once.

4 Place the salsa in a bowl and serve with toasts.

NOTE: This fruit salsa is delicious, and the addition of the cider vinegar reduces the higher glycemic index of the tropical fruits. The acidity of the vinegar slows the absorption of the sugars.

TIP: Try this salsa over grilled chicken breast or fish at lunch or dinner.

VARY IT! Try this recipe with canned mandarin oranges, apricots, or peaches instead of the pineapple, depending on your accompaniments and your taste buds on a given day. But be sure to avoid fruit packed in heavy syrup.

PER SERVING: Calories 264 (From Fat 89); Fat 10g (Saturated 1g); Cholesterol 0mg; Sodium 201mg; Carbohydrate 40g (Dietary Fiber 7g); Protein 9g; Sugars 17g.

Discovering Delicious Dips

Dips don't have to be fat-laden creamy concoctions that add inches to your waist-line and bags to your saddle. With a little creativity, you can create delicious dips that keep you eating healthy and your glucose levels normal.

Whipping up dips with pantry staples

Dips are among the quickest and easiest (not to mention tastiest!) appetizers around. Keep your pantry and fridge stocked with a few dip-making essentials and you'll never be stuck wondering what to whip up when unexpected guests stop by.

REMEMBER

Here are our best bets for quick dip-making essentials to keep on hand:

>> **Any of the ingredients listed under "Stocking essentials for scrumptious salsas" earlier in this chapter:** Adding any of the salsa ingredients to any of the items in this list makes for a terrific dip. In fact, one of our favorite quick dips blends a can of black beans (rinsed and drained, of course) with ½ cup of salsa. Whip the mixture in a food processor, and you have an instant party treat.

>> **Beans:** Pureed beans make a great base for a dip, and they're high in fiber and low in fat. Blend them in a food processor and season them with your favorite spices. Look for fat-free, low-sodium canned beans, and try cannellini beans, black beans, pinto beans, black-eyed peas, garbanzo beans, great Northern beans, navy beans, and kidney beans.

TIP

Unless a recipe says otherwise, rinse and drain canned beans before adding them to a dip. Often, the liquid they're canned in is salty or flavored in some way. Rinse and drain and season them your way.

>> **Fancy olives:** Olives impart great flavor and texture to dips. Use some of the olive juice to blend into the dip, too. If olives perk up a martini, just think what they can do for some ho-hum dips!

>> **Fresh herbs:** Fresh herbs make an instant impression on an otherwise bland dip base. Dill, basil, and cilantro are excellent choices for keeping on hand.

>> **Lowfat sour cream:** Use sour cream to add a little body and creamy texture to your dips.

>> **Plain yogurt and Greek yogurt:** This staple is a natural partner to fresh herbs and a touch of lemon juice. Keep it handy to mix in a soon-to-be bean dip.

>> **Spice blends:** Look for prepackaged, salt-free spice blends. These healthy spices can take the guesswork out of seasoning.

Adding dips and salsas to snacks

Of all the snacks out there, dips (and salsas) are probably the most popular. Whether you're watching TV, enjoying a snack with others, or eating on the go, having a few good snacking options in your repertoire is important. Best of all, you can make these recipes in advance and serve them as appetizers as a part of lunch or dinner.

Dips (and salsas) are another great way to sneak legumes, fresh vegetables, and fruit into the diets of people who don't normally get enough of them. Easy and economical, let these wholesome dishes become new staples in your home.

WHAT TO SERVE WITH DIPS

Many people shy away from dips when they are trying to eat healthfully because they can be a hiding place for unwanted ingredients as well as extra fat, sodium, and sugar. When made with nutritious ingredients like the recipes in this chapter, though, nothing is farther from the truth. These dips can be enjoyed on a daily basis. The key is to serve them with the proper dipping vessel that will add health benefits. Instead of prepared tortilla chips and white bread, serve these items with your favorite dip:

- Carrot and bell pepper sticks are beautiful in color — red, yellow, green, and orange — have a crunchy texture, and add antioxidants to your meal.

- Cucumber slices are a great, low-calorie way of adding hydrating compounds and crunch.

- Use the individual spears of endive lettuce leaves to dip into your favorite dips.

- Be sure to follow the serving size suggestions of 100 percent whole-wheat pita.

- Yucca Chips from this chapter add unique flavor and satisfying texture.

- Roasted sweet potatoes wedges are another great option.

🍅 Red Lentil Dip with Crudites

PREP TIME: 5 MIN   COOK TIME: 20 MIN   YIELD: 6 SERVINGS

INGREDIENTS

1 cup (192g) dried red lentils, sorted, rinsed, and drained

1 cup (240ml) Homemade Vegetable Stock (see Chapter 10)

1 tablespoon (44.5g) tomato paste

5 cloves garlic, chopped

¼ teaspoon (1.2g) salt

Pepper to taste

1 tablespoon (5g) ground coriander

¼ cup (56g) Greek yogurt

¼ cup (4g) fresh, finely chopped cilantro for garnish

3 cups (362g) crudites (mixture broccoli florets, celery sticks, carrot sticks, bell pepper strips, and cherry tomatoes)

DIRECTIONS

1   Combine the lentils, stock, tomato paste, garlic, salt, and pepper in a medium saucepan and bring to boil over high heat.

2   Stir, reduce the heat to low, add the coriander, and cover. Simmer for about 20 minutes, or until lentils are tender and all the liquid is absorbed.

3   Using a potato masher or large fork, mash the red lentil mixture into a paste (the consistency should be similar to refried beans).

4   If serving immediately, place the mixture in a shallow serving bowl. Make a dent in the center and fill with the Greek yogurt.

5   Sprinkle with the cilantro and serve with the fresh vegetables for dipping.

NOTE: Lentils are the hero of this dish with a good amount of protein and fiber to keep you feeling full. B vitamins and folate are in high concentration as well as iron and selenium, which makes them an important staple for people who are vegetarian.

TIP: This red lentil mixture also tastes great as a base for wraps. Just spread out a whole-wheat tortilla, lavash bread, or pita and slather with a serving of the red lentil dip. Top with sliced cucumbers, bell peppers, and lettuce or other greens. Add a dollop of Greek yogurt. Roll up, slice in half, and serve.

VARY IT! You can prepare brown lentils or beans the same way — it just takes them longer to cook.

PER SERVING: *Calories 167 (From Fat 14); Fat 2g (Saturated 0g); Cholesterol 0mg; Sodium 117mg; Carbohydrate 30g (Dietary Fiber 6g); Protein 11g; Sugars 6g.*

Fresh, Creamy Hummus with Vegetables

PREP TIME: 10 MIN	COOK TIME: 0 MIN	YIELD: 6 SERVINGS

INGREDIENTS

2 cups (328g) cooked or no-salt added canned chickpeas, peeled

1 clove minced garlic

⅓ cup (79g) tahini

2 ice cubes

Dash chili flakes, if desired

Juice of 2 lemons

Water, as needed

2 teaspoons (10ml) Amy Riolo Selections or extra-virgin olive oil

Dash smoked paprika, if desired

2 cucumbers, sliced into rounds

6 celery stalks, trimmed and cut into quarters

2 cups (142g) broccoli florets

DIRECTIONS

1 Place the chickpeas (reserving a few for garnish), garlic, tahini, ice cubes, chili flakes, and lemon juice into a food processor. Pulse on and off a few times to begin mixing ingredients. Process on high for 5 minutes, stopping and swiping down the sides with a spatula every minute or two.

2 Add the water, a tablespoon at a time through the spout if mixture isn't creamy enough. Continue to pulse until smooth and creamy. Taste and add a touch of salt if necessary.

3 Carefully remove the blade from food processor and transfer the hummus to a serving plate. With the back of a spoon, smooth the surface and make a dent in the center. Add the reserved chickpeas.

4 Drizzle the olive oil in the dent. Sprinkle with paprika, if desired, and serve with vegetables.

NOTE: Hummus has been praised for its health benefits for thousands of years, with sesame to make tahini coming from Ethiopia all the way to the Fertile Crescent in ancient times. The fiber and vitamins from chickpeas combine with the healthy sesame paste along with the bioactive compounds from ingredients like garlic and EVOO. And the best thing is that you can dip your vegetables in it!

TIP: Peeling the chickpeas (see Figure 7-5) is traditional in making hummus, and peeling really makes a difference in the consistency. Although peeling chickpeas isn't fun when you're in a hurry, you can take your time and do it when you're watching TV, talking with a friend, and so on. If you can't peel the chickpeas, use them whole and continue to process longer. The consistency won't be as smooth, but the dip will still be delicious and healthful.

VARY IT! Even though it's not traditional, I sometimes add ½ cup plain Greek yogurt to the hummus and top it with pomegranate seeds. Especially at holiday time, this dish can be a festive and nutritious appetizer to serve.

PER SERVING: *Calories 222 (From Fat 94); Fat 10g (Saturated 1g); Cholesterol 0mg; Sodium 189mg; Carbohydrate 27g (Dietary Fiber 7g); Protein 9g; Sugars 6g.*

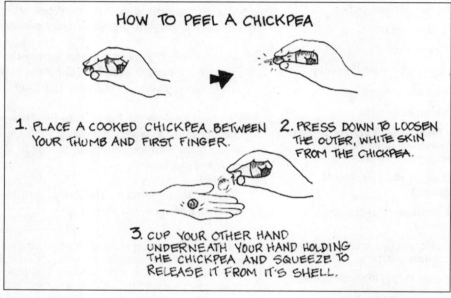

HOW TO PEEL A CHICKPEA

1. PLACE A COOKED CHICKPEA BETWEEN YOUR THUMB AND FIRST FINGER.

2. PRESS DOWN TO LOOSEN THE OUTER, WHITE SKIN FROM THE CHICKPEA.

3. CUP YOUR OTHER HAND UNDERNEATH YOUR HAND HOLDING THE CHICKPEA AND SQUEEZE TO RELEASE IT FROM IT'S SHELL.

FIGURE 7-5: How to peel chickpeas.

Illustration by Liz Kurtzman

THE MANY DIMENSIONS OF DIPS

Making a batch or two of different pureed bean dips gives you an advantage throughout the week. You can use them for snacking, as a part of a light lunch or dinner, and also as a simple and nutritious appetizer for when guests arrive. They're a great way to achieve the Mediterranean diet recommendation of a serving of beans/legumes per day.

You can also turn dips into creamy soups by adding them to a stockpot and adding stock to cover. Bring to a boil, uncovered, reduce the heat to low, and simmer a few minutes to warm through. Taste and adjust the seasonings and finish with your favorite herbs and a drizzle of good-quality extra-virgin olive oil.

☙ White Bean Dip

PREP TIME: 10 MIN PLUS 3 TO 4 HR CHILL TIME	COOK TIME: 5 MIN	YIELD: 4 SERVINGS

INGREDIENTS

1 teaspoon (5ml) Amy Riolo Selections or extra-virgin olive oil

½ cup (80g) chopped onions

2 garlic cloves, minced

2 cups (358g) cooked cannellini beans or one 15-ounce can cannellini beans, drained and rinsed

½ teaspoon (.34g) chopped fresh sage

1 teaspoon (5ml) Amy Riolo Selections White Balsamic or balsamic vinegar

1 teaspoon (5ml) water

⅛ teaspoon (.6g) salt

⅛ teaspoon (.6g) pepper

Crudites to serve (2 red bell peppers, 2 green bell peppers, both sliced, 4 carrots, peeled and cut into sticks, 1 English cucumber, sliced into rounds, ½ cup (75g) grape tomatoes)

DIRECTIONS

1 Place a medium skillet over medium heat and coat it with olive oil. Add the onions and cook until they're soft and translucent, about 3 to 5 minutes. Add the garlic and continue to cook for about 30 seconds.

2 Place the beans in a food processor and add the cooked onions and garlic as well as the sage, vinegar, water, salt, and pepper. Process until smooth, about 1 to 2 minutes.

3 Transfer the mixture to a bowl, cover it, allow to cool, and serve with crudites.

NOTE: Different types of beans give different profiles of polyphenols along with fiber, vitamins and minerals. They offer so many added nutrients, and when prepared with ingredients like garlic, onions, and EVOO, they become even better for you!

PER SERVING: *Calories 212 (From Fat 20); Fat 2g (Saturated 0g); Cholesterol 0mg; Sodium 109mg; Carbohydrate 40g (Dietary Fiber 14g); Protein 10g; Sugars 9g.*

Choosing healthy dippers

TIP

What's a good dip without something to dip into it? Rather than ruining all your hard work of choosing healthy dips by dipping fried chips into them, we offer you the following alternatives to keep you moving in the right direction:

>> **Bagel chips:** Look for these chips in the specialty bread section of your grocery store but read the label because some are high in fat and sodium. You also can make your own by slicing off slivers of a bagel and then baking them until they're crisp.

>> **Fresh veggies:** Choose broccoli florets, cauliflower florets, carrot sticks, celery sticks, zucchini slices, red pepper spears, endive scoops, or any of your favorites. Any veggie can be a dip delivery system.

>> **Pita wedges:** Make your own by quartering pitas and then baking them until they're crisp.

>> **Whole-wheat crackers:** Kashi makes a line called TLC, Tasty Little Crackers, made with whole-grain flour from seven different grains. Ry-Krisp is a filling and tasty choice as well.

>> **Yucca chips:** This root vegetable has great health benefits. Check out the following recipe.

Yucca Chips

| PREP TIME: 10 MIN | COOK TIME: 45 MIN | YIELD: 4 SERVINGS |

INGREDIENTS

⅛ teaspoon (.6g) salt

⅛ teaspoon (.6g) pepper

1 tablespoon (4.2g) za'atar spice mix, or your favorite dry spice

2 large yucca (about 400g), peeled and cut into wedges, approximately ⅜-inch cut

2 tablespoons (30ml) Amy Riolo Selections or extra-virgin olive oil, divided

DIRECTIONS

1 Preheat the oven to 375 degrees F.

2 In a small bowl, combine the salt, pepper, and za'atar. In a large bowl, coat the yucca wedges with the olive oil and then toss in the spices.

3 Coat a baking sheet with the olive oil and arrange the yucca wedges on the sheet. Bake about 30 to 45 minutes, or until the yucca is cooked through and lightly browned.

NOTE: Yucca is a Latin American alternative to a standard french fry. The mild, somewhat nutty flavor adds a nice depth to the taste. Yucca is also known as cassava, which is a great low GI carbohydrate particularly noted for its vitamin and mineral content. It offers significant amounts of vitamin C, thiamine, and niacin.

VARY IT! You can prepare sweet potatoes, rutabaga, or carrots this way.

PER SERVING: Calories 228 (From Fat 65); Fat 7g (Saturated 1g); Cholesterol 0mg; Sodium 117mg; Carbohydrate 40g (Dietary Fiber 2g); Protein 2g; Sugars 2g.

Making Base Recipes to Use As Needed

Many recipes in this book call for cooked beans, lentils, roasted red peppers, and breadcrumbs. We always recommend making them yourself, once a week if possible, so that you can enjoy the healthiest versions of base ingredients which are eaten often.

Preparing bread-related basics

The recipes in this section are great to keep on hand because they save you calories, time, and money while increasing the flavor quotient in your meals. You can use leftover bread to create breadcrumbs, crostini, and bruschetta.

Homemade croutons and crostini taste better as well because they're fresher than what you buy in the store. In addition, homemade versions of these everyday items are free from unwanted chemicals and additives, so they're better for your health, too.

TIP

None of these recipes have any added ingredients like stabilizers and artificial colorants. You can incorporate EVOO with its unique polyphenols into baking recipes as an ingredient or include it afterward to reduce the glycemic rise, improve insulin performance, and to add flavor and health.

🍅 Fresh Breadcrumbs

INGREDIENTS

One 8-ounce (227g) loaf dense, day-old country-style bread

DIRECTIONS

1 Cut the loaf of bread into 1-inch cubes and, working in batches, if necessary, place them in a food processor, being careful not to fill it more than halfway. Pulse on and off until the crumbs are as fine as possible.

2 If not using immediately, freeze the breadcrumbs in a plastic freezer bag for up to a month.

NOTE: Try using the Homemade Whole-Grain Bread in Chapter 6 to make breadcrumbs. Store-bought bread may take a few days for the bread to get hard enough to process into breadcrumbs. If so, either leave the bread uncovered overnight to dry out or place it in a 200-degree oven until it hardens and begins to turn color (golden). Allow it to cool and then grind it.

PER SERVING: *Calories 164 (From Fat 9); Fat 1g (Saturated 0g); Cholesterol 0mg; Sodium 369mg; Carbohydrate 32g (Dietary Fiber 1g); Protein 7g; Sugars 1g.*

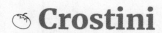 Crostini

PREP TIME: 5 MIN	COOK TIME: 5 MIN	YIELD: 4 SERVINGS

INGREDIENTS

Eight ¼-inch slices (¾ ounce each) whole-wheat baguette loaf dense, day-old

DIRECTIONS

1 Preheat the broiler to high.

2 Cut slices of baguette–style bread into thin, ¼–inch–wide slices on the diagonal and place them on a baking sheet.

3 Place under the boiler and toast until golden, about 1 to 2 minutes on each side.

NOTE: Some people get crostini and bruschetta confused. The main difference between them: Crostini are usually smaller (hence the suffix "ini" at the end of the word) and thinner. They're toasted without the addition of EVOO, which is drizzled on bruschetta after they're toasted.

VARY IT! The sky is the limit with crostini toppings you can have. Leftover bits of meat, cheese, seafood, and vegetables make excellent crostini toppers. Chopped fresh tomatoes with garlic, basil, and EVOO are a classic. Marinated seafood, mascarpone cheese with sausage or grilled vegetables, eggplant or bean purees with tomatoes or greens, salt-cod mousse, pesto with octopus, chicken livers, and caramelized onions with pecorino cheese are all great combinations.

PER SERVING (2 CROSTINI): *Calories 115 (From Fat 12); Fat 1g (Saturated 0g); Cholesterol 0mg; Sodium 208mg; Carbohydrate 22g (Dietary Fiber 2g); Protein 4g; Sugars 2g.*

☙ Bruschetta

INGREDIENTS

4 ½-inch (1.25cm) slices ciabatta or other light, crusty, country bread

2 tablespoons (30ml) Amy Riolo Selections or extra-virgin olive oil

DIRECTIONS

1 Preheat broiler to high or grill to medium–high.

2 Brush the olive oil on both sides of the bread.

3 Grill the bread slices on both sides until grill marks appear or place under the broiler until golden brown, about 2 to 3 minutes per side.

NOTE: Bruschetta is said to be the most mispronounced of all Italian words. The correct pronunciation is broos-*keht*-tah (not broo-*sheh*-tah). Italian words that end with the vowel "a" change to an "e" ending for the plural form. Bruschetta becomes bruschette when plural, pizza becomes pizze, and so on.

TIP: Prepare your toppings ahead of time so you can place them on the hot bread and enjoy the bruschette immediately.

VARY IT! If you use good-quality bread and olive oil, then plain, simple bruschetta can be a decadent snack or accompaniment to soup or salad. To serve them as an appetizer, use your favorite combinations of ingredients. I (Amy) like to use ricotta cheese, grilled vegetables, or tomatoes and eggplant most often, but you can choose from many other options.

PER SERVING: *Calories 106 (From Fat 63); Fat 7g (Saturated 1g); Cholesterol 0mg; Sodium 104mg; Carbohydrate 9g (Dietary Fiber 0g); Protein 2g; Sugars 0g.*

Cooking your own beans and legumes

Throughout the centuries, beans and lentils were often dismissed as poor man's food and even nowadays are considered vegetarian protein sources that are meat substitutes. However, when you consider how good beans are for your health, how good they are for the environment, and the fact that they lend themselves to so many cooking applications, why not enjoy them more often?

I (Amy) like to cook beans once a week at the same time I'm using my leftover bits to make stock, breadcrumbs, and crostini. That way, I know that I have them on hand for the week to add to soups, salads, and pasta dishes, to puree and use to top crostini, or to create a bed for vegetables or seafood.

Beans and lentils come in many varieties. All dried beans need to be soaked overnight (or covered in boiling water for an hour) before you can cook them. Lentils come in red, green, brown, and black varieties and don't require soaking before cooking. The red varieties can cook up in as little as 5 minutes — making them one of the most ancient forms of fast food.

⊙ Dried Beans

PREP TIME: 1 HR	COOK TIME: 30 MIN	YIELD: 8 SERVINGS

INGREDIENTS

1 cup (202g) dried beans (any variety)

¼ teaspoon (1.2g) salt

DIRECTIONS

1 Place the beans in a medium stockpot and cover with cold water; leave to soak overnight.

2 Drain the soaked beans and place them in a medium saucepan. Add the salt, cover the beans with water, and bring to a boil, uncovered, over high heat.

3 Reduce the heat to medium-low, cover, and let cook until the beans are tender, about 25 to 50 minutes. (It may take longer depending on the size of the beans.)

4 Drain and cool. If not using right away, store in an airtight container in the refrigerator for up to one week.

TIP: If you're short on time, in Step 1, place the beans in a stockpot, cover with boiling water, and leave to soak for 1 hour instead.

PER SERVING: *Calories 84 (From Fat 2); Fat 0g (Saturated 0g); Cholesterol 0mg; Sodium 63mg; Carbohydrate 15g (Dietary Fiber 4g); Protein 6g; Sugars 1g.*

🍅 Cooked Beans

PREP TIME: 5 MIN PLUS 8 HRS SOAKING	COOK TIME: 40 MIN	YIELD: 8 SERVINGS

INGREDIENTS

1 cup (202g) dried cannellini or other beans

4 rosemary sprigs, divided

1 tablespoon (15ml) Amy Riolo Selections or extra-virgin olive oil

¼ teaspoon (1.2g) salt

DIRECTIONS

1 In a large bowl, add the beans and enough cold water to cover them by 4 inches. Let them soak in a cool place or in the refrigerator for at least 8 hours or overnight.

2 Drain the beans and transfer them to a 2-quart saucepan. Pour in enough water to cover by 1 inch and drop in two rosemary sprigs. Bring the water to a boil, and then lower the heat so the water is barely at a simmer. Cook, uncovered, until the beans are tender but not mushy, with just enough liquid to cover them, about 30 to 40 minutes. (If necessary, add more water, 1 tablespoon at a time, to keep the beans covered as they simmer.)

3 Remove the beans from the heat and gently stir in the olive oil, salt, and the remaining two rosemary sprigs. Let the beans stand to cool and absorb the cooking liquid. If you're not using them right away, store the beans in an airtight container in the refrigerator up to one week.

NOTE: The end result should be tender beans with a creamy consistency in just enough liquid to coat them.

PER SERVING: *Calories 99 (From Fat 17); Fat 2g (Saturated 0g); Cholesterol 0mg; Sodium 63mg; Carbohydrate 15g (Dietary Fiber 4g); Protein 6g; Sugars 1g.*

☺ Lentils

INGREDIENTS

1 cup (192g) dried lentils (any variety)

¼ teaspoon (1.2g) salt

¼ teaspoon (1.2g) pepper

1 bay leaf

DIRECTIONS

1 Rinse the lentils in a colander.

2 Place the lentils in a medium saucepan and add enough water to cover them twice (you should have twice as much water as lentils). Add the salt, pepper, and bay leaf.

3 Bring to a boil over high heat. Reduce the heat to low, and simmer, uncovered, until the lentils are tender, about 5 to 30 minutes, depending on the variety of lentil.

4 If you're not using them right away, store the cooked lentils in an airtight container in the refrigerator up to one week.

NOTE: Red lentils are the quickest-cooking variety, followed by green, brown, and then black.

PER SERVING: *Calories 113 (From Fat 3); Fat 0g (Saturated 0g); Cholesterol 0mg; Sodium 80mg; Carbohydrate 19g (Dietary Fiber 10g); Protein 8g; Sugars 1g.*

☺ Roasted Red Peppers

PREP TIME: 5 MIN	COOK TIME: 40 MIN	YIELD: 4 SERVINGS

INGREDIENTS

4 red bell peppers (keep whole)

1 tablespoon (15 ml) Amy Riolo Selections or extra-virgin olive oil

DIRECTIONS

1 Preheat the oven to 500 degrees F.

2 On a baking sheet, place the whole bell peppers. Bake until the skins are wrinkled and the peppers are charred, about 30 to 40 minutes, being sure to turn them each time a side is charred (approximately twice during cooking).

3 Remove from the oven and cover tightly with aluminum foil to create steam. Set aside.

4 When the peppers are cool enough to handle, after about 30 minutes, cut into quarters, peel off the skin, and remove the seeds. Add to your favorite recipe or, if not eating immediately, place the pepper pieces in a jar, cover with the olive oil for additional flavor and nutrition, and seal with a lid; refrigerate up to 2 weeks. Before using, drain the oil from the peppers; reserve the oil in the refrigerator for another use.

NOTE: Called *pepperoni rossi arrostit* in Italian, they're often added to antipasto platters, pastas, soups, and sauces.

NOTE: Bell peppers are a great source of vitamin C, containing approximately three times as much vitamin C as an orange. They also contain the bioactive compound lycopene that's also found in tomatoes and is shown to be active against prostrate and lung cancer. Cooking in EVOO increases the absorption of the lycopene in the peppers.

TIP: You don't need to purchase jarred peppers when you can make them easily at home. Stock up on peepers when they're on sale. You can roast them and freeze them for later use.

PER SERVING: *Calories 67 (From Fat 34); Fat 4g (Saturated 0g); Cholesterol 0mg; Sodium 5mg; Carbohydrate 7g (Dietary Fiber 2g); Protein 1g; Sugars 5g.*

Chapter **8**

Small Plates on the Go

mall plates on the go are perfect for people with a busy lifestyle. They're also a great solution for people who are eating four to six smaller meals each day instead of three larger ones. Although these recipes and the notion of food on the go is simplistic, these kinds of food are often one of the most overlooked aspects of diet plans.

In this chapter, we get you started with the basics of preparing smaller meals to enjoy on the go. You discover how to prepare for simple recipes that are also diverse, nutritious, and satisfying. Whether you're in the mood for a fun board, a portable box, a quick bite, a wrap, or a bountiful bowl, this chapter proves that good taste and good nutrition can go hand in hand.

Although people tend to think of sit-down meals at home when the term "meal planning" comes to mind, the meals that you eat on the go can actually derail your diets most drastically. That's why planning ahead and always having meals ready to go is a great idea.

Be sure to read the Note in each recipe to find out about its nutritional values. Also refer to the book's Introduction for some recipe conventions we use.

Planning Ahead — Preparation Is Key

Have you ever been to a fast-casual restaurant that has packaged meals ready to go? Or perhaps a supermarket with a refrigerator case of prepared items. Nowadays prepared meals take up a significant percentage of people's shopping. Dedicate a shelf or a portion of a shelf in your refrigerator for these types of meals that you make yourself. Keeping the recipes in this chapter on hand can save you from a lot of pitfalls and ensure that you're nourished the proper way.

Being prepared in the kitchen plays an important role in helping you stay on track with your eating plan. If you're new to the kitchen or currently not used to preparing meals, you don't need to be intimidated. Think of this exercise in organization and planning ahead as a way to enjoy your meals more and feel better while saving time and money. You don't need to be a professional chef to reap the benefits of kitchen organization. Borrowing a few tips from restaurants and from the housekeeping traditions from the last century though, can really help you, the modern home cook and meal prepper.

I (Amy) used to create 90-second Mediterranean meals for a televised series geared toward athletes. The goal was to offer recipes that sports enthusiasts could make to fuel themselves before and replenish themselves after workouts. The project sponsors chose the extremely fast time limit because they wanted to show that it's possible putting together a nutritious meal or snack in the same amount of time that it takes to wait in line at a fast-food restaurant.

In order to pull off the meals in that short of a time period, I created a checklist of items that the athletes should keep on hand each week. You can apply many of these suggestions. Just dedicate an hour a week to making a meal plan/menu, another hour to shopping, and a third hour to prep the following foods:

» Hardboiled eggs

» Crudites (cleaned and cut into strips bell peppers, cauliflower, broccoli, celery, carrots)

» Cooked edamame

» Cooked lentils and beans of choice

» Cooked quinoa, barley, or whole grain of choice

TIP

Wash, dry, and store greens and any other vegetables in airtight containers so that they're ready to go when needed.

REMEMBER

You don't need to write your grocery list, shop, and prep the food all on the same day. Look at your schedule at the beginning of the week and find time to do those three things or help getting them done; that way planning everything won't seem so difficult.

With these prepared items on hand, grabbing a snack or making a meal within minutes is in reach. This time savings is particularly beneficial to people with diabetes because they need to avoid spikes in blood sugar. This strategy is also extremely helpful to people who don't have much time to prepare meals on a daily basis.

REMEMBER

Keeping a well-stocked pantry, freezer, and fridge full of nutritious options can help you stay on track and prevent junk food binges.

Creating Boards, Boxes, and Bites

Food should be fun. Just because you're dealing with a diabetes diagnosis doesn't mean that you can't enjoy taste, presentation, and the preparation of the foods that you're supposed to eat. This section proves that healthful meals can be exciting and contemporary. In addition to being great portable dishes, we recommend using the recipes in this section as appetizers at parties and as pot-luck contributions that everyone will love.

TIP

Throughout this chapter, each recipe discusses how to store the dishes so you can enjoy them on the go. That's why stocking up on different sized containers to store them is a good idea. We suggest purchasing the following:

>> Small containers with lids to store dressings and sauces

>> Individual serving size bowls with lids

>> Rectangular individual serving size containers with lids

>> Large containers with lids for storing full recipes

REMEMBER

The serving sizes in this chapter are usually 2 or 4. The reason: The 2 serving size recipes usually don't stay fresh long, so the recipes have been created to share immediately or use the next day. The recipes with a serving size of 4 make four separate meals. You can stack them in your refrigerator and pull them out when needed, or you can use them to serve two people twice or four people once.

Purple Power Cheese Board

INGREDIENTS

1 head purple cauliflower, florets only

1 cup (151g) purple grapes

1 cup (148g) blueberries

1 cup (144g) blackberries

1 cup (138g) toasted almonds

2 cups (179g) Pink Beet Hummus (see Chapter 6)

2 plums, sliced

A handful of purple edible flowers, such as pansies, for garnish, if desired

DIRECTIONS

1 Place the cauliflower in four corners of a large rectangular platter, cutting board, or transportable container.

2 Arrange the grapes, blueberries, and blackberries around each of the four cauliflower sections.

3 Place the almonds and pink hummus in small bowls and arrange in the middle.

4 Arrange plum slices in missing holes on the platter. Cover and store in the refrigerator until serving.

NOTE: Purple plant foods are often rich in flavonoid polyphenols that include anthocyanins. These polyphenols have antioxidant properties and may contribute to a healthy, anti-inflammatory diet. They're often present in ingredients with other benefits with plenty of fiber and vitamins.

TIP: Serve this recipe at a party or bring it to a party. You can store it in 4 separate containers for a portable snack.

VARY IT! Use whatever combination of purple fruits and vegetables that you enjoy.

NOTE: Refer to the color insert for a photo of this dish.

PER SERVING: *Calories 421 (From Fat 249); Fat 28g (Saturated 3g); Cholesterol 0mg; Sodium 222mg; Carbohydrate 37g (Dietary Fiber 11g); Protein 15g; Sugars 21g.*

Vegetable Box with Spiced Chickpeas, Tahini, and Olives

PREP TIME: 10 MIN	COOK TIME: 20 MIN	YIELD: 4 SERVINGS

INGREDIENTS

1 cup (164g) cooked chickpeas

½ (1g) teaspoon smoked paprika

⅛ (.6g) teaspoon salt

¼ teaspoon (.45g) ground ginger

¼ teaspoon (.45g) cumin

1 teaspoon (5ml) Amy Riolo Selections or extra-virgin olive oil

¼ cup (60g) tahini

Juice of ½ lemon

Water, as needed

1 celery sticks cut into sticks

4 carrots, cut into sticks

1 English cucumber, sliced thinly and divided into quarters

1 cup (149g) cherry tomatoes

⅓ cup (49g) jarred green or black olives, drained and rinsed

DIRECTIONS

1 Heat the oven to 425 degrees F. Place the chickpeas on a baking sheet and combine the paprika, salt, ginger, and cumin in a small bowl, and mix well. Drizzle with olive oil and mix well to combine. Bake for 20 minutes, or until golden and crispy.

2 In another small bowl, combine the tahini and the lemon juice, stirring well. Then add water, a tablespoon at a time, and continue to whisk with a fork until you obtain a smooth sauce (this may take up to a ¼ cup of water).

3 Prepare 4 boxes, using takeout containers or plastic containers with airtight lids.

4 Divide the cooled chickpeas, celery, carrots, cucumber, cherry tomatoes, and olives into each box. Place 2 tablespoons of the tahini in small plastic condiment containers and add to the boxes.

NOTE: This dish combines a variety of vegetables and provides an array of vitamins, minerals, and bioactive compounds including carotenoids and polyphenols with B vitamin–rich tahini, also an excellent source of minerals. Olives contain numerous antioxidants including maslinic acid, which researchers have shown interest for potential anticancer properties.

TIP: Prepare the tahini and chickpeas in advance and in large quantities.

PER SERVING: *Calories 229 (From Fat 109); Fat 12g (Saturated 2g); Cholesterol 0mg; Sodium 360mg; Carbohydrate 26g (Dietary Fiber 8g); Protein 8g; Sugars 7g.*

Hardboiled Egg, Crudites, and Pita Box

PREP TIME: 5 MIN | COOK TIME: 5 MIN | YIELD: 4 SERVINGS

INGREDIENTS

4 eggs

4 carrots, cut into sticks

1 English cucumber, sliced thinly and divided into quarters

1 cup (149g) cherry tomatoes

2 whole white pita, cut into quarters, and toasted if desired

1 teaspoon (1.4g) za'atar spice mix

DIRECTIONS

1 Bring a small pot of water to a boil over high heat. Add the eggs, reduce heat to medium–high, and cook for 10 minutes, or until just cooked through. Drain the eggs and allow to cool.

2 Divide the vegetable and pita pieces into 4 plastic or other portable containers with an airtight lid.

3 Season the eggs with za'atar or your favorite seasoning and place one in each box.

4 Seal and store in the refrigerator.

NOTE: Combined with other healthy ingredients, za'atar spices stand out in this recipe. The Middle Eastern herbs and spices of za'atar, which include thyme, oregano, marjoram, sesame, and sumac, add a distinctive flavor and deliver powerful, concentrated antioxidant compounds.

TIP: Make this meal and take it with you any time of the day.

VARY IT! Vegans can substitute the egg with a cup of edamame or tofu.

PER SERVING: *Calories 140 (From Fat 51); Fat 6g (Saturated 2g); Cholesterol 212mg; Sodium 189mg; Carbohydrate 15g (Dietary Fiber 3g); Protein 9g; Sugars 5g.*

Edamame, Almonds, Cucumber, and Tomato Box

INGREDIENTS

¼ cup (35g) whole, unsalted almonds

4 Persian cucumbers, or
2 English cucumbers, sliced

1 cup (149g) cherry tomatoes

1 recipe Spiced Edamame and Chickpeas (see Chapter 7)

DIRECTIONS

1 Divide the almonds, cucumbers, and cherry tomatoes evenly in 4 portable containers with fitted lids.

2 Add ¼ of the edamame mixture to each box.

NOTE: Plenty of evidence supports the benefits of legumes such as edamame and chickpeas. They're a great source of protein as well as a low-glycemic and fiber-rich carbohydrate along with B vitamins and minerals.

TIP: Serve this recipe before a meal or as nibbles to accompany a glass of wine.

VARY IT! Instead of edamame, use a serving of plain Greek yogurt or 2 ounces of goat cheese in each box.

PER SERVING: *Calories 297 (From Fat 116); Fat 13g (Saturated 1g); Cholesterol 0mg; Sodium 868mg; Carbohydrate 34g (Dietary Fiber 10g); Protein 12g; Sugars 15g.*

Bagel Bakery Bag

PREP TIME: 5 MIN | COOK TIME: 2 TO 3 MIN | YIELD: 2 SERVINGS

INGREDIENTS

2 whole-wheat bagels

2 tablespoons (31g) cream cheese

4 ounces (113g) smoked salmon

1 cup (20g) arugula or baby spinach

2 clementines or mandarin oranges

DIRECTIONS

1 Slice the bagel in half and toast until desired doneness. Slather each bagel half with ½ tablespoon of cream cheese.

2 Top with the smoked salmon and arugula or baby spinach.

3 Cover with the bagel top and slice in half.

4 Wrap each bagel in parchment or wax paper. Place in a bag with a clementine or mandarin orange.

5 Enjoy immediately or store in the fridge until serving.

NOTE: Salmon contains healthy omega-3 fats. Meanwhile the clementines not only add a flavorsome dose of vitamin C, which is a powerful antioxidant, but the acidity of vitamin C also reduces the glycemic index of the bagel's carbohydrate.

TIP: To make this recipe ahead of time, wrap the bagel, smoked salmon, and greens individually in plastic wrap. Place the cream cheese in a small portable container and store in the fridge until serving. Assemble at the last minute.

VARY IT! Almond butter and flaked almonds, feta cheese and avocado, scrambled eggs, and hummus with radish and cucumbers are all great alternatives.

PER SERVING: *Calories 427 (From Fat 78); Fat 9g (Saturated 4g); Cholesterol 27mg; Sodium 1118mg; Carbohydrate 69g (Dietary Fiber 11g); Protein 24g; Sugars 10g.*

🍅 Mediterranean Medley Box

INGREDIENTS

Fresh, Creamy Hummus with Vegetables (see Chapter 7)

1 cup (226g) Greek yogurt

⅓ cup (49g) green or black olives, drained and rinsed

2 whole-wheat pita, cut into quarters, and toasted if desired

2 tablespoons (30ml) Amy Riolo Selections or extra-virgin olive oil

DIRECTIONS

1 Spoon ¼ of hummus and ¼ of Greek yogurt (separately) into plastic or other portable containers with fitting lids.

2 Place the vegetables, olives, and pita around the hummus and yogurt.

3 Drizzle each hummus and yogurt with ¼ tablespoon of olive oil. Cover and store in the fridge until serving.

NOTE: This box is especially good for your gut microbiome, which includes prebiotic olives and hummus with probiotic Greek yogurt.

TIP: You can also bring the hummus and yogurt in separate containers.

VARY IT! Substitute 2 ounces of feta cheese or goat cheese for the yogurt.

PER SERVING: *Calories 347 (From Fat 162); Fat 18g (Saturated 3g); Cholesterol 0mg; Sodium 370mg; Carbohydrate 37g (Dietary Fiber 8g); Protein 14g; Sugars 7g.*

Rainbow Crudites with White Bean and Feta Dip

PREP TIME: 15 MIN   **YIELD: 4 SERVINGS**

INGREDIENTS

1½ cups (269g) cooked cannellini beans (see Chapter 7)

⅓ cup (75g) plain feta

Juice and zest of 1 lemon

¼ cup (60ml) Amy Riolo Selections or extra-virgin olive oil, divided

¼ cup (6g) fresh mint

Pepper to taste

4 radishes, trimmed and sliced

2 heads Belgian endive, trimmed and leaves separated

1 cup (149g) cherry tomatoes, whole

1 head broccoli, cut into florets

4 carrots, cut into sticks

DIRECTIONS

1 Combine the cannellini beans, feta, lemon and zest, most of the olive oil (leave a teaspoon for garnish), and mint in a food processor.

2 Pulsing on and off, puree until smooth.

3 Taste and season with pepper. Serve with the crudites.

4 Stir and plate in a shallow dish. Make a hole in the center and drizzle with olive oil.

NOTE: Broccoli is a source of the sulfur-containing antioxidant compounds classed as glucosinolates. Along with polyphenols and carotenoids, they're important bioactive compounds that are important for maintaining health (see Chapter 4). Beans and feta add protein and healthy fats from fermented sheep and goat cheese. Mint contains interesting antioxidant polyphenols including eriocitrin and rosmarinic acid (which appear also in rosemary).

TIP: You can serve this tasty dip in many ways. Top toasted bread with it and stir it into hot pasta.

VARY IT! Substitute your favorite beans for the cannellini beans.

PER SERVING: *Calories 308 (From Fat 162); Fat 18g (Saturated 5g); Cholesterol 17mg; Sodium 177mg; Carbohydrate 28g (Dietary Fiber 7g); Protein 11g; Sugars 5g.*

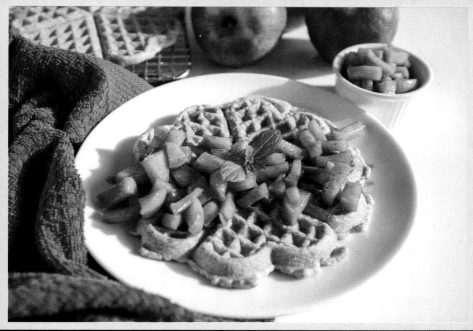

The Whole-Grain Waffles with Warm Apple Spice Compote from Chapter 6 are a nutritious spin on a comforting breakfast classic.

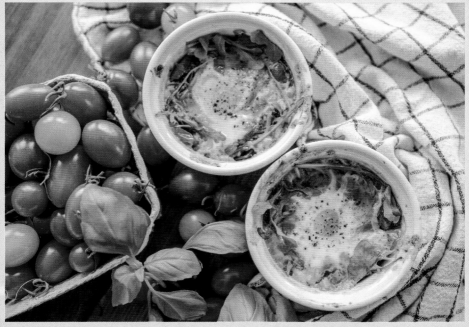

You can eat the Baked Italian Eggs with Tomatoes, Garlic, and Herbs from Chapter
for breakfast or with a salad for a light Italian-style dinner

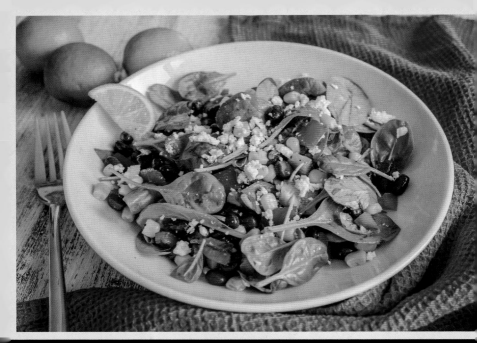

The Black Bean, Corn, and Red Pepper Sunshine Salad from Chapter 7 is the perfect way to get your veggies and nutrients while on the go.

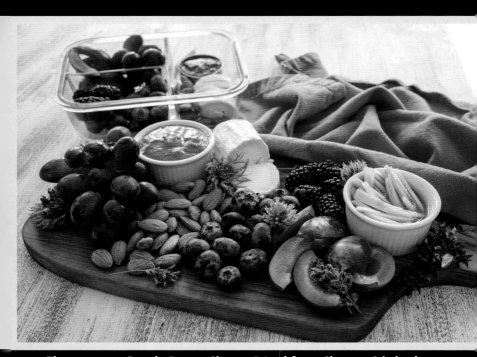

The gorgeous Purple Power Cheese Board from Chapter 8 is both a

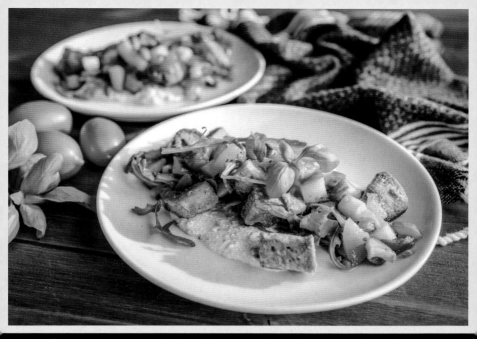

The Tuscan Panzanella Salad over Basil Ricotta Cream from Chapter 9 is a delicious and filling way to enjoy summer's bounty.

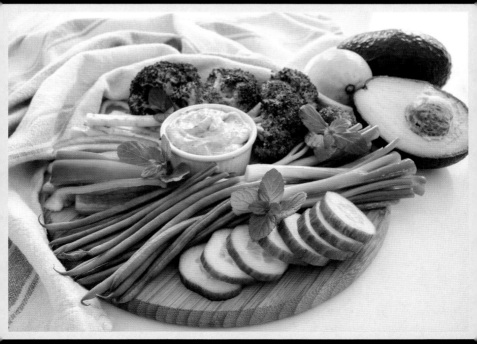

The Green Goddess Vegetable Platter from Chapter 9 can do double duty

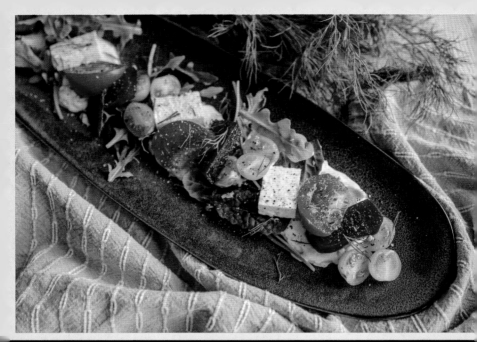

The Enchanted Garden Salad over Tzatziki from Chapter 9 adds nutrition and wonderful Mediterranean flair at any time of day.

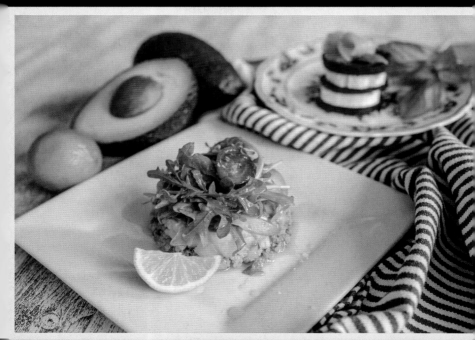

Napoleons with Smoked Salmon, Greek Yogurt and Basil from Chapter 10 and C

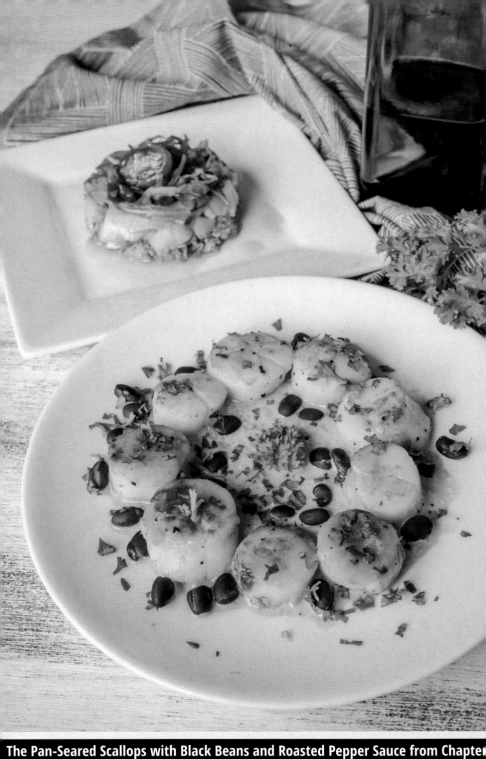

The Pan-Seared Scallops with Black Beans and Roasted Pepper Sauce from Chapter and Quinoa paired with the Mango and Avocado Timbale from Chapter 11 make an impressive and healthful meal perfect for entertaining.

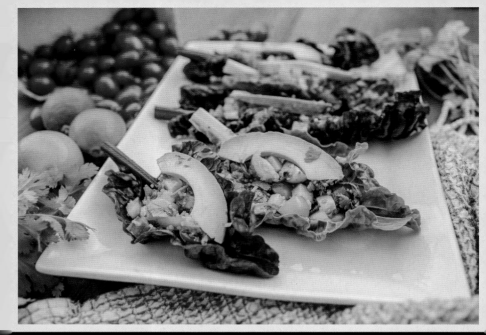

Swiss Chard and Vegetable Confetti "Tacos" from Chapter 10 are a creative, colorful, and healthful way to begin lunch or dinner.

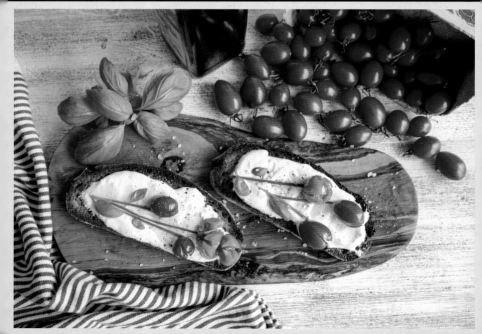

Tulip Bruschetta recipe from Chapter 10 offers an artistic spin on an Italian classi

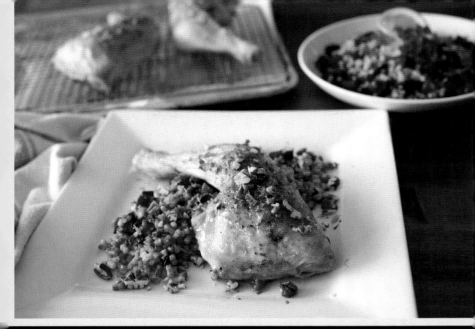

Beet Couscous with Orange Glazed Chicken and Pecans from Chapter 11 adds bright Middle Eastern flavor and colors to the dinner table.

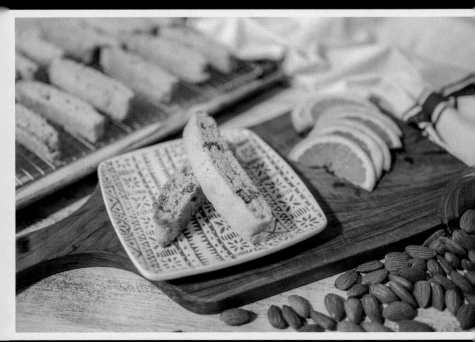

Almond and Orange Biscotti from Chapter 12 incorporates the aromas of Calabr here Chef Amy's family hails from and add authentic Italian flair to the end of a

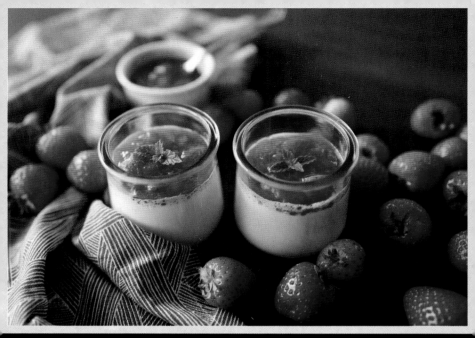

Strawberry Almond Panna Cotta from Chapter 12 is a healthful and pleasing dessert to serve to your guests.

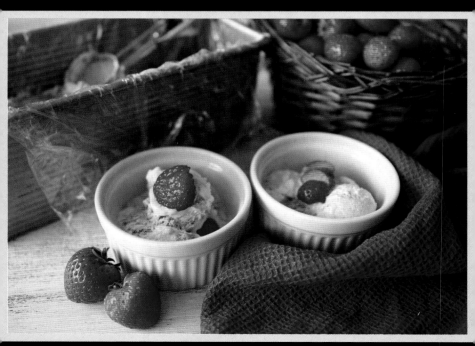

The Strawberry Swirl Ice Cream from Chapter 12 is a mouthwatering, wholesome alternative to commercially prepared ice cream.

☕ Caprese Bites with Mushrooms

PREP TIME: 10 MIN	YIELD: 4 SERVINGS

INGREDIENTS

4 tablespoons (60ml) Amy Riolo Selections or extra-virgin olive oil, divided

12 large button mushrooms or baby portobello mushrooms, stems removed and cleaned

¾ cup (85g) diced fresh mozzarella cheese

12 grape tomatoes, halved

2 tablespoons (5g) freshly chopped basil

2 tablespoons (5g) freshly chopped parsley

⅛ teaspoon (.6g) salt

¼ teaspoon (1.2g) pepper

4 cups (80g) mixed greens or lettuce of your choice

2 tablespoons (30ml) Amy Riolo Selections White Balsamic or balsamic vinegar, for drizzling, optional

DIRECTIONS

1 Preheat the oven to 425 degrees F. Line a baking sheet with parchment paper and drizzle with 1 tablespoon olive oil.

2 Using the back of a spoon, clean out the insides of the mushrooms to leave room for the filling.

3 Place the mozzarella, half of the tomatoes, basil, parsley, 2 tablespoons olive oil, salt, and pepper in a small bowl and mix to combine. Set aside for 10 minutes to marinate.

4 Fill each mushroom with 1 tablespoon of the mixture or until full. Top each mushroom with a tomato half, place the mushrooms on the prepared baking sheet, and bake for 20 to 25 minutes, or until the cheese is golden and melted.

5 Remove from the oven and let cool for 5 minutes.

6 Place 1 cup greens in each of the portable boxes and set the mushrooms on top of the greens. Refrigerate and drizzle 2 tablespoons extra-virgin olive oil and balsamic vinegar before serving.

NOTE: Mushrooms are not only rich in minerals like selenium and potassium but also are an important source of vitamin D. Many people are at risk of being deficient of vitamin D, which is important for bone and general health. The human body requires exposure to sunlight to make most of the vitamin D. Mushrooms are good dietary soures of vitamin D. The combination with EEVO is also important to aid the absorption of this fat-soluble vitamin.

NOTE: These stuffed mushrooms make a great appetizer or side dish.

VARY IT! If you're short on time, place the same filling in lettuce or radicchio leaves and eat them raw.

PER SERVING: *Calories 220 (From Fat 168); Fat 19g (Saturated 5g); Cholesterol 17mg; Sodium 205mg; Carbohydrate 7g (Dietary Fiber 2g); Protein 8g; Sugars 5g.*

Wrapping Wraps and Rolling Rolls

Wraps and rolls are a creative and fun way of combining healthful ingredients into a delicious appetizer or small meal. Kids especially love eating foods that they can pick up, and they're a great way for them to eat more vegetables without noticing. Wraps and rolls are also easy to transform for delicious meals on the go.

If you've never made rolls with wonton or rice paper before, don't worry. Figure 8-1 shows you how to do it. After you get the hang of it, you'll find all kinds of tasty combinations to prepare the same way. Another bonus to preparing rolls is that you can make them in advance and store them in the refrigerator prior to serving, so they're great for entertaining.

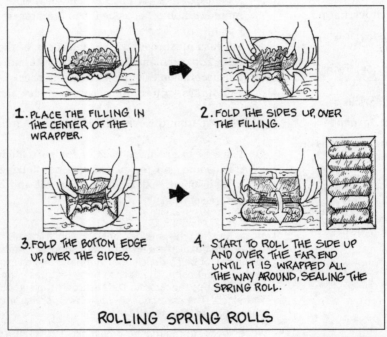

1. PLACE THE FILLING IN THE CENTER OF THE WRAPPER.

2. FOLD THE SIDES UP, OVER THE FILLING.

3. FOLD THE BOTTOM EDGE UP, OVER THE SIDES.

4. START TO ROLL THE SIDE UP AND OVER THE FAR END UNTIL IT IS WRAPPED ALL THE WAY AROUND, SEALING THE SPRING ROLL.

ROLLING SPRING ROLLS

Illustration by Liz Kurtzman

FIGURE 8-1:
How to roll spring rolls.

Fruit and Veggie Rice Paper Rolls

PREP TIME: 20 MIN	YIELD: 4 SERVINGS

INGREDIENTS

12 rice paper wrappers (or large green lettuce leaves)

1 ripe avocado, pitted, and sliced

2 red peppers, seeded and sliced into thin slices

1 cup (110g) shredded carrots

½ cup (124g) tofu (soft or medium), if desired

½ cup (35g) shredded purple cabbage

12 green lettuce leaves

1 mango, sliced into thin strips

DIRECTIONS

1 Soak the rice wrappers in cool water for 5 seconds, drain, and lay on a flat surface.

2 Top with equal parts of all of the remaining ingredients and roll up jelly roll fashion.

3 Slice each wrap in half on the diagonal and place in a shallow dish (or two portable containers standing upright with cut sides exposed). You can place a moist paper towel in between the rolls so that they don't stick.

Dipping Sauce

INGREDIENTS

¼ cup (64g) organic peanut butter

2 tablespoons (30ml) tamari

2 tablespoons (30ml) rice vinegar

1 teaspoon (7g) raw honey

2 tablespoons (30ml) water

1 tablespoon (6g) grated fresh ginger root or ½ teaspoon (.9g) ground ginger

1 clove garlic, minced

DIRECTIONS

1 Place all the dipping sauce ingredients in a blender and emulsify or place in a medium bowl and whisk until smooth.

2 Pour the sauce into separate containers for serving and serve immediately or refrigerate until needed.

TIP: This recipe is a great way to use leftover grilled vegetables and your favorite seasonal fruit.

VARY IT! Use Bibb or Romaine lettuce leaves instead of rice paper wraps.

PER SERVING: *Calories 430 (From Fat 163); Fat 18g (Saturated 3g); Cholesterol 0mg; Sodium 746mg; Carbohydrate 60g (Dietary Fiber 10g); Protein 13g; Sugars 16g.*

Baked Chickpea Fritters with Tomato Jam in Pita Pockets

PREP TIME: 15 MIN | **COOK TIME: 25 MIN** | **YIELD: 4 SERVINGS**

INGREDIENTS

2 tablespoons (30ml) Amy Riolo Selections or extra-virgin olive oil, divided

2 cups (328g) cooked chickpeas (see Chapter 7)

½ cup (46g) chickpea flour or whole-wheat flour

¼ cup (6g) freshly chopped mint or parsley

Juice of 1 lemon

¼ teaspoon (1.2g) salt

⅛ teaspoon (.6g) pepper

4 cups (80g) baby spinach or arugula or other greens

4 whole-wheat pita pockets

DIRECTIONS

1 Place all the ingredients (using only 1 tablespoon of olive oil) into a food processor. Pulse on and off to create a paste.

2 Preheat the oven to 425 degrees F. Line a baking sheet with parchment paper or aluminum foil and grease with the remaining tablespoon of the olive oil.

3 Using a small ice cream scoop, make round fritters out of chickpea mixture. Place on the baking sheet and press lightly. Bake for 20 to 25 minutes or until golden.

4 To serve, slice a pita in half and open. Place ½ cup lettuce in each and top with 3 fritters and jam. Wrap in plastic wrap and refrigerate until serving.

Tomato Jam

INGREDIENTS

2 tablespoons (30ml) Amy Riolo Selections or extra-virgin olive oil, divided

2 Roma tomatoes, diced

Handful of basil, finely chopped

1 teaspoon (7g) raw honey

1 tablespoon (15ml) Amy Riolo Selections White Balsamic or balsamic vinegar

⅛ teaspoon (.6g) salt

DIRECTIONS

1 While the fritters are baking, heat 2 tablespoons of olive oil in a large wide skillet over medium heat.

2 Add the tomatoes and basil and stir to combine. Cover and cook for 5 to 10 minutes or until the tomatoes soften. Carefully remove the lid and stir in the honey, vinegar, and salt. Cover and let cook for another 5 to 10 minutes until the tomatoes form a very chunky sauce–like consistency.

PER SERVING: *Calories 452 (From Fat 163); Fat 18g (Saturated 2g); Cholesterol 0mg; Sodium 630mg; Carbohydrate 61g (Dietary Fiber 13g); Protein 16g; Sugars 9g.*

Smoked Salmon, Arugula, and Mozzarella Sandwich

PREP TIME: 5 MIN   YIELD: 2 SERVINGS

INGREDIENTS

4 thin slices Homemade Whole-Grain Bread (see Chapter 6) or 100 percent whole-grain bread

4 ounces (113g) smoked salmon

2 ounces (57g) fresh mozzarella, sliced thin

1 cup (20g) arugula

1 tablespoon (15ml) Amy Riolo Selections or extra-virgin olive oil

DIRECTIONS

1 Place the bread on a clean surface. Add 2 ounces salmon on top of each of 2 slices. Top with the mozzarella and arugula.

2 Drizzle with the olive oil and top with the remaining 2 slices. Then slice in half. Wrap and serve immediately or store in the refrigerator.

NOTE: Arugula, also known as rocket, is a green leafy vegetable from the same family as broccoli and kale. Its peppery pungency provides the hint that it's rich in polyphenols and glucosinolate bioactive antioxidant compounds. Studies have shown that it may increase glucose uptake by cells thereby improving blood glucose regulation.

TIP: For a gluten-free option, swap the bread for lettuce leaves or grilled portobello mushrooms.

VARY IT! Make pinwheels instead of sandwiches by using 2 tortillas or lavash bread instead of regular bread. Place ingredients on the top of the tortilla, roll up, and slice into pinwheels. They also make cute appetizers.

PER SERVING: *Calories 397 (From Fat 172); Fat 19g (Saturated 6g); Cholesterol 35mg; Sodium 853mg; Carbohydrate 35g (Dietary Fiber 4g); Protein 22g; Sugars 3g.*

Assembling Bountiful Bowls

Bowls are increasingly popular and easy ways of eating healthfully. They offer a variety of delicious flavors and contrasting textures in one dish, without the need to pair several courses together in a meal. Bowls can also be a creative way to repurpose leftovers and are convenient to prepare in advance. Keep beans and legumes, whole grains, and lots of fresh vegetables, spices, and good-quality EVOO, vinegar, and citrus juice on hand to create tasty and nutritious bowls quickly.

TIP

If you've ever been to a fast-casual restaurant you may have noticed how they have counters full of prepared vegetables, proteins, and condiments to choose from. If you're short on time but want to eat well, one of the biggest favors that you can do for yourself is to set up these kinds of bars in your own refrigerator. Here are the steps to convert a shelf in your refrigerator into a restaurant-style prep station:

1. **Determine which vegetables, healthful carbohydrates, and lowfat proteins you want to eat for a week.**

2. **Shop for the ingredients.**

3. **Set aside a 2-hour block of time to prepare food for the week.**

4. **Wash and trim vegetables and store in an airtight container on empty refrigerator shelf.**

5. **Cook proteins (eggs, chicken, fish, beans/legumes, and such)**

6. **Prepare condiments (lemon and/or lime juice, fresh salsa, and so on)**

7. **Prepare quality carbs (quinoa, barley, farro, brown rice, and such)**

8. **Store all the items in separate labelled ontainers in the refrigerator.**

9. **Be sure to use the most perishable items first.**

    Fish should be used the next day, chicken within two days, beef and eggs up to three days; lentils and beans last up to 5 days or you can freeze them.

With this method, by dedicating a few hours to food prep on a Sunday, you can put together healthful meals to your liking all week long. For more meal planning ideas, read our book *Diabetes Meal Planning & Nutrition for Dummies*, 2nd Edition (John Wiley & Sons).

Red Lentil, Couscous, Tomato, and Eggplant Bowl

PREP TIME: 5 MIN	COOK TIME: 15 TO 20 MIN	YIELD: 4 SERVINGS

INGREDIENTS

1 cup (192g) red lentils, rinsed and sorted

5 cups (1.18L) water

1 clove garlic, minced

1 tablespoon (15g) tomato puree

½ teaspoon (2.4g) salt, divided

¼ teaspoon (1.2g) pepper

2 cups (.5L) water

1 cup (173g) couscous

4 tablespoons (60ml) Amy Riolo Selections or extra-virgin olive oil, divided

1 medium eggplant cut into 1-inch pieces

2 Roma tomatoes, diced

1 lemon, quartered

DIRECTIONS

1 Place the lentils in a medium saucepan and add 3 cups water. Add the garlic, tomato puree, ¼ teaspoon salt, and pepper. Bring to a boil over high heat and reduce heat to low. Cover and cook for 5 to 10 minutes until the water has absorbed and the lentils are soft and cooked through.

2 Place 2 cups water in another medium saucepan. Add ¼ teaspoon salt. Bring to a boil over high heat, stir, and add the couscous. Stir and cover immediately, allowing it to sit for 5 minutes with the heat off. Remove the lid, add the remaining ¼ teaspoon salt, and fluff the couscous with a fork and a tablespoon of olive oil.

3 Place the eggplant slices on a greased baking sheet and coat, tossing with your fingers, with 2 tablespoons olive oil.

4 Place under the broiler heated to high and broil for a few minutes, carefully turning once, until cooked through.

5 In 4 portable bowls, layer the lentil puree, couscous, tomatoes, and eggplant. Drizzle with the remaining tablespoon olive oil. Seal and drizzle with the lemon juice before serving.

NOTE: Lentils and couscous are wonderful fibrous sources of plant proteins and have plenty of vitamins and minerals, especially selenium. The minerals copper and manganese are especially concentrated in eggplant, which also has antioxidant polyphenols providing its deep colors.

VARY IT! Swap out brown or green lentils for red lentils and mushrooms for eggplant. You can also substitute quinoa for couscous.

PER SERVING: Calories 490 (From Fat 136); Fat 15g (Saturated 2g); Cholesterol 0mg; Sodium 247mg; Carbohydrate 72g (Dietary Fiber 12g); Protein 19g; Sugars 4g.

Arborio Rice, Fresh Tuna, Vegetables, and Lemon–Herb Dressing

PREP TIME: 10 MIN	COOK TIME: 20 MIN	YIELD: 4 SERVINGS

INGREDIENTS

1 cup (185g) arborio rice

3 tablespoons (45ml) Amy Riolo Selections or extra-virgin olive oil, divided

½ teaspoon (2.4g) salt

Two 4-ounce (113g) fresh tuna steaks

⅛ teaspoon (.6g) pepper

1 cup (91g) broccoli, cut into small florets

1 medium red pepper, diced

2 carrots, peeled and shredded

1 lemon, zested and juiced

½ cup (30g) fresh herbs (parsley, mint, dill, oregano or your favorite), minced

DIRECTIONS

1 Preheat the oven to 425 degrees F. Line a baking sheet with a tablespoon of olive oil and place the tuna on top. Drizzle with another tablespoon of olive oil and season with salt and pepper. Bake the tuna for 10 to 15 minutes or until the desired doneness.

2 Combine the broccoli, red pepper, and carrots in a large bowl.

3 In a small bowl whisk the remaining tablespoon of olive oil and lemon juice and fresh herbs together until emulsified. Drizzle the dressing over the vegetables. Add the cooled rice and toss to coat well.

4 When the tuna is done, remove from the oven and allow to rest for 5 minutes. Slice the tuna thinly and place slices on top of rice salad.

NOTE: Tuna is an oily fish and a good source of healthy omega-3 fats. The lemon in the dressing adds delicious flavor and also slows the absorption of the carbohydrate from the rice, resulting in a healthier, lower rise and fall in blood glucose with a meal. Arborio rice undergoes less milling than other types of rice, which means it retains more healthy fiber.

TIP: Make this salad a day ahead of time and dress it at the last moment.

VARY IT! You can substitute leftover chicken, fish, or vegetables instead of those called for in the recipe. You can also use quinoa, black rice, or barley instead of arborio rice.

PER SERVING: *Calories 355 (From Fat 101); Fat 11g (Saturated 2g); Cholesterol 26mg; Sodium 292mg; Carbohydrate 45g (Dietary Fiber 3g); Protein 18g; Sugars 3g.*

Chilled Rice Noodles with Vegetables and Peanut Sauce

PREP TIME: 15 MIN	COOK TIME: 10 MIN	YIELD: 4 SERVINGS

INGREDIENTS

½ pound (227g) rice or soba noodles or whole-wheat linguine

2 cups (142g) broccoli florets

2 eggs

3 medium cucumbers, halved and sliced

2 scallions, thinly sliced

¼ cup (4g) fresh cilantro, minced

DIRECTIONS

1 Bring a large pot of water to a boil over high heat. Add the noodles and broccoli and cook until al dente.

2 Bring a small saucepan of water to a boil over high heat, add the eggs, and cook about 10 minutes or until cooked through. Remove from the heat, drain and rinse with cold water, and set aside.

3 Drain and rinse the noodles with cold water. Toss the noodles with tongs to prevent clumping. Transfer the noodles to the sauce bowl and toss with the sauce to coat. Stir in the cucumbers, scallions, and cilantro.

4 Peel and chop the eggs and toss them into the noodle mixture to combine.

5 Allow to cool and transfer to 4 individually sized containers with fitting lids. Store in the refrigerator.

Peanut Sauce

INGREDIENTS

¼ cup (64g) organic peanut butter

1 tablespoon (18g) tamari

3 tablespoons (45ml) rice vinegar

1 teaspoon (7g) raw honey

1 tablespoon (6g) grated fresh ginger root or ½ teaspoon (.9g) ground ginger

1 clove garlic, minced

2 tablespoons (30ml) water

DIRECTIONS

1 Combine all the ingredients in a large bowl and whisk well. Set aside.

PER SERVING: *Calories 382 (From Fat 103); Fat 11g (Saturated 3g); Cholesterol 106mg; Sodium 826mg; Carbohydrate 29g (Dietary Fiber 2g); Protein 19g; Sugars 7g.*

🍅 Whole–Wheat Pasta with Tomatoes, Olives, and Mozzarella

PREP TIME: 10 MIN	COOK TIME: 10 MIN	YIELD: 4 SERVINGS

INGREDIENTS

½ pound (227g) whole-wheat pasta (ziti, rigatoni, penne) or lentil pasta

1 pound (454g) fresh mozzarella, diced

Handful of fresh basil, finely chopped

1 cup (149g) cherry tomatoes, halved

¼ cup (37g) kalamata or other olives, pitted and chopped

2 tablespoons (30ml) Amy Riolo Selections or extra-virgin olive oil

DIRECTIONS

1 Cook the pasta until al dente and drain.

2 Combine the mozzarella, basil, tomatoes, and olives in a large bowl.

3 Drizzle with the olive oil and toss to combine with the cooked pasta.

4 Divide into 4 portable containers and store in the refrigerator.

NOTE: This recipe illustrates another important combination that regulates and optimizes carbohydrate metabolism and blood glucose control. The generous addition of EVOO helps lessen the glycemic load carbohydrate in the pasta and increases insulin sensitivity.

TIP: Add leftover vegetables, fresh vegetables, and chicken or shrimp to this dish.

VARY IT! Try the same dish warm. Heat the olive oil in a large skillet. Add the tomatoes and olives and cook for 5 minutes until the tomatoes are soft. Stir in the mozzarella until melted. Add the hot pasta, toss to combine, and serve.

PER SERVING: *Calories 615 (From Fat 306); Fat 34g (Saturated 16g); Cholesterol 90mg; Sodium 817mg; Carbohydrate 47g (Dietary Fiber 1g); Protein 34g; Sugars 2g.*

Sweet Potato, Black Bean, and Cashew Bowl

PREP TIME: 10 MIN	COOK TIME: 5 MIN	YIELD: 2 SERVINGS

INGREDIENTS

1 medium sweet potato, scrubbed

2 cups (60g) baby spinach

1 cup (185g) cooked Black Beans (see Chapter 7) or canned, no-sodium black beans, rinsed

½ cup (75g) cherry tomatoes, halved

¼ cup (34g) plain cashews, chopped

½ cup (112g) Greek yogurt

2 tablespoons (30ml) extra-virgin olive oil

1 lime, halved

⅛ teaspoon (.6g) salt

DIRECTIONS

1 Prick a sweet potato with a fork several times, place on a plate, and cook it in the microwave for 4 to 5 minutes on high speed or until done.

2 Divide the spinach, black beans, tomatoes, and cashews into the bottom of two bowls.

3 Cut the sweet potato in half and then quarters and place the pieces on top of the salad mixture and salt them.

4 Top with the Greek yogurt and olive oil and squeeze half of the lime in each bowl. Refrigerate until serving.

NOTE: Sweet potatoes are high in fiber, and their orange color indicates that they're an excellent source of carotenoids, especially important for vitamin A production, which plays a role in eye health and supports immune system. The protein and fiber in black beans and cashew nuts also help to fill you up.

TIP: To serve this recipe as a side dish, just sauté the spinach and toss in the other ingredients, topping with Greek yogurt.

VARY IT! Swap out sweet potato for quinoa or another whole grain.

PER SERVING: Calories 461 (From Fat 102); Fat 222g (Saturated 25g); Cholesterol 0mg; Sodium 189mg; Carbohydrate 47g (Dietary Fiber 8g); Protein 18g; Sugars 8g.

Baked Avocado Eggs with Mixed Greens

PREP TIME: 5 MIN	COOK TIME: 15 MIN	YIELD: 2 SERVINGS

INGREDIENTS

1 medium to large avocado

1 lime or lemon, halved

2 eggs

2 cups (40g) mixed greens

2 tablespoons (30ml) Amy Riolo Selections or extra-virgin olive oil

1 lemon, halved

⅛ teaspoon (.6g) salt

Pepper to taste

DIRECTIONS

1 Preheat the oven to 425 degrees F. Slice the avocado in half, remove the pit, and place on a baking sheet. Drizzle juice of ½ lemon or lime over avocado.

2 Break an egg into each half. Bake for 10 minutes, or until the egg is set. Place the greens on the bottom of 2 portable bowls or fitted lids.

3 Scoop the avocado out of the shell and place on top of greens. Drizzle with olive oil and place a half of a lemon in the bowl. Season with salt and pepper to taste.

NOTE: Eggs once or twice a week eaten alongside other healthy ingredients are a great way to enjoy a multitude of vitamins including the important B vitamins in a protein-rich and satisfying recipe. Pepper is a great flavor enhancer with egg dishes and adds the polyphenol peperine, which has antioxidant and anti-inflammatory properties as well as possibly improving blood glucose regulation and increasing the absorption of important minerals.

NOTE: This recipe also works well at brunch.

VARY IT! Bake the eggs in Portobello mushroom caps.

PER SERVING: *Calories 362 (From Fat 300); Fat 33g (Saturated 6g); Cholesterol 12mg; Sodium 200mg; Carbohydrate 12g (Dietary Fiber 7g); Protein 9g; Sugars 2g.*

Chapter **9**

Sensational Salads for All Occasions

Salads are the easiest and fastest way to fill yourself with the nutrients that you need. They're chock-full of delicious and antioxidant-rich vegetables with complex carbohydrates that help people with diabetes manage their glucose levels. Depending on what you add to them, dress them with, or pair them with, they can be a snack, meal, appetizer, or even a terrific last course. Stuff them in a pita pocket for a quick sandwich. Fill up a portable plastic container with them for an easy brown-bag lunch. Or toss them with a light vinaigrette for an easy meal.

In this chapter, we show you how to make the most from your salad choices. We give you excellent ideas for fun salads and tips for whipping up great homemade dressings to match your nutritional needs. We explain how to add fruit to your salads for a sweet, refreshing twist. And finally, we offer recipes for protein-packed salads, a perfect meal solution for just about any nutritional quandary.

Be sure to read the Notes after the recipes to find out about its nutritional values. Also refer to the book's Introduction for some recipe conventions we use.

Feasting on Great Salad Greens

Whether greens are an important part of the salad you're making or added just for garnish, using special and novel greens makes your salad stand out. Skip the pale green iceberg lettuce and buy some darker green lettuces like romaine and leaf lettuce instead. Kale, arugula, dandelion greens, cabbage, and others all make great choices. The greener the leaf, the more nutrients it contains, especially magnesium, a mineral important for heart and bone health.

Here we discuss what greens to choose for you next salad and how you can elevate your greens to create tasty and healthful salads.

Picking fresh greens at the store

We recommend purchasing local and organic produce as often as possible. Always choose the freshest vegetables you can find. When you go shopping, consider picking up some of these types of greens (see Figure 9-1):

» Arugula	» Mizuna
» Boston butter lettuce	» Radicchio
» Dandelion greens	» Red leaf lettuce
» Endive	» Romaine
» Escarole	» Spinach
» Frisée	» Swiss chard
» Kale	» Watercress

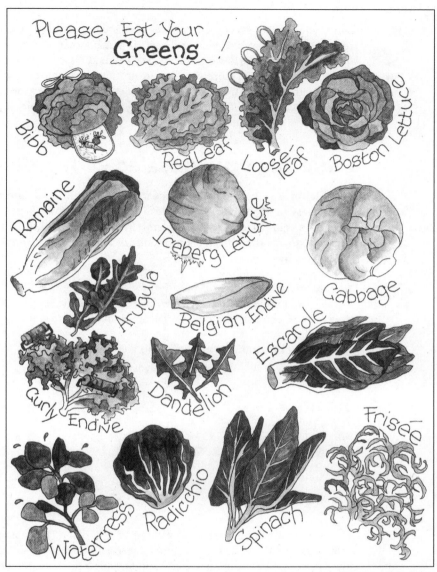

FIGURE 9-1: A sampling of tasty greens to try for your next salad.

Illustration by Liz Kurtzman

Store your salad greens in the vegetable compartment of your fridge. Store romaine and radicchio with the head intact because the outer leaves keep the inner leaves moist. However, loose-leaf lettuce, like arugula and spinach, has a shorter shelf life. To store this type of lettuce, remove the leaves and wash and drain them. Gather and wrap them in a clean, damp paper towel or two and then store in a container. The leaves will stay fresh for a couple days, but not much longer.

Punching up your salad with protein

Eggs, leftover or grilled chicken, meat, fish, shrimp, nuts, and small amounts of goat cheese or aged sheep milk cheese and fresh mozzarella are great ways to add protein to your salads. Combining protein and good-quality fat with your vegetables transforms them from a simple side or appetizer to a complete meal that you can enjoy anytime.

Nuts have an undeserved reputation for being fattening. Not so! In moderation, nuts are an excellent source of fiber and monounsaturated fat, the good fat. Plus, they provide you with long-lasting protein that helps to stabilize your blood sugar.

Here's a list of seeds and nuts to try in your next salad:

>> Almonds

>> Cashews

>> Pecans

>> Pine nuts

>> Sunflower seeds

>> Walnuts

You can toast nuts before adding them to any dish. The toasting process really brings out the flavor of the nuts, making them much more satisfying to eat. Simply place them in a sauté pan over medium-high heat, shaking them occasionally to ensure they don't burn. They're done when they become fragrant and slightly darker in color.

☺ Roasted Beet, Citrus, and Watercress Salad with Asparagus

PREP TIME: 15 MIN	COOK TIME: 45 MIN	YIELD: 4 SERVINGS

INGREDIENTS

¾ pounds (340g) medium red and golden beets

1 head garlic

¼ cup (240ml) extra-virgin olive oil, divided

1 bunch fresh asparagus, trimmed

⅛ teaspoon (.6g) salt

Pepper to taste

Juice and zest of 1 orange

2 tablespoons (30ml) Amy Riolo Selections White Balsamic or your favorite balsamic vinegar

4 cups (136g) fresh watercress

4 ounces (110g) fresh goat cheese or feta, crumbled

4 tablespoons (30g) toasted walnuts, finely chopped

DIRECTIONS

1 Preheat the oven to 425 degrees F.

2 Place the beets in a small baking dish and cover it with foil. Cut off the top third of the garlic and drizzle it with 1 teaspoon of olive oil and wrap it in foil. Bake the beets and garlic until tender, about 45 minutes, and allow to cool enough to handle.

3 Place the asparagus on a lined baking sheet on a rack under the beets during the last 15 minutes of cooking and cook until tender. Remove the asparagus to cool.

4 Remove the beets, peel them, cut them into wedges, and place them in a large bowl.

5 Squeeze the garlic cloves into a bowl and mash with a fork. Stir in the remaining olive oil and season with salt and pepper.

6 In a bowl, whisk together the orange juice, zest, and vinegar.

7 Toss the beets, dressing, asparagus, and watercress in a large bowl. Sprinkle with the goat cheese and walnuts and serve immediately.

NOTE: Beets are full of natural nitrates, compounds that help to lower blood pressure, especially when combined with the heathy fats of olive oil. The peppery watercress adds flavor but also is rich in minerals and vitamins, especially vitamin K as well as more than 40 varieties of flavonoid polyphenols.

TIP: Roast beets ahead of time and keep them on hand to use in salads whenever the mood strikes.

VARY IT! In addition to watercress, arugula, mixed greens, and baby spinach also work well in this salad.

PER SERVING: *Calories 351 (From Fat 242); Fat 27g (Saturated 8g); Cholesterol 22mg; Sodium 260mg; Carbohydrate 19g (Dietary Fiber 5g); Protein 12g. Sugars 11g.*

🍅 Heirloom Tomato, Arugula, and Mozzarella Salad

| PREP TIME: 10 MIN | YIELD: 4 SERVINGS |

INGREDIENTS

10 to 12 ounces (284 to 340g) baby arugula, washed and drained

1 or 2 garlic cloves, mashed with salt (.6ml or ⅛ tsp)

2 tablespoons (30ml) Amy Riolo Selections White Balsamic or balsamic vinegar

3 tablespoons (45ml) Amy Riolo Selections or extra-virgin olive oil

⅛ teaspoon (.6g) salt

Pepper to taste

2 medium heirloom tomatoes, peeled and cut in bite-size pieces

4 ounces (113grams) fresh mozzarella balls, drained

DIRECTIONS

1 Place the arugula on a serving dish.

2 In a small bowl, whisk together the garlic, balsamic vinegar, olive oil, salt, and pepper. Pour over the arugula and toss.

3 Top with the tomatoes and mozzarella.

NOTE: Heirloom tomatoes are a little more expensive than regular tomatoes because they're raised more intensively. In general, plants that are grown in more traditional ways have to work harder to protect themselves from the stresses of their environment and therefore are more likely to be higher in antioxidant and anti-inflammatory bioactive compounds. In the case of tomatoes these compounds include carotenoids and polyphenols, which may be 30 percent higher in heirloom tomatoes grown in organic conditions.

TIP: Enjoy this salad in the summertime or when tomatoes are at their peak.

VARY IT! Fresh peaches make a great alternative to tomatoes when they're in season. You can also use beets in the winter.

PER SERVING: *Calories 210 (From Fat154); Fat 17g (Saturated 5g); Cholesterol 22mg; Sodium 322mg; Carbohydrate 7g (Dietary Fiber 2g); Protein 9g. Sugars 4g.*

🍅 Radish and Orange Salad with Bulgur and Pistachios

PREP TIME: 10 MIN	COOK TIME: 5 MIN	YIELD: 4 SERVINGS

INGREDIENTS

⅔ cup (92g) uncooked bulgur wheat, cooked and cooled

1 bunch radishes, washed, trimmed, and thinly sliced.

1 large orange, peeled and chopped (approximately ¾ cup) (135g)

1 cup (164g) cooked chickpeas

1 cup (60g) Italian parsley, finely chopped

2 tablespoons (15ml) orange juice

2 tablespoons (15ml) Amy Riolo Selections or extra-virgin olive oil

⅛ teaspoon (.6ml) salt

Pinch of pepper to taste

½ cup (62g) shelled unsalted pistachios, finely chopped

DIRECTIONS

1 Place the bulgur in a large bowl and add the radishes, orange pieces, chickpeas, and parsley.

2 Combine the orange juice, olive oil, salt, and pepper in a small bowl and whisk until emulsified.

3 Pour the dressing over the bulgur mixture and toss to coat.

4 Sprinkle the pistachios on top and serve.

NOTE: Radishes are an example of a vegetable with a pungent flavor and vibrant colors that indicate the presence of many bioactive compounds and varieties of carotenoids and polyphenols. The ancient Greeks and Romans used radishes as medicines, and researchers are now studying their anti-inflammatory effects. Pistachios, in common with other nuts, are satiating with protein, minerals, vitamins, fiber, and numerous antioxidants.

TIP: Make this salad a day in advance and dress it before serving.

VARY IT! Swap brown rice, quinoa, couscous, or barley for the bulgur, if desired.

PER SERVING: *Calories 348 (From Fat 143); Fat 16g (Saturated 2g); Cholesterol 0mg; Sodium 227mg; Carbohydrate 44g (Dietary Fiber 12g); Protein 12g. Sugars 9g.*

🍅 Purple Potato Salad with Edamame and Dill

PREP TIME: 15 MIN	COOK TIME: 15 TO 20 MIN	YIELD: 4 SERVINGS

INGREDIENTS

4 ounces (110g) frozen or fresh edamame (soybeans) in the pod, thawed

Bowl of ice water

10 ounces (283g) purple potatoes, or your favorite potato, cut into large chunks

1 teaspoon (5g) salt, divided

½ pound (227g) haricots verts or regular green beans, trimmed

¼ cup (56g) Greek yogurt

¼ cup (2g) finely chopped fresh dill

¼ cup (60ml) Amy Riolo Selections White Balsamic Vinegar or balsamic vinegar

¼ cup (60ml) Amy Riolo Selections or extra-virgin olive oil

⅛ teaspoon (.6g) pepper

DIRECTIONS

1 Bring a large pot of salted water to a boil over high heat. Add the edamame and boil, uncovered, for 1 to 3 minutes, until tender but still crisp on the outside. Transfer with a slotted spoon to a bowl of ice water and leave the pot to boil potatoes in.

2 When cool enough to handle, shell the edamame (if they're already shelled, skip this step.)

3 Bring the pot of water back to a boil over high heat and add the potatoes. Cook until fork-tender and drain, about 10 minutes.

4 Bring a separate pot of water to a boil and add ½ teaspoon salt. Add the green beans and cook until tender, about 3 to 4 minutes. Drain when slightly tender and place in the ice water.

5 In a small bowl, mix the yogurt, dill, balsamic vinegar, and extra-virgin olive oil and whisk until smooth.

6 Combine the edamame, potatoes, green beans, remaining ½ teaspoon salt in a large bowl. Add the pepper and mix until combined well. Refrigerate until serving.

NOTE: Choosing vegetables with colorful skins, in this case potatoes, adds antioxidant and anti-inflammatory polyphenols in both the outer layer and the flesh. Polyphenols act to increase insulin sensitivity and balance blood glucose levels, which is probably the reason that the glycemic index of purple potatoes is lower than standard potatoes.

VARY IT! If you can't find purple potatoes, you can use sweet potatoes, russet potatoes, or red-skinned baby potatoes. You can also use lima beans instead of edamame.

PER SERVING: *Calories 249 (From Fat 141); Fat 16g (Saturated 2g); Cholesterol 0mg; Sodium 487mg; Carbohydrate 22g (Dietary Fiber 4g); Protein 7g. Sugars 6g.*

Going beyond greens with tomatoes

For many people, salad and lettuce are synonymous. When tomatoes are in season, they can add a great deal more of visual appeal, flavor, and nutrients. Trying your hand at other salads that highlight other terrific vegetables, like tomatoes and cucumbers, is fun. Flavor them with various types — different shapes and sizes of tomatoes for a fun visual effect.

As you can see from the different types of salads in this chapter, greens don't have to be boring. If they're prepared with the same amount of detail as the rest of the meal, there's no reason why they can't be a highlight.

REMEMBER

Here are some simple formulas to keep your salads interesting and to ensure that you're getting the adequate amounts of fresh produce in your daily diet:

>> Greens + fruit + nuts or other protein

>> Cooked whole grains + roasted vegetables + nuts

>> Beans or lentils + fresh herbs + carrots + fruit

>> Mixture of three to four types of leafy greens

>> Protein (chicken, turkey, fish) + whole grains + greens

>> Roasted pears or apples + leafy greens + goat cheese

>> Cucumbers + tomatoes + leafy greens + feta cheese

TIP

Don't forget that leftover grilled and roasted vegetables and meat, poultry, or fish take on a whole new flavor when tossed with leafy greens, good-quality EVOO, and a good-quality balsamic vinegar or lemon juice.

Tuscan Panzanella Salad over Basil Ricotta Cream

PREP TIME: 10 MIN	COOK TIME: 5 MIN	YIELD: 4 SERVINGS

INGREDIENTS

1 English cucumber, halved lengthwise and cut into small pieces

2 Roma tomatoes, diced

2 ripe peaches (if in season), cut into bite-size pieces, or 1 cup yellow cherry tomatoes, halved

1 cup (20g) arugula, or your favorite greens

2 pieces day-old whole-wheat bread, cubed

¼ cup (60ml) Amy Riolo Selections or extra-virgin olive oil

2 tablespoons (30ml) Amy Riolo Selections White Balsamic or balsamic vinegar

¼ teaspoon (1.2g) salt

⅛ teaspoon (.6g) pepper

2 cups (492g) whole-milk ricotta

1 bunch fresh basil

DIRECTIONS

1 Combine the cucumber, tomatoes, peaches, and arugula in a large bowl.

2 Place the bread cubes on a baking tray under the broiler heated at high for 1 to 2 minutes, or until golden. Remove from the oven, turn over the cubes, and return for another minute. Remove from the oven and allow to cool.

3 Drizzle the olive oil, balsamic vinegar, salt, and pepper over the vegetables. Add the bread and toss to coat.

4 Pulse to combine the ricotta and basil in a food processor or blender, or finely chop the basil and stir it into the ricotta.

5 Spoon the ricotta mixture onto the bottom of a platter and smooth it with a spatula. Add the salad over the top in a mound, leaving room for the ricotta to show.

NOTE: Ricotta cheese is a particular type of whey cheese that's lower in saturated fat and salt than other cheeses. Whenever possible, choose ricotta made from sheep or goat milk, which contains saturated fats that are less likely to affect LDL cholesterol levels and is more sustainably produced.

NOTE: Refer to the color insert for a photo of this recipe.

VARY IT! You can add leftover meat, chicken, shrimp, or salmon to this dish, which transforms it into what Italians call a "Monday salad" — a salad that's made with the leftover items from a large Sunday supper.

PER SERVING: *Calories 434 (From Fat 277); Fat 31g (Saturated 12g); Cholesterol 63mg; Sodium 284mg; Carbohydrate 25g (Dietary Fiber 3g); Protein 17g. Sugars 11g.*

Enjoying Entree Salads

Entree salads are popular restaurant menu options, but for some reason a lot of people don't consider them when cooking at home. The idea of having a salad or serving a salad to guests might not seem like enough to people. Traditionally they weren't popular in the Mediterranean region, but that's beginning to change. On recent trips to Greece, I (Amy) have noticed many more entree salad options, even in traditional restaurants. In Italy, a lot of people that I know have started eating them as a light dinner because the heavier meal is traditionally served at lunch.

TIP

The key to making a delicious yet nutritious entree salad is to use the freshest ingredients possible. Be sure to include the three macronutrients (good-quality protein, fat, and complex carbohydrates) in your salad. Load up on lots of leafy greens and cruciferous vegetables for antioxidants and fiber. Finally, be sure to use good-quality EVOO and vinegars or lemon juice instead of sugar and sodium-laden commercial dressings that are full of unwanted additives, calories, and fat.

Entree salads are a great way to incorporate leftovers into a portable lunch or dinner, too. I find that even those who aren't salad fans tend to change their opinion when the salads are made with their favorite proteins and tossed with flavorful EVOO, vinegar, and citrus juice. Best of all, they can be prepared in a few minutes and fill you up without making you feel sluggish or heavy after the meal.

Tomato, Radish, and Red Onion Salad with Citrus and Shrimp

INGREDIENTS

4 tablespoons (60ml) Amy Riolo Selections or extra-virgin olive oil, divided

1 pound (455g) shrimp, peeled and deveined

Pinch of crushed red chili flakes

⅛ teaspoon (.6g) salt

Juice and zest of 2 lemons, divided

1 medium red onion, thinly sliced

8 radishes, trimmed and thinly sliced

4 Roma tomatoes, finely chopped

1 bunch fresh cilantro or Italian parsley, finely chopped

DIRECTIONS

1 Heat 1 tablespoon of the olive oil in a large skillet over medium–high heat. Add the shrimp and crushed chili flakes and allow to cook 1 to 2 minutes per side or until the shrimp change color and begin to shrink. Remove from the heat and season with the salt and half of the lemon juice. Set aside.

2 Place the red onion, radishes, tomatoes, and cilantro in a large bowl. Toss to coat.

3 Combine the remaining half of the lemon juice and olive oil in a small bowl and whisk to emulsify. Pour the dressing over the vegetables and toss to coat. Top the salad with the warm shrimp.

NOTE: Red onions are an example of higher levels of antioxidant polyphenols in colored vegetables. The polyphenols, quercetin, and anthocyanins, which have been the subject of research for possible anticancer effects, are found in greater amounts. Shrimp is a great source of iodine that's important for brain and thyroid gland health.

TIP: You can add cooked quinoa to this salad to make it an even more filling meal.

VARY IT! Use chicken or fish, such as salmon, cod, or tuna, rather than shrimp.

PER SERVING: *Calories 274 (From Fat 142); Fat 16g (Saturated 2g); Cholesterol 172mg; Sodium 244mg; Carbohydrate 9g (Dietary Fiber 2g); Protein 25g. Sugars 4g.*

Smoked Salmon, Avocado, and Egg Salad

| PREP TIME: 5 MIN | COOK TIME: 5 MIN | YIELD: 4 SERVINGS |

INGREDIENTS

4 eggs

4 cups (80g) baby lettuce or greens of your choice

2 avocados, sliced

4 ounces (110g) smoked salmon, sliced

1 lemon, juiced

2 tablespoons (30ml) Amy Riolo Selections or extra-virgin olive oil

⅛ teaspoon (.6g) salt

Pepper to taste

DIRECTIONS

1 Place the eggs in a medium saucepan and cover with water. Boil over high heat for 4 minutes. Remove from the heat and drain.

2 Divide the lettuce onto 4 plates and arrange the avocado slices on each place.

3 Carefully wrap one slice of salmon at a time around your pinky finger into the shape of a rosette and place on top of lettuce. Place the eggs in the middle of each plate.

4 Pour the lemon juice over each plate, drizzle with the olive oil, and season with the salt and pepper.

NOTE: Combining the salmon's protein and fish omega-3 fats with the satiating egg proteins and the monounsaturated fats of EVOO and avocado produces a lower carbohydrate snack that will keep you satisfied for longer.

TIP: To make this salad ahead of time, wait until serving to top with the avocado, olive oil, and lemon juice.

VARY IT! Substitute the salmon for leftover chicken, meat, or shrimp if desired. You can also add 2 cups of whole grains such as barley, whole wheat, or quinoa.

PER SERVING: *Calories 333 (From Fat 250); Fat 28g (Saturated 5g); Cholesterol 218mg; Sodium 363mg; Carbohydrate 11g (Dietary Fiber 7g); Protein 14g. Sugars 2g.*

⏲ Roasted Cauliflower with Chickpeas and Hazelnut Dressing

PREP TIME: 10 MIN	COOK TIME: 30 MIN	YIELD: 4 SERVINGS

INGREDIENTS

1 head cauliflower

3 tablespoons (45ml) Amy Riolo Selections or extra-virgin olive oil, divided

1 cup (164g) cooked chickpeas

1 teaspoon (.6g) dried coriander

1 teaspoon (.6g) smoked paprika

⅛ teaspoon (.6g) salt

Pepper to taste

1 teaspoon (5ml) hazelnut oil

¼ cup (29g) shelled hazelnuts, toasted and finely chopped

2 tablespoons (30ml) sherry vinegar

DIRECTIONS

1 Preheat oven to 425 degrees F. Slice the cauliflower into four ¾-inch steaks (see Figure 9-2). Oil a baking sheet with 1 tablespoon of olive oil. Add the cauliflower steaks and brush both sides with 1 tablespoon of olive oil.

2 Combine the chickpeas, 1 tablespoon of olive oil, coriander, paprika, salt, and pepper.

3 Spread the chickpeas on the baking sheet with the cauliflower and place in the oven until crispy and golden, approximately 15 minutes. Remove from the oven, flip the cauliflower, and toss the chickpeas.

4 Return to the oven and bake for another 15 minutes or until golden. When done, transfer to a plate.

5 Combine the hazelnut oil, hazelnuts, and sherry vinegar in a small bowl. Mix well with a fork to combine and drizzle over the cauliflower and chickpeas.

PER SERVING: *Calories 258 (From Fat 161); Fat 18g (Saturated 2g); Cholesterol 0mg; Sodium 106mg; Carbohydrate 20g (Dietary Fiber 7g); Protein 8g. Sugars 5g.*

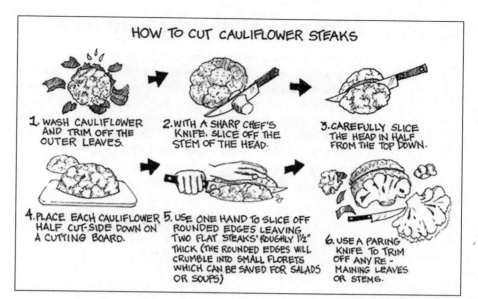

FIGURE 9-2:
Slicing a
cauliflower.

Illustration by Liz Kurtzman

Adding fresh fruit to your salad

Everyone knows how refreshing fruit salad can taste, made with three or four of the season's best crops. But people with diabetes need to enjoy fruit, which is full of natural and easily absorbed sugars, in moderation. How can you still include the juicy pleasures of fruit in a diabetic diet? By creating meals with small amounts of fruit and combining it with other macronutrients such as quality protein and fat, such as those recipes in this section. Remember that even though some of these ingredients — eggplant, avocados, and tomatoes — are often considered vegetables, they're actually fruit.

Pear and Butternut Squash Salad with Roasted Pecans

PREP TIME: 20 MIN	COOK TIME: 25 MIN	YIELD: 4 SERVINGS

INGREDIENTS

1 small butternut squash, peeled and chopped into ½-inch (1.25cm) pieces

¼ cup plus 2 tablespoons (60ml + 30ml) Amy Riolo Selections or extra-virgin olive oil, divided

1 cup (30g) baby spinach

1 large Bosc pear, sliced into quarters

¼ cup (38g) feta or gorgonzola cheese

1 cup (198g) cooked lentils

¼ cup (27g) pecans, toasted and chopped

Juice of 1 lemon

⅛ teaspoon (.6g) salt

Pepper to taste

DIRECTIONS

1 Preheat the oven to 425 degrees F. Place the squash on a baking sheet and drizzle with 2 tablespoons olive oil. Turn to coat well. Roast, uncovered, until cooked through and lightly browned, about 20 minutes, stirring halfway through. Allow to cool (you can do this step a day in advance).

2 Add the spinach, pear slices, cheese, lentils, and pecans to a large bowl.

3 Whisk well to combine the lemon juice, ¼ cup olive oil, salt, and pepper into a medium bowl.

4 Top the salad with the squash. Pour the dressing over the salad and serve immediately.

NOTE: Pears are rich in dietary fiber and antioxidants, which promote digestive health and reduce the risk of chronic diseases. Butternut squash is packed with vitamins, minerals, and fiber, which support eye health and immune function and help with digestion.

TIP: Purchase fresh, peeled butternut squash to save time with preparation.

VARY IT! You can substitute carrots or other root vegetables instead of butternut squash.

PER SERVING: *Calories 373 (From Fat 243); Fat 27g (Saturated 5g); Cholesterol 8mg; Sodium 174mg; Carbohydrate 30g (Dietary Fiber 8g); Protein 8g. Sugars 9g.*

Thai Mango Salad

INGREDIENTS

1 large ripe mango, peeled and sliced into thin strips

1 medium green onion, finely chopped

1 medium sweet red pepper, diced

1 cup (129g) fresh bean sprouts

⅛ teaspoon (.6g) salt

Pepper to taste

½ cup (73g) unsalted peanuts, finely chopped

1 tablespoon (.02g) chopped fresh cilantro

1 teaspoon (5ml) sweet chili sauce

Juice of 1 lime

1 teaspoon (2g) grated fresh ginger

DIRECTIONS

1 Place the mango, onion, red pepper, bean sprouts, salt, pepper, peanuts, and cilantro in a large bowl and mix well.

2 Combine the chili sauce, lime juice, and fresh ginger in a medium bowl.

3 Whisk until combined and then pour over the salad and toss to combine.

NOTE: Mangoes, a great source of vitamins A and C, help with immune support, vision, and skin health.

TIP: To make the salad in advance, store the salad and dressing separately in the refrigerator. When you're ready to serve, toss them to combine. Make a double batch of the dressing to use as a marinade for chicken.

VARY IT! Use shrimp or hardboiled eggs for additional protein, if desired.

PER SERVING: *Calories 162 (From Fat 84); Fat 9g (Saturated 1g); Cholesterol 0mg; Sodium 64mg; Carbohydrate 17g (Dietary Fiber 4g); Protein 6g. Sugars 11g.*

Asparagus and Strawberry Salad with Fresh Mozzarella

PREP TIME: 15 MIN	COOK TIME: 10 MIN	YIELD: 4 SERVINGS

INGREDIENTS

1 bunch kale leaves, rinsed and stems trimmed

2 tablespoons (15g) walnuts, toasted

1 cup (166g) strawberries, hulled and sliced thinly

1 ounce (28g) fresh mozzarella cheese, cut into small pieces

1 bunch asparagus, trimmed

2 tablespoons (30ml) Amy Riolo Selections or extra-virgin olive oil

2 tablespoons (30ml) balsamic vinegar

Pepper to taste

DIRECTIONS

1 Preheat oven to 425 degrees F.

2 Massage the kale by removing the fibrous ribs, taking the bunches into both hands, and rubbing together for 5 minutes. Chop the kale into thin ribbons and place in a large bowl.

3 Chop the walnuts and add the walnuts, strawberries, and mozzarella to the kale.

4 Place the asparagus on a lined baking sheet and bake for 5 to 10 minutes, turning after the first three minutes, or until barely soft. Allow to cool.

5 Whisk and combine the olive oil, balsamic vinegar, and pepper in a small bowl. Pour the dressing over the kale, add the cooked asparagus, and toss until coated. Serve immediately.

NOTE: Asparagus, low in calories and high in nutrients, supports heart health and provides essential vitamins and minerals. Strawberries, high in polyphenol antioxidants, vitamin C, and fiber, contribute to heart health and reduce inflammation.

TIP: Add leftover protein, if desired to this salad.

VARY IT! Swap the kale for another green and the strawberries for tomatoes.

PER SERVING: Calories 146 (From Fat 97); Fat 11g (Saturated 2g); Cholesterol 6mg; Sodium 62mg; Carbohydrate 10g (Dietary Fiber 3g); Protein 4g. Sugars 4g.

Cucumber Rolls Filled with Avocado, Tomato, and Baby Kale

| PREP TIME: 20 MIN | YIELD: 4 SERVINGS |

INGREDIENTS

⅓ cup (80g) whole-milk ricotta

2 tablespoons (5g) fresh basil, finely chopped

Juice and zest of 1 lemon

⅛ teaspoon (.6g) salt

Pepper to taste

1 large English cucumber, ends trimmed

9 grape tomatoes, sliced in halves

1 avocado, thinly sliced

½ cup (34g) baby kale

DIRECTIONS

1 Combine the ricotta, basil, lemon juice and zest, salt, and pepper in a medium bowl and stir until creamy, approximately 5 minutes.

2 With a vegetable peeler, remove and discard the peel from one side of the cucumber. Peel the cucumber lengthwise into 16-inch long, thin ribbons.

3 Spread 1 side of each slice with approximately ¾ tablespoon of the ricotta mixture. Place a ½ tomato on one end of each cucumber slice followed by 1 avocado slice and ⅛ cup of baby kale.

4 Roll up the cucumber slices, flat side down to make 8 rollups.

NOTE: Cucumbers are hydrating and low in calories and assist in hydration and provide many essential vitamins and minerals. Kale, a nutrient powerhouse, rich in vitamins A, K, and C, promotes bone health, vision, and immune function.

TIP: Make them in advance for a party or special event.

VARY IT! If you want to include variations, you can. None of these ingredients is required.

PER SERVING: *Calories 141 (From Fat 92); Fat 10g (Saturated 3g); Cholesterol 10mg; Sodium 86mg; Carbohydrate 11g (Dietary Fiber 4g); Protein 4g. Sugars 3g.*

Green Goddess Vegetable Platter

PREP TIME: 15 MIN	COOK TIME: 5 MIN	YIELD: 4 SERVINGS

INGREDIENTS

16 stalks asparagus, trimmed

4 cups (364g) broccoli, florets only

1 small bunch spring onions

1 teaspoon (5ml) Amy Riolo Selections or extra-virgin olive oil

1 bunch fresh mint

2 medium green peppers, cored and cut into strips

¼ teaspoon (1.2g) salt

DIRECTIONS

1 Brush the asparagus, broccoli, and spring onions with the olive oil and place on a preheated grill pan or on a pan placed under the broiler. Grill for 3 to 5 minutes on each side or until tender. Sprinkle with salt.

2 Arrange the mint and green peppers on a large platter. Add the grilled vegetables.

Green Goddess Dressing

INGREDIENTS

1 cup (226g) Greek yogurt

1 avocado, peeled, destoned, and flesh removed

Handful of fresh parsley

Handful of fresh cilantro

¼ cup (60ml) Amy Riolo Selections or extra-virgin olive oil

Juice of 1 lemon

⅛ teaspoon (.6g) pepper

DIRECTIONS

1 Place all the dressing ingredients in a blender and puree until smooth.

2 Pour the dressing into a small bowl and place in the center of the platter.

NOTE: Broccoli, high in fiber and vitamins C and K, helps with digestion, immune support, and bone health. It's also a rich source of glucosinolate bioactive compounds. See the color insert for a photo.

TIP: Serve this platter in individual containers for a snack, on a large board at dinner, or as part of a buffet.

VARY IT! You can swap these green vegetables for red, yellow, or purple ones.

PER SERVING: Calories 330 (From Fat 228); Fat 25g (Saturated 5g); Cholesterol 0mg; Sodium 184mg; Carbohydrate 21g (Dietary Fiber 9g); Protein 11g. Sugars 7g.

🍅 Enchanted Garden Salad over Tzatziki

| PREP TIME: 15 MIN | COOK TIME: 30 MIN | YIELD: 4 SERVINGS |

INGREDIENTS

2 small beets

2 medium yellow or green tomatoes, cut into wedges

2 medium red tomatoes, cut into wedges

1 cup (67g) baby kale, baby spinach, or microgreens

4 ounces (110g) plain feta cheese (preferably sheep/goat milk), cut into 1-inch (2.5cm) pieces

DIRECTIONS

1 Preheat the oven to 450 degrees F. Prick the beets with a fork and place them on a baking sheet lined with aluminum foil. Bake approximately 30 minutes, or until tender, and then remove from the oven.

2 When the beets are cool, peel them and chop them into 1-inch pieces.

3 Place the vegetables in a decorative fashion in the middle of a serving plate. Begin with a slice of yellow tomato and follow with a piece of feta, a red tomato, a beet, continuing this pattern until you've used all the vegetables.

4 Scatter the kale, spinach, or microgreens over the top of the vegetables.

5 Serve immediately or store the tzatziki and vegetables and feta in separate containers until using.

Tzatziki

INGREDIENTS

2 cups (226g) Greek yogurt

1 English cucumber, trimmed and shredded with a box grater

¼ teaspoon (1.2g) salt

¼ cup (2g) finely chopped fresh mint or dill

1 clove garlic, minced

1 small yellow onion, grated

DIRECTIONS

1 Place the yogurt, cucumber, salt, herbs, garlic, and onion in a medium bowl. Mix well to combine. Spoon the tzatziki in the middle of a serving plate surrounded by the vegetables.

NOTE: Tzatziki, made with yogurt and cucumbers, provides probiotics for gut health. The variety of colored vegetables adds the rainbow of polyphenol varieties that have broad anti-inflammatory and antioxidant effects. Refer to the color insert for a photo.

PER SERVING: *Calories 272 (From Fat 60); Fat 7g (Saturated 7g); Cholesterol 37mg; Sodium 581mg; Carbohydrate 28g (Dietary Fiber 4g); Protein 28g. Sugars 12g.*

⊙ Lentil, Pomegranate, and Citrus Salad

INGREDIENTS

4 cups (120g) mixed field greens or spinach

1 cup (198g) cooked lentils

¼ cup (44g) pomegranate arils

1 orange, sliced

½ cup (120ml) pomegranate juice

1 tablespoon (15ml) Amy Riolo Selections or extra-virgin olive oil

⅛ teaspoon (.6g) salt

Pepper to taste

DIRECTIONS

1 Place the greens on a platter. Top with the lentils, pomegranate arils, and orange slices.

2 Combine the pomegranate juice with the olive oil, salt, and pepper in a small bowl and whisk to combine.

3 Place the dressing in a small pitcher and serve with the salad.

NOTE: Pomegranates, rich in polyphenol antioxidants such as ellagitannins and flavanols, support heart health and reduce oxidative stress.

TIP: Serve this fun salad during the winter holidays. In Italy, lentils are eaten on New Year's for prosperity, and pomegranate symbolizes good luck in Greece for the New Year.

VARY IT! Substitute lentils for cooked beans of your choice.

PER SERVING: *Calories 135 (From Fat 35); Fat 4g (Saturated 1g); Cholesterol 0mg; Sodium 86mg; Carbohydrate 21g (Dietary Fiber 6g); Protein 6g. Sugars 10g.*

Parmesan-Crusted Brussels Sprouts Caesar Salad

PREP TIME: 10 MIN	COOK TIME: 30 MIN	YIELD: 4 SERVINGS

INGREDIENTS

1 cup (88g) Brussels sprouts, trimmed and quartered

1 tablespoon (5g) grated Parmigiano-Reggiano cheese

3 cups (141g) chopped romaine

½ cup (15g) homemade whole-wheat croutons

¼ cup (56g) Greek yogurt

1 tablespoon (15g) tahini

Juice of 1 lemon

⅛ teaspoon (.6g) pepper

DIRECTIONS

1 Preheat the oven to 425 degrees F. Line a baking sheet with aluminum foil or parchment paper. Place the Brussels sprouts on it and cook for 20 minutes or until tender and golden.

2 Remove from the oven and sprinkle with Parmigiano-Reggiano. Place back in the oven for another 10 minutes, or until golden. Carefully remove and allow to cool.

3 Place in a bowl, top with the croutons, and toss in the Brussels sprouts when cool.

4 Whisk to combine the Greek yogurt, tahini, lemon juice, and pepper in a medium bowl. Before serving, toss the dressing into the salad and mix well to combine.

NOTE: Brussels sprouts, high in fiber and vitamins C and K, promote digestive health and bone strength.

VARY IT! Add leftover protein or avocado to the salad.

VARY IT! Swap romaine for kale or spinach.

PER SERVING: *Calories 72 (From Fat 25); Fat 3g (Saturated 1g); Cholesterol 3mg; Sodium 65mg; Carbohydrate 8g (Dietary Fiber 2g); Protein 5g. Sugars 1g.*

☙ Apple, Beet, and Carrot Salad over Arugula

PREP TIME: 15 MIN	YIELD: 4 SERVINGS

INGREDIENTS

1 medium red beet, peeled and shredded

2 medium carrots, peeled and shredded

1 large Granny Smith apple, peeled and shredded

3 cups (60g) arugula

¼ cup (29g) chopped walnuts

4 tablespoons (15g) chopped fresh flat-leaf parsley or dill, or a combination

Juice of 1 blood orange

⅛ teaspoon (.6g) salt

Pepper to taste

2 tablespoons (30ml) Amy Riolo Selections or extra-virgin olive oil

DIRECTIONS

1 Place the beets, carrots, and apple in a large mixing bowl and mix to combine.

2 Place the arugula on a large serving platter and top with the beet mixture.

3 Add the walnuts and green herbs on top of the mixture.

4 In a small bowl whisk to combine the orange juice, salt, pepper, and olive oil, and toss into the salad.

NOTE: Apples, a good source of fiber and vitamin C, as well as important antioxidant polyphenols such as flavanols, phenolic acid, and anthocyanins, help with digestion and support immune function.

TIP: If you omit the arugula, this salad makes a delicious slaw.

VARY IT! Add hardboiled eggs for additional protein.

PER SERVING: *Calories 171 (From Fat 108); Fat 12g (Saturated 1g); Cholesterol 0mg; Sodium 102mg; Carbohydrate 16g (Dietary Fiber 3g); Protein 3g. Sugars 11g.*

🍅 Fennel, Orange, and Arugula Salad

PREP TIME: 5 MIN	YIELD: 4 SERVINGS

INGREDIENTS

2 large fennel bulbs (about 1½ pounds) (680g), thinly sliced

2 large oranges, peeled and sliced into segments

4 tablespoons (15g) fresh flat-leaf parsley, chopped

Juice of 1 lemon

Juice of 1 orange

2 tablespoons (30ml) Amy Riolo Selections or extra-virgin olive oil

⅛ teaspoon (.6g) salt

Pepper to taste

4 hardboiled eggs, halved

DIRECTIONS

1 Place the fennel, oranges, and parsley on a large platter.

2 In a small bowl, whisk to combine the lemon juice, orange juice, and olive oil.

3 Pour the dressing over the salad, season with the salt and pepper, and top with the eggs.

NOTE: Fennel, low in calories and rich in fiber, promotes digestive health and provides essential nutrients. It contains numerous types of polyphenols that contribute to its unique taste and powerful antioxidant capacity. Refer to Figure 9-3 to see how to slice fennel.

NOTE: This salad, without the eggs, is usually served after large meals in Southern Italy because fennel is believed to aid digestion.

VARY IT! Swap the eggs for nuts or mozzarella cheese.

PER SERVING: Calories 231 (From Fat 112); Fat 12g (Saturated 3g); Cholesterol 212mg; Sodium 184mg; Carbohydrate 23g (Dietary Fiber 6g); Protein 9g. Sugars 11g.

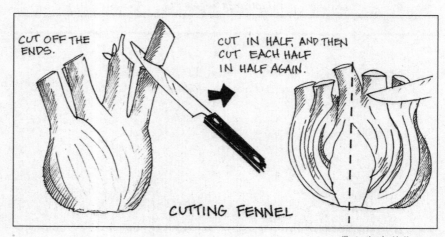

CUT OFF THE ENDS.

CUT IN HALF, AND THEN CUT EACH HALF IN HALF AGAIN.

CUTTING FENNEL

FIGURE 9-3: Cutting fennel.

Illustration by Liz Kurtzman

⏾ Celery, Cranberry, and Walnut Salad with Gorgonzola

PREP TIME: 10 MIN	YIELD: 4 SERVINGS

INGREDIENTS

4 stalks celery, finely sliced

¼ cup (28g) unsweetened dried cranberries

½ cup (59g) walnuts, finely chopped

1 cup (240g) Italian parsley, finely chopped

¼ cup (34g) gorgonzola cheese

2 tablespoons (30ml) Amy Riolo Selections or extra-virgin olive oil

2 tablespoons (30ml) Amy Riolo Selections White Balsamic or balsamic vinegar

DIRECTIONS

1 Combine the celery, cranberries, walnuts, parsley, and gorgonzola in a medium bowl and stir to combine.

2 Top the salad with the oil and balsamic and toss to coat. Serve immediately.

NOTE: Cranberries have been studied for possible benefits for bladder and kidney health. Walnuts are an excellent plant source of healthy unsaturated fats including omega-3 fats as well as fiber and polyphenols. Celery is an ultralow calorie vegetable that provides numerous vitamins and minerals.

TIP: Eat this salad alone or alongside roasted or grilled meat.

VARY IT! Swap cranberries for cherries and walnuts for almonds.

PER SERVING: *Calories 198 (From Fat 158); Fat 18g (Saturated 3g); Cholesterol 6mg; Sodium 162mg; Carbohydrate 7g (Dietary Fiber 2g); Protein 4g. Sugars 3g.*

Boning up on bagged salad blends

Fortunately, produce manufacturers are taking convenience foods to a healthy level for a change. Look in your produce section for prewashed, ready-to-use salad greens and blends. You can open a bag and have a delicious meal in a matter of minutes. For super easy and quick salads, pick up prewashed salad blends like these:

» **American blend:** This familiar blend usually includes iceberg lettuce, carrot shreds, radish slices, and red cabbage.

» **Baby lettuce mix:** This blend contains baby field and spring greens that are tender and taste great with just a homemade lemon vinaigrette.

» **European blend:** This mix is great to try if your salad experience stops at iceberg lettuce. It includes mild green leaf lettuce, romaine, iceberg, curly endive, and a bit of radicchio. It goes well with just about any dressing, toasted nuts, and any kind of cheese, including blue cheese and goat cheese.

» **Italian blend:** This blend is terrific for simple protein-based salads, dressed with good-quality EVOO and lemon juice. It usually consists of a blend of romaine and radicchio.

» **Spring mix:** This tasty mixture is a staple at most fine restaurants. It's usually a blend of baby greens that include baby spinach, radicchio, and frisée. It may also be called mesclun, spring greens, or field greens. It makes a gorgeous garnish or bed for serving fresh fish or steak.

Different manufacturers call different mixes by different trademarked names. Many blends also include other veggies, like radishes, carrots, and even snow peas. We recommend buying organic blends when possible. All blends should include a description or listing of the greens (and other tasty veggies) included in their package, so find what suits your fancy and get munching!

WARNING

Although these salad greens blends are great, many manufacturers also sell salad kits, which include the salad greens, dressing, cheese, and croutons. And remember, you don't have to eat it just because it comes in the kit. Feel free to toss that full-fat dressing in the trash and substitute good-quality EVOO and vinegar or lemon juice instead. Swap out the croutons for a small piece of whole-wheat pita or bread if desired.

Growing your own greens

Growing fresh baby greens is incredibly simple, no matter where you live. Their shallow root systems make them ideal for indoor gardening. All you need is a shallow bowl or planter, high-quality potting soil, lettuce seeds, and a nice sunny window.

Here's how you do it:

1. **Fill a shallow container that has good drainage with high-quality potting soil.**

2. **Gently press seeds into the soil.**

   Because you'll be harvesting your baby greens when they're, well, babies, you don't need to space out the seeds. Go ahead and just sprinkle them around rather than make nice neat rows.

3. **Water your seeds.**

   Keep the seeds moist but not soggy. Light but frequent watering produces the best leafy greens.

4. **Set the container in a sunny window.**

   Most greens *germinate,* or sprout seeds, within a few weeks. Feel free to start harvesting when the greens are a few inches tall. Just trim off what you need with kitchen shears.

TIP

To keep a constant supply of greens on hand, sow a second container two weeks later. Use a mixture of different seeds to create your own spring mix. For more information on growing lettuce or other vegetables in containers, check out *Container Gardening For Dummies* by Bill Marken, Suzanne DeJohn, and the editors of the National Gardening Association, (John Wiley & Sons, Inc.).

Creating sensational homemade dressings

Until recently, bottled salad dressings didn't offer much in the way of flavor unless they were full of fat, salt, sugar, and other no-nos for a diabetic diet. Some of the newer light dressings have improved flavor, are less detrimental to your health, and are convenient. But there's really no substitute for making dressings yourself. And believe it or not, the process is pretty simple.

To make basic diabetes-friendly vinaigrette, take a Mediterranean approach and vow to only top salads with the best quality EVOO and fresh lemon juice or your favorite vinegar. Doing so not only avoids consuming unwanted sugar, chemicals, and calories that many bottled dressings contain, but it also ensures that you get even additional nutritional benefits from your salad.

TIP

To add a truly professional touch, combine all your ingredients (except the oil) in a food processor or blender. With the appliance running, slowly pour the oil into the other ingredients. The dressing will *emulsify,* or blend, really well.

> » **Creating diabetes-friendly seafood, dips, and soup recipes**
>
> » **Making homemade stocks**

Chapter 10

Savory Starters

Planning multi-course meals can be complicated, especially if you have diabetes. Deciding which portion sizes, macronutrients, and minerals are necessary confuses many people. In restaurants, starters tend to be heavy with fats and carbs, which can also be problematic. If you love appetizers but don't know where to start when putting a meal together, we have you covered.

In this chapter, we show you how to include starters in multi-course meals and how to transform them into complete meals. Whether you're a lover of seafood, dips, creative vegetable dishes, or savory soups, you'll be able to enjoy creating, serving, and eating these recipes while still getting the most nutritional bang for your buck.

TIP

Be sure to read the Notes after the recipes for suggestions on how to pair the starter if it's meant to be eaten as a first course in a multi-course meal. Also refer to the book's Introduction for some recipe conventions we use.

Enjoying Simple Starters

Starters, often called appetizers, antipasti, and hors d'oeuvres, can be a great way to pack more nutrients into your diet. When prepared with the right ingredients needed for a diabetes-friendly diet, they can both satisfy your appetite and ensure that you don't overeat during and after the main course. We focus on seafood and plant-based recipes in order to give you more creative ways of enjoying them. Even children will love the fun and creative presentation of these dishes. Note that these portions are meant to be appetizer-sized, but you can easily increase the amount on each recipe to transform it into a meal. The Vary It! at the end of the recipes tells you how.

Succulent seafood

Seafood is especially beneficial to people with diabetes. In many places in the world, however, people don't eat enough of it. Consuming fish and seafood a minimum of two times per week is recommended in the Mediterranean diet (see Chapter 2 for more about this diet). Fish is high in protein and low in calories while being an excellent choice for anyone trying to gain muscle, lose weight, or increase brain function. Furthermore, seafood is full of omega-3 fatty acids, — something the body needs to function but can't produce on its own. Consuming them helps to lower triglycerides and blood pressure while reducing the risk of heart failure and stroke — risks that increase with diabetes.

Seafood also contains essential nutrients such as zinc (immune system support), potassium (heart health), selenium (anticancer protection), and iodine (thyroid function), along with vitamins A (vision, organ function, and immune support) and D (bone strength, nutrient absorption, and disease prevention). Additional benefits of omega-3 and fish consumption have been shown to do the following:

>> Prevent inflammation and improve rheumatoid arthritis

>> Enhance mood

>> Protect the vision of those suffering from age-related macular degeneration

>> Potentially lower the risk of Alzheimer's disease, dementia, and decreased cognitive function

>> Help reverse ultraviolet (UV) damage from sun exposure

>> Relieve and prevent asthma symptoms

>> Lessen the symptoms of ADHD, poor concentration, and negative behavior

You can also find seafood recipes sprinkled in Chapters 8, 9, and 11.

TIP

Many people are concerned about the health of the fish that they're buying. Always choose the freshest fish possible. If you live in the United States and are concerned about toxicity of fish, consult the Environmental Defense Fund's Seafood Selector or Monterey Bay Aquarium's Seafood Watch program online to check guidelines and ensure that you're eating sustainable and healthful seafood. Many organic and health food stores have this type of information available at the seafood counter in the United States.

Pan-Seared Scallops with Black Beans and Red Pepper Sauce

PREP TIME: 10 MIN	COOK TIME: 20 MIN	YIELD: 4 SERVINGS

INGREDIENTS

1 pound (454g) dry sea scallops, muscle removed, if applicable

2 tablespoons (30ml) Amy Riolo Selections or extra-virgin olive oil

¼ teaspoon (1.2g) salt

⅛ teaspoon (.6g) pepper

1 cup (172g) cooked black beans (refer to Chapter 7) or no salt-added canned beans

DIRECTIONS

1 Dry the scallops with paper towels. Season with salt and pepper. Heat the olive oil over high heat in a large skillet. As soon as it's warm, add the scallops and cook for approximately 2 to 3 minutes, or until the scallops have browned on one side.

2 Turn over and cook a minute or two on the other side until both sides are golden. Add the black beans to the pan with the scallops and turn to coat.

Roasted Red Pepper Sauce

INGREDIENTS

1 recipe Roasted Red Peppers (see Chapter 7)

2 tablespoons (30ml) Amy Riolo Selections or extra-virgin olive oil

¼ cup (56g) Greek yogurt

2 tablespoons (7g) freshly chopped parsley

DIRECTIONS

1 Place the red peppers and olive oil in a blender and puree on high until smooth and stir in the Greek yogurt to make a creamy sauce.

2 Pour the red pepper sauce onto the bottom of a platter. Top with the scallops and black beans in the center. Garnish with the parsley.

NOTE: Scallops are an excellent source of vitamins, especially B12 as well as minerals from the sea, and include phosphorous and a high percentage of daily recommended amount of selenium, essential for thyroid function and making your DNA. It also reduces oxidative stress.

TIP: Serve this show-stopping appetizer as a first course to fish or a vegetable-based main course.

PER SERVING: *Calories 357 (From Fat 171); Fat 19g (Saturated 3g); Cholesterol 37mg; Sodium 311mg; Carbohydrate 21g (Dietary Fiber 6g); Protein 25g. Sugars 5g.*

Salmon Pops with Creamy Dill Sauce

PREP TIME: 10 MIN	COOK TIME: 10 MIN	YIELD: 4 SERVINGS (2 EACH)

INGREDIENTS

1 pound (454g) thick sliced skinless salmon fillet, cut into 24 (1-inch) cubes

2 tablespoons (30ml) Amy Riolo Selections or extra-virgin olive oil

1 tablespoon (9g) sesame seeds

¼ teaspoon (1.2g) salt

1 large lemon, thinly sliced

DIRECTIONS

1 Preheat the oven to 425 degrees F. Place the salmon in a bowl and coat with olive oil, sesame seeds, and salt; toss to coat.

2 Line a baking sheet with parchment paper and set aside.

3 Thread the salmon onto a skewer, alternating with folded lemon slices (3 pieces of salmon and 2 pieces of lemon for each skewer), leaving a bit of space between each, and place them onto the baking sheet. Place in the oven and bake for approximately 8 to 10 minutes, or until the salmon is slightly golden and fully cooked. Remove from the oven, set aside, and cover with aluminum foil to keep warm, if desired.

Creamy Dill Sauce

INGREDIENTS

2 tablespoons (1g) finely chopped fresh dill

¼ cup (56g) Greek yogurt

Pepper to taste

1 large lemon, juiced and zested

DIRECTIONS

1 Combine the dill, yogurt, and pepper along with the lemon juice in a medium bowl and whisk until smooth.

2 Spoon the sauce on the platter. Place the salmon skewers on top in a decorative pattern. Garnish with lemon zest and lemon slices and serve warm.

NOTE: Use 8 bamboo skewers, soaked in water for 20 minutes, or 5-inch stainless steel skewers.

NOTE: Salmon is rich in omega-3 fatty acids, which are potentially at risk of breakdown when heated. Coating fish and cooking with EVOO, which has a higher tolerance of heat, ensures a glaze of protective oil around the fish, preserving and enhancing the availability of the healthy omega-3 fats.

PER SERVING: *Calories 250 (From Fat 141); Fat 16g (Saturated 3g); Cholesterol 62mg; Sodium 173mg; Carbohydrate 2g (Dietary Fiber 0g); Protein 24g. Sugars 1g.*

Spiced Salmon Sushi "Muffins"

PREP TIME: 15 MIN	COOK TIME: 15 MIN PLUS 30 MINS MARINADE TIME	YIELD: 4 SERVINGS

INGREDIENTS

2 sheets nori paper

½ pound (227g) salmon, skin removed and diced

1 tablespoon (15ml) Amy Riolo Selections or extra-virgin olive oil

1 tablespoon (18g) tamari

1 tablespoon (21g) raw honey

2 scallions, diced

1 garlic clove, minced

¼ teaspoon (.7g) each: cumin, cinnamon, dried ginger mixed together

⅛ teaspoon (.6g) unrefined sea salt

½ cup (102g) cooked sushi rice

Black sesame seeds, for garnish, if desired

DIRECTIONS

1 Preheat the oven to 400 degrees F. Cut the nori paper into 4 equal squares each.

2 Toss the salmon in a bowl with the olive oil, tamari, honey, scallions, garlic, spices, and salt, and turn to coat. Allow to marinade for 30 minutes.

3 Add a heaping tablespoon of rice to each nori square and transfer it to a muffin well in a muffin tin. Push down the center carefully so that the edges cover the sides of the well. Repeat with the remaining muffin wells.

4 Place the salmon on the rice equally in the 8 wells. Transfer to the oven and bake until the rice is slightly golden and salmon is cooked through, 10 to 13 minutes.

5 Cool and place on a serving tray. Garnish with sesame seeds and serve with the dip.

Dip

INGREDIENTS

½ ripe avocado

1 tablespoon (14g) siracha sauce

¼ cup (56g) Greek yogurt

DIRECTIONS

1 Combine the avocado, siracha, and Greek yogurt in a blender and process until smooth and creamy. Place in a small bowl.

TIP: Serve with the Cucumber Rolls Filled with Avocado, Tomato, and Baby Kale in Chapter 9.

PER SERVING: *Calories 221 (From Fat 103); Fat 11g (Saturated 2g); Cholesterol 31mg; Sodium 436mg; Carbohydrate 15g (Dietary Fiber 2g); Protein 15g. Sugars 5g.*

Smoked Salmon, Avocado, and Brown Rice Sushi Cubes

PREP TIME: 30 MIN	COOK TIME: 20 MIN	YIELD: 4 SERVINGS

INGREDIENTS

½ pound (227g) cooked brown rice

1 tablespoon (15ml) rice vinegar

2 teaspoons (10ml) toasted sesame oil, divided

2 Persian or mini cucumbers, thinly sliced

1 ripe avocado, diced

2 ounces (57g) smoked salmon

1 chive, finely chopped

DIRECTIONS

1 While the rice is still warm, mix it with the vinegar and 1 tablespoon sesame oil. Allow to cool enough to handle.

2 Line an 8x8-inch square baking dish or container with large sheets of plastic wrap that extend a few inches beyond the sides of the dish to mold the sushi.

3 Add the rice to the container by using the back of a spoon to press down, ensuring the grains stick together. Pull the sides of the plastic wrap over the rice and press down with your fingers to make sure that it's compact. Cover with additional plastic wrap and transfer to the refrigerator to cool overnight.

4 Carefully lift the rice out of the dish and place it on the counter. Using a small rectangular mold, or a knife, cut 12 rectangular-shaped and equal-sized pieces (dip the mold or the knife into water so that it doesn't stick to the rice).

5 Top with a layer of cucumber slices, avocado pieces, and smoked salmon.

6 Heat the remaining 1 tablespoon of sesame oil in a small saucepan and drizzle on top of the cubes. Garnish with chive and serve.

NOTE: Rice vinegar supports weight management and blood glucose regulation. Sesame oil is a healthy fat with polyphenols with potential antioxidant and anti-inflammatory properties.

NOTE: Serve this appetizer before the Roasted Fresh Tuna and Vegetables Tower in Chapter 11 or the fish dish of your choice.

TIP: If you want to make this dish more substantial and enjoy it as a full meal, increase the serving size of the squares and serve them alongside the Spiced Edamame and Chickpeas from Chapter 7.

PER SERVING: *Calories 192 (From Fat 97); Fat 11g (Saturated 2g); Cholesterol 3mg; Sodium 119mg; Carbohydrate 20g (Dietary Fiber 5g); Protein 6g. Sugars 2g.*

Delicious dips

Dips are fun, interactive, and delicious. They allow you to use your fingers and enjoy crunchy and creamy textures at the same time. Fortunately, dips are easy to prepare and can be done in advance. You don't have to reserve the following dips for parties and special occasions because they're nutritious enough to enjoy daily.

Tzatziki is a classic Greek dip enjoyed in various forms all over the Mediterranean region. The combination of Greek yogurt, cucumbers, garlic, and fresh herbs is actually a complete meal (from a nutrition perspective) in a bowl. You can enjoy it any time of day and know that it's doing your body good. The Roasted Red Pepper, Walnut, and Pomegranate Dip is one that hails from the Middle East and is also known as a "beauty dip" because it contains nutrients that are particularly beneficial to the skin. Baba Ghanouj is another classic Arab appetizer that combines roasted eggplant with tahini, lemon juice, and garlic for a wonderfully rich flavor and wide range of nutrients in a single vegan dish.

TIP

We recommend making large batches of the dips and keeping them on hand to enjoy as a light meal or snack when you're short on time. Or you can serve all three together for a vegetarian meal or when entertaining. Whole-grain pita, peppers, and other vegetables make the perfect dipping partners.

🍅 "Carrot" Peppers with Tzatziki

PREP TIME: 10 MIN	COOK TIME: 10 MIN	YIELD: 4 SERVINGS

INGREDIENTS

12 orange mini bell peppers

1 batch of Tzatziki (Enchanted Garden Salad in Chapter 9)

1 bunch fresh dill

DIRECTIONS

1 Lay the peppers on a cutting board and slice off the tops. Then slice them parallel to the cutting board lengthwise. Remove the rib and seeds (if any) and discard.

2 Using a teaspoon or a piping bag, fill the pepper halves with the tzatziki.

3 Place the peppers on a serving platter and garnish the top with dill to look like carrots.

NOTE: Dill is an interesting herb packed with vitamins and minerals. Scientists have studied it for possible benefits for insomnia, though the evidence isn't yet convincing.

NOTE: Because this recipe contains vegetables, herbs, and dairy, it pairs well with meat, chicken, and other vegetable dishes. I (Amy) especially like serving it before the Turkish Vegetable Stew with Brown Basmati Rice or the Egyptian Okra Stew with Brown Rice Pilaf (both in Chapter 11).

VARY IT! To make a meal, serve it with lettuce greens and the protein of your choice.

PER SERVING: *Calories 195 (From Fat 54); Fat 6g (Saturated 3g); Cholesterol 0mg; Sodium 172mg; Carbohydrate 24g (Dietary Fiber 5g); Protein 13g. Sugars 16g.*

Roasted Red Pepper, Walnut, and Pomegranate Dip with Pita Chips

PREP TIME: 5 MIN	COOK TIME: 10 MIN	YIELD: 4 SERVINGS

INGREDIENTS

3 tablespoons (45ml) Amy Riolo Selections or extra-virgin olive oil, divided

1 tablespoon (15ml) lemon juice

6 ounces (170g) roasted red peppers, drained, rinsed, and dried

4 tablespoons (27g) Fresh Breadcrumbs (recipe in Chapter 7) or plain breadcrumbs, or almond flour

¼ cup (31g) walnuts, plus a few extra for garnish

2 cloves garlic, minced

3 tablespoons (45ml) pomegranate molasses or pomegranate juice, divided

3 whole-wheat pita, cut into 2-inch pieces

DIRECTIONS

1 Combine 2 tablespoons of the olive oil, lemon juice, red peppers, breadcrumbs, walnuts, garlic, and 2 tablespoons pomegranate molasses in a food processor or high-speed mixer and blend on high to form a paste.

2 Heat the oven to 500 degrees F. Line a baking sheet with parchment paper or aluminum foil.

3 Place the pita pieces on the baking sheet and drizzle with the remaining 1 tablespoon of olive oil. Bake in the oven until slightly golden, flipping once at 2 to 3 minutes, until lightly golden, approximately 4 to 6 minutes.

4 Place the dip in a shallow bowl or a plate. Using the back of a spoon, smooth it onto the bottom leaving a border around the sides. Drizzle the remaining tablespoon of pomegranate molasses on top and garnish with a few walnuts in the middle. Serve with pita chips.

NOTE: Pomegranate is particularly high in polyphenols called ellagitannins and anthocyanins. The molasses concentrates these powerful antioxidants, though we advise that you monitor your blood sugar if the syrup contains added sugars.

TIP: In Step 1, if the paste is too thick to spread, add water, a tablespoon at a time, until you have the consistency of a spreadable sauce.

NOTE: The Arabic name for this dish is *M'hammara,* which means "to make red," but it's also used in place of the English cooking term "to brown." The predecessor to this dip is a pomegranate-walnut sauce served over duck in Iranian kitchens. If you want to pair this dish with a second course, I (Amy) suggest the Mediterranean-Stuffed Eggplant or the Beet Couscous with Orange-Glazed Chicken and Pecans in Chapter 11.

PER SERVING: *Calories 269 (From Fat 144); Fat 16g (Saturated 2g); Cholesterol 0mg; Sodium 401mg; Carbohydrate 27g (Dietary Fiber 3g); Protein 6g. Sugars 4g.*

🍅 Sweet Potatoes with Dill Dip

PREP TIME: 5 MIN	COOK TIME: 30 MIN	YIELD: 4 SERVINGS

INGREDIENTS

2 large sweet potatoes, scrubbed

⅛ teaspoon (.6g) salt

2 tablespoons (30ml) Amy Riolo Selections or extra-virgin olive oil

¼ cup (31g) walnuts, finely chopped (optional)

DIRECTIONS

1 Preheat the oven to 425 degrees F. Line a baking tray with parchment paper.

2 Slice the sweet potatoes into 1/8-inch-thin slices and place on baking sheet. Drizzle with olive oil and sprinkle with salt; turn to coat well. Place in the oven and roast until tender and golden, approximately 15 to 20 minutes, flipping halfway through .

3 Place the dip in a small bowl in the middle of a platter. Spoon potatoes onto the platter around bowl. Garnish the potatoes with the remaining tablespoon of dill and the dip in the walnuts and serve.

Dill Dip

INGREDIENTS

½ cup (112g) Greek yogurt

1 tablespoon (15g) tahini

1 tablespoon (15ml) fresh lemon juice

2 tablespoons (1g) finely chopped fresh dill, divided

DIRECTIONS

1 Combine the Greek yogurt, tahini, lemon juice, and 1 tablespoon of dill in a medium bowl. Using a fork, whisk well to combine into a smooth dip.

NOTE: Tahini, produced from sesame, is a good way to get healthy unsaturated fats as well as plenty of vitamins, minerals, and polyphenols. Sweet potatoes are loaded with vitamin A and beta-carotene and have been shown to reduce LDL cholesterol.

NOTE: I (Amy) like to serve this dish as an appetizer before the Citrus Chicken, Strawberry, and Avocado Salad in Chapter 11, but any greens and protein are a great pairing.

VARY IT! To make a meal, serve the sweet potatoes in a bowl with a serving of beans, greens, and the dill dip. Add grilled chicken or a hardboiled egg for extra protein.

PER SERVING: Calories 239 (From Fat 134); Fat 15g (Saturated 2g); Cholesterol 0mg; Sodium 106mg; Carbohydrate 22g (Dietary Fiber 4g); Protein 7g. Sugars 7g.

Baba Ghanouj with Crudites

PREP TIME: 10 MIN	COOK TIME: 20 MIN	YIELD: 4 SERVINGS

INGREDIENTS

2 medium eggplants

2 tablespoons (30g) tahini

¼ cup (60ml) Amy Riolo Selections or extra-virgin olive oil, divided

Juice of 1 lemon

1 garlic clove, minced

⅛ teaspoon (.6g) salt

2 tablespoons (7g) finely chopped fresh parsley

1 English cucumber, cut into julienne strips

2 medium bell peppers, mixed colors, cut into strips

4 celery stalks, cut into strips

DIRECTIONS

1 Preheat the broiler to 500 degrees F. Cover a baking sheet with aluminum foil.

2 Pierce the eggplants with a fork and set them on the baking sheet. Place the baking sheet on the highest rack in the oven and roast the eggplants until they start to char and turn black, approximately 10 to 15 minutes.

3 When done, remove the eggplants from the oven and use tongs to put them in a colander over a bowl to drain until cool.

4 As soon as the eggplants are cool enough to touch, cut off the tops and remove the skins. Allow all the liquid to drain from them.

5 Transfer the eggplant pulp to a cutting board and chop/mash it a bit. Transfer it to a large bowl where you add the tahini sauce, all but 1 tablespoon olive oil, lemon juice, and salt. Stir vigorously with a fork to combine. Taste and salt if needed.

6 Transfer the baba ghanouj to a bowl and dent the center. Pour the remaining olive oil into the center and sprinkle with parsley. Serve with crudites arranged decoratively on a plate or platter.

TIP: In Step 2, if the eggplants haven't turned at least partially black and aren't tender to the touch, they need to cook more. Be sure to watch them carefully.

NOTE: The ingredients in this traditional Levantine dish speak for themselves. Combining the eggplant with the lemon juice and healthy fats of the tahini and EVOO makes the glucose rise following the meal more controlled and improves insulin performance.

PER SERVING: *Calories 269 (From Fat166); Fat 18g (Saturated 3g); Cholesterol 0mg; Sodium 110mg; Carbohydrate 26g (Dietary Fiber 12g); Protein 5g. Sugars 11g.*

Creating Crostini

The Italian cousins of toast, crostini, and bruschetta are easy, elegant, and versatile appetizers that you can make minutes before meals. You can switch it up and add different toppings, especially depending on what you have on hand or left over. Crostini are usually made with smaller pieces of bread whereas bruschetta tend to be larger like toasts. If you're short on time, a single piece of bruschetta or a few pieces of crostini and a salad enriched with proteins like the ones in Chapter 9 make a great dinner. Chapter 7 has basic crostini and bruschetta recipes.

CROSTINI COMBINATIONS

In Italy crostini are eaten as snacks, appetizers, and, depending on the amount served, a light dinner when served with soup or salad. They're a great way to repurpose day-old bread and leftovers as well as showcase prized ingredients and good-quality olive oil.

Here are a few of my (Amy) favorite combinations:

- Cooked sautéed greens and goat cheese
- Sautéed mushroom with herbs and Parmigiano cheese
- Fresh, diced tomatoes, garlic, and basil
- Goat cheese or fresh mozzarella and smoked salmon
- Fresh figs, gorgonzola cheese, walnuts
- Tzatziki and grilled, shredded chicken
- Pureed beans or lentils with sautéed greens or peppers

🍅 Tulip Bruschetta

PREP TIME: 10 MIN	COOK TIME: 5 MIN	YIELD: 4 SERVINGS

INGREDIENTS

1 tablespoon (15ml) Amy Riolo Selections or extra-virgin olive oil

4 thin slices Homemade Whole-Grain Bread from Chapter 6 or 100 percent whole-grain bread

One 4-ounce (113g) log goat cheese

1 tablespoon (15ml) water

12 chives

12 red and yellow cherry tomatoes

Handful of fresh small basil or Italian parsley

DIRECTIONS

1 Heat the broiler to high. Brush the olive oil over both sides of each piece of bread. Broil 1 to 2 minutes per side, or until golden, watching carefully so that the bread doesn't burn. Remove from the oven and set aside.

2 Place the goat cheese in a small bowl and add 1 tablespoon of water. Mash with a fork and stir to create a creamy, spreadable consistency. Add additional water a tablespoon at a time if needed.

3 Using a skewer, make an indentation in the center of the part of the tomato that's attached to a stem. Then place a piece of chive inside to resemble an actual stem.

4 Using a paring knife, make a cross indentation on the other end (top) of the cherry tomato. Open the indentation slightly to resemble a flower.

5 Lay the 3 tomato tulips on top of each slice of bread with the stems overlapping as in a bunch of flowers.

6 Tear off the basil and parsley leaves and place a few around 3 chive "stems" to look like the leaves on a flower stem. Repeat with remaining ingredients.

7 To serve, scatter remaining herbs on the bottom of a platter and place the bruschetta on top.

TIP: Choosing a healthy bread is key to enjoying this meal. Go for whole grain, ancient grain, sourdough, or a combination of these ingredients to ensure, with the addition of plenty of EVOO, that the glycemic load is lowered and the benefits of the fiber, vitamins, and minerals in the bread are maximized.

NOTE: Refer to the color insert for a photo of this dish.

PER SERVING: *Calories 236 (From Fat 122); Fat 14g (Saturated 6g); Cholesterol 22mg; Sodium 238mg; Carbohydrate 20g (Dietary Fiber 3g); Protein 10g. Sugars 3g.*

Pear Crostini with Blue Cheese, Honey, and Walnuts

PREP TIME: 5 MIN	COOK TIME: 5 MIN	YIELD: 4 SERVINGS

INGREDIENTS

8 thin slices of bread from a whole-wheat baguette

2 pears, cored, and cut into quarters

¼ cup (34g) blue cheese or gorgonzola, crumbled

1 teaspoon (7g) raw honey

2 tablespoons (16g) finely chopped walnuts

DIRECTIONS

1 Preheat the broiler to high. Place the bread on a baking sheet and broil (with pan at least 3 inches under the heat) for 1 to 3 minutes, watching carefully, until it turns golden. Carefully remove the sheet from under the broiler and set aside to cool slightly.

2 Cut each of the pear quarters into 4 thin slices.

3 When the bread is cool enough to touch, turn it over and top with the cheese. Place back under the broiler for 1 or 2 minutes until it melts.

4 Remove the crostini from the oven and carefully transfer the crostini to a serving platter using tongs.

5 Place 2 pear slices on top of each piece. Drizzle with the honey and garnish with walnuts to serve.

NOTE: Blue cheeses are excellent probiotics that support a healthy and diverse gut microbiome and help manage and reduce the risks of type 2 diabetes. Raw (unprocessed) honey adds sweetness with natural sugars in a form that is better for blood glucose control than added, refined sugars.

TIP: Serve this recipe with the Purple Sweet Potato and Herb Soup with Cashews or the Cream of Broccoli and Celery Soup in this chapter, or your favorite fall soup.

VARY IT! If you want to make this recipe as a meal, serve the crostini with thinly sliced meat over greens. Pear Crostini also makes a great breakfast, snack, or dessert.

PER SERVING: Calories 200 (From Fat 49); Fat 5g (Saturated 2g); Cholesterol 6mg; Sodium 320mg; Carbohydrate 33g (Dietary Fiber 4g); Protein 7g. Sugars 11g.

Adding Vegetables to Your Starters

Incorporating vegetables into starters is an easy way to get more flavor and nutrients into your diet. You have many ways you can use them, so it's easy to be creative. By choosing a wide variety of vegetables with different colors, and choosing what's in season, you can get the most out of them while saving money and supporting the environment.

If you're looking to add visual appeal to your food and impress those you eat with, the recipes in this section do just that. With careful presentation and gourmet concepts, even humble vegetables get elevated to new heights. If you're serving them to guests, the emphasis is on their creativity and taste, not on the fact that they're so good for you.

REMEMBER

Not only are these recipes as pleasing for the eyes as they are for the palate, but they also provide as many nutrients as possible. Here are some vegetables that we recommend keeping on hand while in season:

>> Asparagus

>> Bell peppers of all colors

>> Carrots

>> Chicories, such as radicchio and lettuces of all types

>> Cruciferous vegetables, such as broccoli, cauliflower, Brussels sprouts

>> Fresh beets

>> Green leafy vegetables, such as Swiss chard, kale, spinach, dandelion greens

🍅 Polenta with Asparagus and Lemon Cream

PREP TIME: 10 MIN	COOK TIME: 20 MIN	YIELD: 4 SERVINGS

INGREDIENTS

3 cups (710ml) water

1 cup (932g) cornmeal or polenta

2 tablespoons (30ml) Amy Riolo Selections or extra-virgin olive oil, divided

¼ teaspoon (1.2g) salt

½ pound (227g) asparagus spears, trimmed, and cut into thirds

Zest of and juice of 1 lemon

½ cup (112g) Greek yogurt

¼ cup (10g) finely chopped fresh basil

DIRECTIONS

1 Bring 3 cups of water to a boil over high heat in a large saucepan. Whisk in the polenta and reduce the heat to medium–low. Switch to a wooden spoon and stir the polenta often as it thickens.

2 Reduce the heat to low and continue to cook, stirring occasionally, until the polenta is thick and creamy, approximately 15 minutes. Remove from the heat and stir in 1 tablespoon of olive oil and salt.

3 Heat the remaining tablespoon of olive oil in a large wide skillet. Add the asparagus. Cook, stirring often, until the asparagus is a bit charred but still crunchy, approximately 5 minutes.

4 Make the sauce by combining the lemon juice and zest in a bowl, the yogurt, and basil, and whisking well.

5 Spoon the polenta onto a platter and smooth to cover. Place the asparagus in the center of the platter and dollop the yogurt on top.

NOTE: Polenta, made from cornmeal, is low in fat and gluten-free, providing a good source of complex carbohydrates, fiber, and essential minerals that support digestive health and provide sustained energy. Asparagus is low in calories and rich in vitamins A, C, and K, as well as folate and fiber, which supports heart health, aides in digestion, and promotes healthy skin and bones.

NOTE: This recipe tastes best in early spring when it's still cool enough to enjoy polenta but when fresh asparagus is in season. Serve as a precursor to Roasted Spice-Dusted Chicken with Veggies (Chapter 11), or your own favorite roasted protein and vegetable recipe.

TIP: If you use instant polenta, Step 2 only takes a few minutes.

VARY IT! To make this recipe into a complete meal, amp up the protein quotient by adding thinly sliced pieces of meat or cheese to this dish.

PER SERVING: *Calories 320 (From Fat 83); Fat 9g (Saturated 2g); Cholesterol 0mg; Sodium 643mg; Carbohydrate 51g (Dietary Fiber 4g); Protein 8g. Sugars 3g.*

Beet Napoleons with Smoked Salmon, Greek Yogurt, and Basil

INGREDIENTS

3 large beets

Approximately 2 ounces (60g) smoked salmon, cut into 3 slices for garnish, if desired

½ cup (112g) Greek yogurt, strained in a colander for 1 hour

Handful fresh basil, finely chopped

DIRECTIONS

1 Preheat the oven to 425 degrees F. Wash and dry the beets, pierce them with a fork, place them on a baking sheet, and roast for 30 to 40 minutes or until tender. Reduce the heat and set aside.

2 Prepare roses with the salmon by slicing each salmon slice in half lengthwise by cutting a piece that's approximately 5 inches long and 1 inch wide. Fold it in half and gently roll it around your pinky finger into a rose shape. Make 5 more and store in the refrigerator.

3 Allow the beets to cool for 15 minutes, then peel them and slice them into 6 evenly sized pieces. Use a small round cookie cutter to cut perfect rounds through each slice. Dry the slices well so that they don't bleed into the yogurt.

4 Place almost all the basil (leaving a bit for garnish) into a small bowl and stir in the Greek yogurt.

5 Fill a pastry bag with the yogurt mixture. To form the Napoleons, place the cookie cutter on a plate and a piece of beet inside of it, pressing it down to the bottom. Cover the slice with approximately 1 teaspoon of the yogurt mixture.

6 Place another layer on top and push it down to distribute the yogurt. Gently pull the cookie cutter up a bit to add another teaspoon of yogurt and top it with another beet slice.

7 Gently lift the cookie cutter off the Napoleon. Repeat the process with the remaining beet slices. Place the finished Napoleons on a serving platter and top with the salmon roses and the remaining basil.

NOTE: Compounds called nitrates in vegetables are especially high in beets. Nitrates can reduce blood pressure and help blood vessel function. The colored polyphenols give beets their reputation as a powerful anti-inflammatory food.

NOTE: Refer to the color insert for a photo of this dish.

PER SERVING: *Calories 48 (From Fat 13); Fat 1g (Saturated 1g); Cholesterol 2mg; Sodium 117mg; Carbohydrate 5g (Dietary Fiber 1g); Protein 4g. Sugars 3g.*

Swiss Chard with Vegetable Confetti "Tacos"

PREP TIME: 10 MIN | COOK TIME: 0 MIN | YIELD: 4 SERVINGS

INGREDIENTS

8 large Swiss Chard leaves, stems left on

1 English cucumber, diced

1 cup (149g) orange and red cherry tomatoes, quartered

1 small bunch cilantro, finely chopped

1 avocado, cored and sliced

1 cup (185g) cooked quinoa

2 tablespoons (30ml) Amy Riolo Selections or extra-virgin olive oil

Juice of 2 limes

½ teaspoon (2.4g) salt

¼ teaspoon (1.2g) pepper

Handful of edible flowers, for garnish, if desired

DIRECTIONS

1 Spread the leaves on a serving platter.

2 Combine the cucumber, tomatoes, cilantro, avocado, and cooked and cooled quinoa on each leaf.

3 Whisk the olive oil, lime juice, salt, and pepper together. Drizzle over the "tacos." Serve immediately, garnished with edible flowers, if desired.

NOTE: Swiss chard is a green, with numerous polyphenols and carotenoids, minerals, and vitamins. It often has added red and purple polyphenols in the stem that increase the diversity of bioactive compounds.

NOTE: Check out the color insert for a photo of this recipe.

TIP: Serve this fun and colorful recipe prior to the Pan-Seared Shrimp with Barley Pilaf over Butternut Squash in Chapter 11.

PER SERVING: *Calories 238 (From Fat 138); Fat 15g (Saturated 2g); Cholesterol 0mg; Sodium 450mg; Carbohydrate 24g (Dietary Fiber 7g); Protein 6g. Sugars 4g.*

⊙ Cashew and Mango Cabbage Wraps with Peanut Sauce

PREP TIME: 20 MIN	COOK TIME: 20 MIN	YIELD: 4 SERVINGS

INGREDIENTS

2 tablespoons (30ml) Amy Riolo Selections or extra-virgin olive oil

¼ pound (113g) raw cashews, chopped

1 teaspoon (3g) minced garlic

2 tablespoons (36g) tamari

¼ cup (60ml) rice vinegar

½ teaspoon (2.5g) siracha or chili paste

1 cup (165g) chopped mango

¼ cup (28g) shredded carrots

¼ cup (18g) finely chopped scallions

1 tablespoon (6g) freshly grated ginger or ½ teaspoon (1g) ground ginger

¼ cup (4g) chopped fresh cilantro or parsley

1 head green cabbage

DIRECTIONS

1 Heat the olive oil in a large skillet over medium-high heat. Add the cashews and cook until they release their aroma, approximately 1 minute. Add the garlic and cook for another minute. Stir and add the tamari, vinegar, siracha, and allow to cook for another minute.

2 Add the mango, carrots, scallions, and ginger and cook for 5 more minutes, stirring occasionally. Remove from the heat and allow to cool slightly. Stir in the cilantro or parsley. Place the cabbage leaves individually on a work surface. Top with 2 tablespoons of this mixture and roll up. Serve warm with the sauce.

Peanut Dipping Sauce

INGREDIENTS

¼ cup (64g) fresh peanut butter

1 tablespoon (18g) tamari

2 tablespoons (30ml) rice vinegar

1 teaspoon (7g) raw honey

2 tablespoons (30ml) water

1 tablespoon (6g) grated fresh ginger root or ½ teaspoon (1g) ground ginger

DIRECTIONS

1 Blend all the ingredients or whisk in a medium bowl until smooth. Pour the sauce into separate containers for serving and serve immediately or refrigerate until needed.

PER SERVING: *Calories 419 (From Fat 249); Fat 28g (Saturated 5g); Cholesterol 0mg; Sodium 893mg; Carbohydrate 36g (Dietary Fiber 9g); Protein 14g. Sugars 19g.*

☙ Rainbow Spring Rolls with Garlic and Asparagus Sauce

PREP TIME: 20 MIN	YIELD: 2 SERVINGS

INGREDIENTS

4 rice paper wrappers (or large green lettuce leaves)

1 ripe avocado, pitted, and sliced

1 red pepper, seeded and sliced into thin slices

½ cup (55g) shredded carrots

½ cup (124g) tofu (soft or medium),crumbled if desired

½ cup (35g) shredded purple cabbage

8 green lettuce leaves

¼ cup (6.4g) finely chopped mint

DIRECTIONS

1 Soak the rice wrappers in cool water for 5 minutes, drain, and lay on a flat surface. Top with equal parts of all the remaining ingredients and roll up jelly roll fashion.

2 Slice each roll in half on the diagonal and place in a shallow dish (or two portable containers standing upright with cut sides exposed).

Asparagus Sauce

INGREDIENTS

¼ cup (64g) fresh peanut butter

2 tablespoons (36g) tamari

2 tablespoons (30ml) rice vinegar

1 teaspoon (7g) raw honey

2 tablespoons (30ml) water

1 tablespoon (6g) grated fresh ginger root or ½ tsp (1g) ground ginger

1 clove garlic, minced

DIRECTIONS

1 Place all ingredients in a blender and emulsify or place in a medium bowl and whisk until smooth.

2 Pour the sauce into separate containers for serving and serve immediately or refrigerate until needed.

NOTE: Adding tofu is a great idea here, especially for vegetarians, because tofu is a complete plant protein providing all the essential amino acids. Some evidence also suggests that it helps glucose control in people with diabetes.

PER SERVING: *Calories 561 (From Fat 307); Fat 34g (Saturated 6g); Cholesterol 0mg; Sodium 1289mg; Carbohydrate 52g (Dietary Fiber 15g); Protein 20g. Sugars 13g.*

Soup-Making Basics

Homemade stocks are the unsung heroes of the kitchen. Whether you want to make an authentic risotto, homemade soup or stew, braised meat, or seafood recipe, having healthful stock on hand enhances the flavor of your recipes.

From a health perspective, homemade stock can't be beat. Purchased stocks contain a great deal of sodium (even the "low-sodium" varieties contain a hefty amount) and additives, but the homemade versions don't. From a flavor perspective, fresh broth can make or break diabetes-friendly recipes.

TIP

The good news is that stock is easy and inexpensive to make. Whenever I (Amy) have leftover skins from onions, carrot or celery tops, shrimp shells, or roasted chicken or meat bones, I place them in double plastic bags and refrigerate or freeze them until I'm ready to make stock. If you make a stockpot at a time, you can freeze portions in gallon containers for later use. Each week, place a gallon or two in your refrigerator so that you have it on hand to make your recipes during the week.

A proverb from Calabria, Italy, where my family hails from, says that soups do seven things:

» Quench thirst

» Satisfy hunger

» Fill your stomach

» Clean your teeth

» Make you sleep

» Help you digest

» Put color in your cheeks

Whether you're making them as a starter or a main, they are an easy and tasty way to enjoy nutritious and satisfying meals. When prepared with the nutritious and easy stock recipes in this section, they can help you save unwanted calories and sodium while adding flavor and versatility to your menus.

Purple Sweet Potato and Herb Soup with Cashews

PREP TIME: 15 MIN | COOK TIME: 20 MINS | YIELD: 4 SERVINGS

INGREDIENTS

3 purple sweet potatoes or orange, if they aren't available, washed and chopped into bite-sized pieces

2 tablespoons (30ml) Amy Riolo Selections or extra-virgin olive oil, divided

1 large yellow onion, finely chopped

2 small zucchini, diced

2 cloves garlic, minced

1 teaspoon (2g) fresh ginger, minced

¼ teaspoon (1.2g) salt

2 tablespoons (3g) finely chopped fresh mint

⅓ cup (45g) cashews, toasted and chopped

DIRECTIONS

1 Preheat the oven to 425 degrees F. Place the sweet potatoes on a baking sheet and drizzle with 1 tablespoon olive oil. Roast for 20 to 30 minutes or until tender.

2 Heat the remaining tablespoon of olive oil in a large pot over medium heat. Add the onion and zucchini and cook for about 4 to 5 minutes. Stir in the garlic and ginger and cook until fragrant, about 1 minute. Add the sweet potatoes, cover with water, and bring to a boil over high heat.

3 After boiling, reduce the heat to medium-low and simmer until the sweet potatoes are very tender, about 15 minutes. Stir occasionally. Add the salt and mint, stir, taste, and adjust the seasoning if needed.

4 Use an immersion blender or carefully transfer the soup to a blender and puree until very smooth.

5 Transfer the soup to serving bowls and garnish with cashews.

TIP: When transferring to the blender in Step 4, be sure to remove the spout in the center of the blender and cover with a folded clean kitchen towel so that it doesn't burst.

VARY IT! Add 2 cups of cooked quinoa to the soup and serve with a green salad for a complete meal.

PER SERVING: *Calories 239 (From Fat 111); Fat 12g (Saturated 2g); Cholesterol 0mg; Sodium 161mg; Carbohydrate 30g (Dietary Fiber 5g); Protein 5g. Sugars 12g.*

☺ Cream of Broccoli and Celery Soup

PREP TIME: 5 MIN | COOK TIME: 25 MIN | YIELD: 4 SERVINGS

INGREDIENTS

2 tablespoons (30ml) Amy Riolo Selections or extra-virgin olive oil

1 large yellow onion, finely chopped

2 cups (240g) diced celery

¾ pound (340g) broccoli florets

3 cups Homemade Vegetable Stock (recipe in this chapter) or water

½ teaspoon (2.4g) salt

⅛ teaspoon (.6g) pepper

DIRECTIONS

1 Heat the olive oil in a large pot over medium heat. Add the onion and sauté, stirring occasionally, for 3 to 5 minutes, or until translucent.

2 Add the celery and the broccoli to the pot and pour the vegetable stock over them. Increase the heat to high, bring to a boil, and then reduce the heat to medium-low.

3 Add the salt and pepper. Bring to a boil and reduce the heat to medium-low. Cover and allow to simmer for 15 to 20 minutes or until the vegetables are tender.

4 Remove from heat and puree until smooth with an immersion blender or by carefully transferring the soup into a blender. Serve with croutons, if desired.

NOTE: Broccoli and celery are vegetables rich in nutrients, although children can sometimes find them too bitter to enjoy. This recipe is a great way to introduce them to these flavors that are milder and smoother in the form of soup.

TIP: I (Amy) like to serve this soup with the Pear Crostini with Blue Cheese, Honey, and Walnuts from this chapter or before serving roasted chicken or meat.

VARY IT! Add cooked tofu or shredded chicken to the soup and serve with whole-grain bread.

PER SERVING: *Calories 125 (From Fat 65); Fat 7g (Saturated 1g); Cholesterol 0mg; Sodium 417mg; Carbohydrate 14g (Dietary Fiber 4g); Protein 3g. Sugars 7g.*

Homemade Vegetable Stock

INGREDIENTS

1 medium yellow onion, halved (not peeled)

1 carrot, trimmed and halved

1 stalk celery, trimmed and halved (can include leaves, if desired)

4 ounces (113g) cherry tomatoes

4 sprigs fresh basil, with stems

1 small bunch (approximately ¾ cup) (45g) fresh flat-leaf parsley, with stems

16 cups (3.7L) water

½ teaspoon (2.4g) salt

DIRECTIONS

1 In a large stockpot, place the onion, carrot, celery, tomatoes, basil, and parsley. Cover with the water. Bring to a boil over high heat. Reduce the heat to medium-low. Add the salt, and simmer, uncovered, for 30 minutes.

2 Drain the stock, reserving the liquid. Discard the rest. If you're not using it right away, allow to cool and then store in the refrigerator for up to a week or freeze it for up to a month.

PER SERVING: *Calories 24 (From Fat 2); Fat 0g (Saturated 0g); Cholesterol 0mg; Sodium 117mg; Carbohydrate 6g (Dietary Fiber 2g); Protein 0g. Sugars 1g.*

Homemade Seafood Stock

PREP TIME: 15 MIN	COOK TIME: 30 MINS	YIELD: 8 SERVINGS

INGREDIENTS

1 medium yellow onion, halved (not peeled)

1 carrot, trimmed and halved

1 stalk celery, trimmed and halved

Shells from 2 pounds (907g) shrimp or fish bones, or a combination

16 cups (3.7L) water

½ teaspoon (2.4g) salt

1 dried bay leaf

1 tablespoon (9g) whole black peppercorns

DIRECTIONS

1 In a large stockpot, place the onion, carrot, celery, and shrimp shells/fish bones. Cover with the water. Bring to a boil over high heat. Reduce the heat to medium–low.

2 Skim off the residue that forms on top of the stock and discard. Add the salt, bay leaf, and peppercorns. Simmer, uncovered, for about 30 minutes.

3 Drain the stock, reserving the liquid, and discard the rest. If you're not using it right away, allow the stock to cool, and then store it in the refrigerator for three days or freeze for up to a month.

TIP: Whenever I (Amy) cook shrimp, I buy the ones in the shell. They're fresher and cost less. Then I shell them, place the shells in a sealed plastic bag in the freezer until I'm ready to make stock. This is the easiest, cheapest way to make seafood stock and the taste is wonderful.

PER SERVING: *Calories 62 (From Fat 26); Fat 3g (Saturated 1g); Cholesterol 1mg; Sodium 127mg; Carbohydrate 2g (Dietary Fiber 0g); Protein 7g. Sugars 0g.*

Homemade Chicken Stock

INGREDIENTS

1 medium yellow onion, halved (not peeled)

1 medium carrot, trimmed and halved

1 medium stalk celery, trimmed and halved

1¼ pounds (567g) chicken bones or carcass from cooked chicken

1 teaspoon (3g) whole black peppercorns

1 dried bay leaf

16 cups (3.7L) water

½ teaspoon (2.4g) salt

DIRECTIONS

1 In a large stockpot, place the onion, carrot, celery, chicken bones, peppercorns, and bay leaf. Cover with the water. Bring to a boil over high heat. Reduce the heat to medium–low.

2 Skim off the residue that forms on top of the stock and discard. Add the salt and simmer, uncovered, for 40 minutes.

3 Drain the stock, reserving the liquid, and discard the rest. If you're not using the stock right away, allow it to cool, and then store it in the refrigerator or freezer.

PER SERVING: *Calories 82 (From Fat 21); Fat 2g (Saturated 0g); Cholesterol 0mg; Sodium 124mg; Carbohydrate 7g (Dietary Fiber 0g); Protein 5g. Sugars 3g.*

Homemade Meat Stock

PREP TIME: 5 MIN | **COOK TIME: 2 HRS** | **YIELD: 8 SERVINGS**

INGREDIENTS

1 medium yellow onion, halved (not peeled)

1 medium carrot, trimmed and halved

1 medium stalk celery, trimmed and halved

1¼ (567g) pounds roasted meat bones

1 teaspoon (3g) whole black peppercorns

1 dried bay leaf

16 cups (3.7L) water

½ teaspoon (2.4g) salt

DIRECTIONS

1 In a large stockpot, place the onion, carrot, celery, meat bones, peppercorns, and bay leaf. Cover with the water. Bring to a boil over high heat. Reduce the heat to medium-low.

2 Skim off the residue that forms on top of the stock and discard. Add the salt and simmer, uncovered, for 2 hours.

3 Drain the stock, reserving the liquid, and discard the rest. If you're not using the stock right away, allow it to cool, and then store it in the refrigerator or freezer.

TIP: Whenever I (Amy) make meat with bones, I always debone it before serving and save the bones in a sealed plastic bag in the freezer until I'm ready to use them. You can also purchase meat bones at most meat counters or butchers.

PER SERVING: *Calories 62 (From Fat 7); Fat 1g (Saturated 0g); Cholesterol 0mg; Sodium 127mg; Carbohydrate 6g (Dietary Fiber 0g); Protein 9g. Sugars 3g.*

Chapter **11**

Satisfying Main Dishes

Main dishes are the culinary centerpieces of tables. For that reason, newcomers can be intimidated in making them. For individuals who have just been diagnosed with diabetes, who want to prevent it, or who are cooking for a loved one who has recently been diagnosed, the joy of cooking is often replaced by worry and frustration. But you don't need to fret. With a few simple strategies by your side, you can prepare them with ease and satisfaction.

In this chapter, we help you serve mains that the whole family will love in exciting, tasty, and nutritious new ways. We focus on using all vegetables, mushrooms, legumes, and seafood in delicious, restaurant-worthy recipes. We also help you create some special-occasion recipes to enjoy with your guests. And finally, we show you how to pull together complete, mouthwatering vegetarian entrees in minutes. You can serve the recipes in this chapter alone or as part of a larger, multi-course meal on special occasions.

Be sure to read the Note in each recipe to find out about its nutritional values. Also refer to the book's Introduction for some recipe conventions we use.

Making Mains Diabetes Friendly

Creating diabetes–friendly main dishes can be delicious and fun if you follow a few simple guidelines:

» **Adopt a plant-forward mentality.** The human body thrives on the fantastic bioactive compounds, must-have important vitamins and nutrients, and fiber found in vegetables, but most people don't eat enough of them.

» **Enjoy vegetarian entrees.** You can combine vegetables in many satisfying ways in your main dishes: in soups, in salads, pureed in sauces, or as the main event. Whether you eat them cooked or raw or fresh or frozen products, you can improve your health today by increasing the amount of vegetables you eat.

» **Serve seafood more often.** Fish has the healthful omega-3 fats and a potent dose of protein while being low in fat and calories — it's the perfect diabetes-friendly main.

» **Think of meat as an accompaniment instead of the main event.** Thomas Jefferson believed that meat should be regarded as a condiment to a plate of vegetables. Many people decide what animal protein they're going to eat first when planning menus. Then, they serve a larger portion than needed (4 ounces is an actual portion size) with few vegetables. By serving small amounts of meat with more vegetables you're doing yourself a favor.

If you've been following a different diet or lifestyle plan, putting these ideas to use in the kitchen may be difficult. Here are some tips to enjoy the most flavor and nutrition when you eat.

Cooking with macronutrients in mind

We can't overstate the importance of choosing the best quality combinations of healthful fats, protein, and carbohydrates (the three macronutrients) in planning each meal. Including these combinations is exceptionally important with main dishes. If paired together properly, the three micronutrients help to keep you full and performing at your peak while keeping you blood sugar in check.

Here's a simple way to remember them:

>> **Fats:** The best sources of healthful fats that are especially important for people with diabetes are extra-virgin olive oil (EVOO), avocados, raw or roasted (unsalted) nuts, flax, sesame, chia seeds, and omega-3 fatty acids found in fish like salmon and tuna.

>> **Protein:** Lean proteins include soybeans, lentils and beans, fish, seafood, lean poultry, and eggs as well as goat and lean lamb meat.

>> **Carbohydrates:** Carefully portioned quality, low glycemic index (GI) carbohydrates such as whole wheat, bulgur, millet, barley, rice, pasta, potatoes, and starchy vegetables are what you should enjoy in your main dishes.

Expanding your meal options with vegetarian entrees

You don't need to be vegan or even a vegetarian to follow a delicious, diabetes-friendly diet. Many people refrain from serving vegetarian mains, not because they don't like vegetables but because they lack the experience in transforming them into complete meals. The recipes in this section are a treat for vegetarians and meat-lovers alike.

CUTTING BACK ON MEAT

Many people mistakenly believe that meat and animal proteins have always been the center of a well-balanced diet. In reality, however, it wasn't until the 20th century that U.S. doctors and nutrition professionals began spreading that theory among recent immigrants in order to fuel the American beef industry. Many world cultures have survived and thrived on largely plant-based meals.

The Mediterranean diet and lifestyle for example recommends eating meat on occasion. That's not because meat was or is costly in the Mediterranean, but because culturally, meat was only consumed on special occasions when the sacrifice of an animal seemed appropriate. Daily meals traditionally relied on legumes, beans, grains, and greens with some dairy for the majority of nutrients. This formula still applies to modern society and those who eat in a similar way enjoy better health.

(continued)

(continued)

Many high-fiber plant-based ingredients are filling and satisfying and contain protein. We recommend consuming a variety and combination of these foods daily in order to reduce meat:

- Whole grains, especially quinoa and brown rice
- Tofu, tempeh, soybeans, and edamame
- Lentils — red, green, brown, and black
- Beans — cannellini, chickpeas, black beans, navy beans, pinto beans, borlotti beans
- Mushrooms
- Seeds — sunflower, pumpkin, sesame, and flax
- Almonds
- Potatoes
- Plant-based milks (unsweetened)
- Nutritional yeast
- Seaweed
- Broccoli
- Sprouted breads

⊙ Quinoa, Mango, and Avocado Timbale

PREP TIME: 15 MIN	COOK TIME: 15 MIN	YIELD: 4 SERVINGS

INGREDIENTS

1 cup (170g) red quinoa, or white if preferred, rinsed

1½ cups (360ml) water

1 mango

1 shallot, minced

1 lime juiced and zested, divided

¼ teaspoon (1.2g) salt

1 teaspoon (5ml) Amy Riolo Selections or extra-virgin olive oil

1 tablespoon (4g) finely chopped parsley

1 tablespoon (8g) finely chopped almonds

2 ripe avocados

Handful of fresh arugula, spinach, baby kale, or microgreens

2 cherry tomatoes, halved

DIRECTIONS

1 Place the quinoa in a medium saucepan with the water. Bring to a boil over high heat, stir, and reduce heat to medium-low. Simmer for 10 to 15 minutes or until cooked through. Allow to cool and set aside.

2 Make a slit around the mango to cut it open (see Figure 11-1), remove the pit, and score the flesh into small squares without cutting into the skin. Remove from the peel and mix with the shallot and ½ lime juice and zest.

3 Season the quinoa with salt and fluff with a fork. Mix in the olive oil, parsley, and almonds.

4 Cut the avocado open, remove the pit (refer to 11-2), and slice into ½-inch squares into a bowl. Drizzle with the remaining lime juice, add the zest, and stir to coat.

5 Place a 3- to 4-inch cylindrical mold in the center of a dinner plate. Add ¼ of the quinoa to the bottom. Press down with a spoon to make it compact. Then top with ¼ of the mango mix, then ¼ of the avocado. Add ¼ of the fresh greens on top. Carefully remove the mold. Continue three more times with the remaining ingredients on separate plates.

6 Garnish each with a ½ cherry tomato and serve immediately, or refrigerate without the greens, until serving. Add the greens, zest, and cherry tomato at the last minute.

NOTE: Quinoa is a nutrient-dense, low GI grain, rich in protein, fiber, and essential minerals that supports muscle growth, helps with digestion, and provides sustained energy. It contains polyphenols like quercetin and kaempferol, which have antioxidant properties that support cardio-vascular health and reduce inflammation. Mangoes are a tropical fruit rich in vitamins A and C. They contain polyphenols such as mangiferin and catechins, which contribute to antioxidant activity that supports immune function and reduces oxidative stress. The GI of tropical fruits may be higher than others, so if you monitor your individual response to different foods, it may be worth checking that a small amount of mango is fine for you.

NOTE: You can serve a smaller version of this recipe as an appetizer — use 2-inch cylinder molds to make 8 appetizer portions.

NOTE: Refer to the cover for a photo of this recipe.

PER SERVING: *Calories 382 (From Fat 177); Fat 20g (Saturated 3g); Cholesterol 0mg; Sodium 130mg; Carbohydrate 47g (Dietary Fiber 11g); Protein 9g; Sugars 9g.*

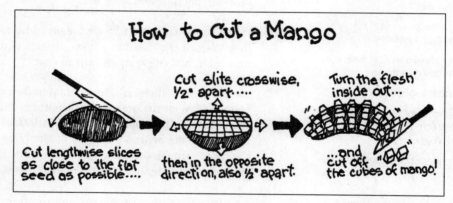

FIGURE 11-1: How to cut a mango.

Illustration by Liz Kurtzman

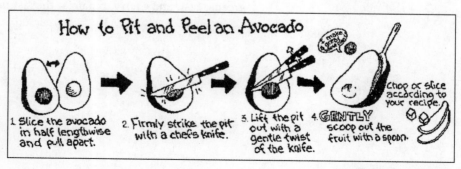

FIGURE 11-2: Pitting an avocado the easy way.

Illustration by Liz Kurtzman

254   PART 2 Healthy Recipes That Taste Great

☙ Turkish Vegetable Stew with Brown Basmati Rice

PREP TIME: 15 MIN	COOK TIME: 1 HR	YIELD: 6 SERVINGS

INGREDIENTS

¼ cup (60ml) Amy Riolo Selections or extra-virgin olive oil, plus 1 teaspoon (5ml), divided

1 medium yellow onion, diced

2 garlic cloves, minced

1 tablespoon (16g) tomato paste

1 teaspoon (5g) spicy chili pepper paste, if desired

5 Roma tomatoes, diced

3½ cups (840ml) water

1 small eggplant, cubed

1 cup (100g) okra, or green beans, trimmed

1 green bell pepper

1 medium zucchini, diced

¼ teaspoon (1.2g) salt

⅛ teaspoon (.6g) pepper

1 bunch fresh parsley, finely chopped

1 cup (192g) brown basmati rice, soaked in water to cover for at least 20 minutes, and drained

DIRECTIONS

1 Heat 3 tablespoons of the olive oil in a large saucepan over medium heat. Add the onion and garlic and sauté until the onion is translucent, about 5 minutes. Add the tomato paste and chili pepper paste and stir to incorporate. Add the tomatoes and 2 cups water. Bring to boil over high heat.

2 Add the eggplant, okra, bell pepper, zucchini, salt, and pepper, stir, and bring to a boil again. Season with salt and pepper. Reduce the heat to low, cover, and cook until vegetables are tender, at least 40 minutes.

3 Heat the remaining teaspoon of olive oil in a medium saucepan with a fitted lid. Add the rice, stir, and add ¼ teaspoon salt. Allow to cook for a few minutes. Add 1½ cups water, stir, and bring to a boil over high heat.

4 Reduce the heat to low and place a paper towel over the top of the pan. Place the lid on top and be sure to trim the paper towel so that it isn't near the fire. Simmer until fluffy, approximately 5 to 10 minutes. Carefully remove the lid from the rice so that the steam doesn't cause a burn. Remove the lid and fluff the rice with a fork.

5 Place the rice and stew in separate serving bowls and garnish both with parsley to serve.

NOTE: Stews are common in the Mediterranean way of eating. When vegetables, rich in nutrients and bioactive compounds are cooked in a stew rather than boiled, the goodness is retained in the juices rather than passing into the water.

TIP: Prepare this dish in advance and serve the next day or freeze in individual portions.

VARY IT! Swap the vegetables for what's in season. You can use quinoa, millet, barley, or another rice instead of basmati.

PER SERVING: *Calories 261 (From Fat 101); Fat 11g (Saturated 1g); Cholesterol 0mg; Sodium 112mg; Carbohydrate 38g (Dietary Fiber 6g); Protein 5g; Sugars 7g.*

MAKING FLUFFY RICE

In order to make the fluffiest basmati rice, it is important that the rice grains don't stick together. Here are three key steps in making your rice fluffy:

1. **Soak the rice.**

   By soaking the rice prior to cooking, it absorbs less water during cooking.

2. **Place a cloth barrier underneath the tight-fitting lid.**

   Many people use clean kitchen towels under the lid (wrapping the ends on top so that they don't touch the burner or fire). Others use a single paper towel, ensuring that the sides are trimmed so that they can't catch flame or touch the burner. This way, as the rice simmers, the steam that touches the lid gets absorbed by the towel and doesn't hit the rice again, which makes it mushy.

3. **Use low heat when cooking rice.**

   Cultures that cook rice often even use flame tamers on their stoves to emit the least amount of heat possible. The lower the temperature, the better the texture of your rice will be.

Cannellini Beans Braised in Tomatoes with Fresh Mozzarella

PREP TIME: 10 MIN	COOK TIME: 20 TO 30 MIN	YIELD: 4 SERVINGS

INGREDIENTS

3 tablespoons (45ml) Amy Riolo Selections or extra-virgin olive oil

2 cloves garlic, thinly sliced

Pinch finely ground red chili flakes

2 cups (298g) red cherry or grape tomatoes, halved

2 cups (298g) yellow cherry or grape tomatoes, halved

¼ teaspoon (1.2g) salt

⅛ teaspoon (.6g) pepper

1 bunch fresh basil, minced

2 cups (358g) cooked cannellini beans (see Chapter 7 for cooking instructions)

6 ounces (170g) fresh mozzarella, shredded

8 thin slices Homemade Whole-Grain Bread (see Chapter 6) or whole-grain bread

DIRECTIONS

1 Heat the olive oil in a large, wide skillet over medium heat. Add the garlic and cook for 2 minutes, or until it releases its aroma. Add the chili flakes and tomatoes to the skillet, stirring well to combine. Season with salt and pepper.

2 Add the basil and cannellini beans and stir to coat. Cover the skillet and allow to cook for 15 minutes or until the tomatoes have broken down and the beans are tender. With a potato masher or the back of a fork, press down on the bottom of the beans to thicken them a bit.

3 Add the mozzarella and cover. Allow to cook for a few minutes or until it melts, approximately 3 minutes.

4 Use the bread to scoop up the bean mixture or slather it onto bread to serve.

NOTE: Cannellini beans are a good source of plant-based protein, fiber, and minerals that support heart health, aid in digestion, and reduce cholesterol. They're a good prebiotic food for your gut microbiome.

TIP: Turn this dish into a soup by transferring the mixture after mashing it in Step 2 to a stockpot or larger saucepan. Add 2 cups chicken or vegetable broth (see Chapter 10), stirring, and cooking for an additional 10 minutes.

VARY IT! Toss this mixture into al dente whole-wheat pasta for a hearty and delicious meal.

PER SERVING: *Calories 555 (From Fat 217); Fat 24g (Saturated 8g); Cholesterol 34mg; Sodium 622mg; Carbohydrate 64g (Dietary Fiber 15g); Protein 24g; Sugars 7g.*

☕ Egyptian Okra Stew with Brown Rice Pilaf

| PREP TIME: 15 MIN | COOK TIME: 45 MIN | YIELD: 4 SERVINGS |

INGREDIENTS

3 tablespoons (45ml) Amy Riolo Selections or extra-virgin olive oil, divided

1 medium yellow onion, finely chopped

3 cups (300g) fresh or frozen okra (baby okra can be left whole), otherwise slice into ¼-inch (.6cm) rounds

2 cups (480ml) Homemade Vegetable Stock (see Chapter 10) or water

½ cup (90g) diced fresh tomatoes, or no-sodium-added canned tomatoes

1 teaspoon (2g) ground coriander

½ teaspoon (1g) ground cumin

¼ teaspoon (1.2g) salt, divided

⅛ teaspoon (.6g) pepper

1 cup (185g) brown rice, rinsed

1¾ cup (415ml) water

½ cup (8g) fresh cilantro, finely chopped

¼ cup (4g) fresh mint, finely chopped

¼ cup (4g) fresh parsley, finely chopped

DIRECTIONS

1 Heat 2 tablespoons olive oil in a large saucepan over medium heat. Add the onion and cook until medium brown, about 7 to 10 minutes. Add the okra and stir to coat. Cover with the stock and tomatoes and add the coriander, cumin, ⅛ teaspoon salt, and pepper.

2 Increase the heat to high and bring to a boil. Then reduce the heat to low, cover, and simmer until tender, approximately 20 minutes.

3 Add the remaining tablespoon of olive oil to a saucepan over medium heat. After the oil is hot, add the rice and stir to coat. Add 1¾ cup water and remaining ⅛ teaspoon salt and stir. Increase the heat to high. After it boils, reduce to low, stir, cover, and allow it to cook until tender, about 20 to 30 minutes. When the rice is cooked through, stir in the cilantro, mint, and parsley and fluff with a fork.

4 To serve, place the rice in a bowl small enough that the rice comes to the top. Using the back of a spoon, press down to make it compact. Place a large platter on top of the bowl and carefully invert to make a mound on the plate.

5 When the stew is finished cooking, spoon all of it around the rice and serve hot.

NOTE: Okra is a great source of fiber, vitamins, including vitamin K and folate, and minerals as well as many polyphenols. In particular, the polyphenol quercetin present in okra has been studied for its capacity to help regulate blood glucose levels.

PER SERVING: *Calories 316 (From Fat 104); Fat 12g (Saturated 2g); Cholesterol 0mg; Sodium 164mg; Carbohydrate 49g (Dietary Fiber 5g); Protein 6g; Sugars 6g.*

Fresh Spinach Crepes filled with Oyster Mushroom Cream

PREP TIME: 10 MIN	COOK TIME: 20 MIN	YIELD: 4 SERVINGS

INGREDIENTS

2 tablespoons (30ml) extra-virgin olive oil

2 cups (172g) oyster mushrooms, roughly chopped, or your favorite mushrooms

¼ tsp (1.2g) salt

Dash of pepper

¼ cup (60ml) water

1 cup (226g) Greek yogurt

1 cup (24g) fresh basil, finely chopped, leave a few leaves for garnish

Zest of 1 lemon

DIRECTIONS

1 Heat a tablespoon of olive oil in a large skillet over medium heat. Add the mushrooms, stir, and add the salt and a bit of pepper. Add the water, increase the heat to high, and bring to a boil.

2 Reduce the heat to low and simmer until the mushrooms are tender. Carefully transfer ½ of the mushrooms to a blender or food processor and process until smooth. Combine pureed mushrooms with mushroom pieces in a bowl. Stir in the yogurt, basil, and remaining tablespoon of olive oil. Stir to combine. Taste, add lemon zest, and adjust seasoning if necessary.

Spinach Crepes

INGREDIENTS

3 cups (90g) fresh baby spinach

1 cup (120g) buckwheat flour

1 teaspoon (5ml) apple cider vinegar

3 tablespoons (45ml) Amy Riolo Selections or extra-virgin olive oil, divided

¼ teaspoon (1.2g) salt

⅛ teaspoon (.6g) pepper

1 cup (240 ml) water

DIRECTIONS

1 Place the spinach in a food processor or blender and pulse on and off until finely chopped. Combine the chopped spinach, flour, apple cider vinegar, 2 tablespoons olive oil, salt, pepper, and water and mix to make a smooth batter.

2 Add a tablespoon of olive oil to a large nonstick skillet over medium heat and swirl to coat the bottom of the pan. Add ¼ cup of the batter and quickly swirl with your wrist to form a circular crepe (you can use the back of a spoon if you want).

3 Cook for approximately 2 to 3 minutes or until bubbles begin to appear on top. Flip over and cook the other side for 30 seconds or until cooked through. Remove from the skillet and place on the counter. Cover with a clean kitchen towel to keep warm and continue with the remaining crepes.

4 To serve, placed a dollop of the mushroom cream mixture on the crepe and roll up to cover the filling. Garnish with basil.

NOTE: Spinach is a nutrient-packed leafy green, rich in iron and vitamins A and K, that support bone health, immune function, as well as a healthy and diverse gut microbiome. It may not guarantee to give you Popeye's muscles, but leafy greens are certainly beneficial for many aspects of health including blood glucose regulation. Spinach is rich in polyphenols like flavonoids and carotenoids that contribute to its anti-oxidant and anti-inflammatory effects, support bone health, and reduce the risk of age-related macular degeneration.

TIP: Make the crepes a day in advance. Store them separately and then reheat the crepes and fill them before serving.

NOTE: Figure 11-3 shows different types of mushrooms that you can use.

VARY IT! Substitute ½ cup finely grated fresh beets for spinach to make beet crepes and swap the mushrooms in the filling for zucchini.

PER SERVING: *Calories 324 (From Fat 187); Fat 21g (Saturated 4g); Cholesterol 0mg; Sodium 283mg; Carbohydrate 27g (Dietary Fiber 5g); Protein 11g; Sugars 3g.*

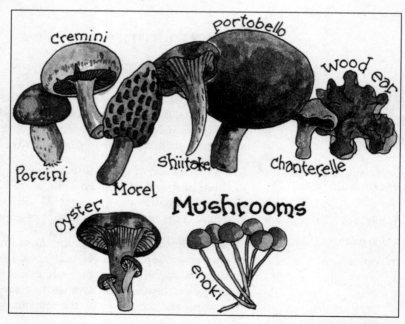

FIGURE 11-3: Mushrooms come in many shapes and sizes.

Illustration by Liz Kurtzman

⊙ Mediterranean-Stuffed Eggplant

PREP TIME: 15 MIN	COOK TIME: 1 HR	YIELD: 4 SERVINGS

INGREDIENTS

4 baby eggplants (approximately ¼ pound each)

3 tablespoons (45ml) Amy Riolo Selections or extra-virgin olive oil, divided

5 ripe Roma tomatoes, diced

1 tablespoon (9g) pitted black kalamata or other olives rinsed

2 cloves garlic, minced

¼ cup (11g) finely chopped fresh basil

¼ cup (11g) finely chopped fresh parsley

¼ teaspoon (1.2g) salt

⅛ teaspoon (.6g) pepper

2 tablespoons (10g) grated pecorino cheese

DIRECTIONS

1 Cut the tops off the eggplants and make boat shapes by cutting the eggplants in half lengthwise. With a corer or grapefruit spoon, carefully remove the flesh from the eggplant, leaving a thin layer next to the skin. Cut the flesh into small cubes and set aside.

2 Heat 2 tablespoons olive oil in a large skillet over medium-high heat and add the eggplant cubes, allowing to cook for about 3 minutes per side or until they begin to soften and change color. Add the tomatoes, olives, garlic, basil, parsley, salt, pepper, and cheese and stir. Reduce the heat to medium-low, cover, and simmer 10 to 20 minutes or until the vegetables are tender.

3 Heat the oven to 400 degrees F. Brush a large baking dish (enough to fit the 8 eggplant halves in a single layer) with 1 tablespoon olive oil. Arrange the eggplant boats in a baking dish. Top with the remaining 2 tablespoons olive oil.

4 When the vegetables have finished cooking, fill the eggplant boats with the vegetable mixture. Bake, uncovered, for 35 to 40 minutes or until the eggplant is tender and the mixture is golden. Serve warm or at room temperature.

NOTE: Eggplant is a deeply colored vegetable with fiber, minerals, and vitamins. Eggplant contains nasunin, a type of anthocyanin polyphenol with antioxidant properties, that contribute to heart health and potentially protect against oxidative stress.

TIP: Make this recipe when eggplants and tomatoes are in season.

VARY IT! During squash season, use squash or zucchini instead of eggplant.

PER SERVING: *Calories 184 (From Fat 106); Fat 12g (Saturated 2g); Cholesterol 2mg; Sodium 189mg; Carbohydrate 19g (Dietary Fiber 10g); Protein 5g; Sugars 9g.*

Poached Eggs over Cauliflower Puree with Sautéed Mushrooms

PREP TIME: 15 MIN	COOK TIME: 30 MIN	YIELD: 4 SERVINGS

INGREDIENTS

4 cups (400g) cauliflower florets

4 tablespoons (60ml) Amy Riolo Selections or extra-virgin olive oil, divided

¼ teaspoon (1.2g) salt, divided

⅛ teaspoon (.6g) pepper

¼ cup (56g) Greek yogurt

1 tablespoon (5g) grated pecorino cheese

2 cups (172g) mixed mushrooms, sliced thinly

¼ cup (120ml) water

1 teaspoon (.8g) finely chopped thyme or your favorite herb

1 tablespoon (15ml) vinegar

4 eggs

2 tablespoons (7.6g) finely chopped fresh parsley

DIRECTIONS

1 Place the cauliflower in a large saucepan and cover with water. Bring to a boil over high heat. Reduce the heat to medium and boil for 10 minutes, or until fork-tender. Drain the cauliflower and transfer to a food processor or blender. Add 2 tablespoons olive oil, ⅛ teaspoon salt, and pepper. Puree until smooth.

2 Carefully spoon the mixture into a bowl and stir in the yogurt and cheese. Cover the bowl with aluminum foil and set aside.

3 Heat the remaining 2 tablespoons olive oil in a large wide skillet over medium heat and add the mushrooms. Stir and add ⅛ teaspoon salt. Add ¼ cup water, increase the heat to high, and bring to a boil. Reduce the heat to medium-low, cover, and simmer for 10 to 15 minutes, or until mushrooms are tender.

4 Bring a saucepan ¾ full with water to a boil on medium-high heat and add the vinegar. Crack each egg into the boiling water one at a time and let them poach until desired doneness, about 3 minutes.

5 Place a quarter of the cauliflower mixture on top of 4 dinner plates and use the back of a spoon to cover the bottom of the plates. Scatter ¼ of the mushroom medley on top and place a poached egg in the middle. Garnish with parsley.

NOTE: Eggs are a good source of choline, which is important for brain health, and they contain lutein and zeaxanthin, carotenoids that support eye health and reduce the risk of age-related macular degeneration.

TIP: The creamy cauliflower makes a great replacement for mashed potatoes.

PER SERVING: *Calories 245 (From Fat 178); Fat 20g (Saturated 4g); Cholesterol 213mg; Sodium 246mg; Carbohydrate 8g (Dietary Fiber 3g); Protein 11g; Sugars 4g.*

☙ Hearty Lentil Soup with Sourdough Croutons and Goat Cheese

PREP TIME: 10 MIN	COOK TIME: 50 MINS	YIELD: 4 SERVINGS

INGREDIENTS

2 tablespoon (30ml) Amy Riolo Selections or extra-virgin olive oil, divided

2 carrots, peeled and diced

1 onion, diced

2 celery stalks, diced

1 cup (192g) brown lentils, rinsed and sorted

¼ (1.2g) teaspoon salt

⅛ teaspoon (.6g) pepper

4 cups (960 ml) Homemade Vegetable Stock (see Chapter 10)

¼ cup (15g) finely chopped Italian parsley

¼ cup (15g) fresh basil, finely chopped

4 ounces (113g) plain goat cheese

2 slices sourdough bread, cubed

DIRECTIONS

1 Heat 1 tablespoon olive oil in a large saucepan over medium heat. Add the carrots onion, and celery. Sauté until translucent, about 3 to 5 minutes, stir, and add the lentils. Stir and cook for 1 minute. Season with salt and pepper to taste.

2 Add the stock and parsley, stir, and increase the heat to high. When the stock begins to boil, reduce the heat to medium-low. Stir, cover, and simmer, about 45 minutes to 1 hour or until the lentils are tender. Taste and adjust seasoning if necessary.

3 Preheat the oven to 500 degrees F. In a small bowl, combine the basil and the goat cheese. Using two soup spoons, form the mixture into *quenelles* (football-shaped balls) and place in the middle of the soup.

4 Line a baking sheet with parchment paper and coat with the remaining 1 tablespoon olive oil.

5 Bake 2 to 3 minutes per side until golden. Add to soup and serve.

NOTE: Lentils contain polyphenols, such as flavonoids, which have antioxidant and anti-inflammatory properties, that support heart health and regulate blood sugar levels. Sourdough is a great type of bread because of its relatively low glycemic index in comparison to other breads.

TIP: Puree this soup to make a smooth and satisfying lentil cream.

VARY IT! Cook this soup in 10 minutes by swapping the red lentils for brown ones.

PER SERVING: *Calories 469 (From Fat 146); Fat 16g (Saturated 7g); Cholesterol 22mg; Sodium 492mg; Carbohydrate 58g (Dietary Fiber 18g); Protein 24g; Sugars 8g.*

Surveying Superior Shellfish and Fish

Seafood is one of the most underused sources of protein in many parts of the world. Even in places where there's plenty of fish to be had, many people have the misconception that it's difficult to prepare or is an expensive splurge. We recommend buying the freshest fish possible. Try stocking up on your favorite fish when it's on sale. You can freeze it to prepare on other occasions. This section includes recipes so you can put fish and seafood to good use for optimizing flavor and nutrition.

You can use an array of herbs and spices to add delicious tastes to your dishes. As for fish, you have numerous choices, including the following:

- Atlantic mackerel
- Bluefish
- Cod
- Herring
- Mussels
- Pacific oysters
- Rainbow trout
- Sablefish
- Sardines
- Salmon
- Shrimp
- Squid
- Tuna

TIP

Choosing fresh fish that's free from toxic elements can be confusing. *Note:* The larger fish that have spent the most amount of time in the water is most at risk. If you eat tuna or other fish that's known for its mercury levels, be sure to buy it from a source that practices sustainable fishing methods. Some markets list the sources where fish and seafood are caught. If you're unsure, we recommend checking with your local fishing authorities. In the United States, Seafoodwatch.org is a great resource to consult while shopping. The site lists seafood in four categories: Best Choice, Certified, a Good Alternative, or Avoid. Studies have shown that the phenols in EVOO prevent negative effects of mercury exposure, so we recommend always dressing seafood with good-quality EVOO.

Linguine with Seafood and Zucchini Cream Sauce

PREP TIME: 5 MIN	COOK TIME: 20 MINS	YIELD: 6 SERVINGS

INGREDIENTS

2 zucchini, washed and cut into halves and quarters

¼ cup (60ml) Amy Riolo Selections or extra-virgin olive oil, divided

¼ cup (25g) Parmigiano-Reggiano cheese

⅛ teaspoon (.6g) pepper

1 pound (454g) linguine

2 cloves garlic, peeled and sliced thinly

1½ pounds (680g) mussels, scrubbed well and debearded if necessary

1 pound (454g) shrimp, peeled and deveined

½ cup (120ml) Seafood Stock, divided (see Chapter 10)

¼ teaspoon (1.2g) salt, for flavor

2 tablespoons (7g) finely chopped fresh flat-leaf Italian parsley

1 lemon, cut into 6 wedges

DIRECTIONS

1 Place the zucchini on a baking sheet and preheat the broiler on high. Brush 1 tablespoon olive oil over both sides of the zucchini and top with the cheese and pepper. Broil for 2 to 3 minutes per side, watching carefully until golden. Remove and allow to cool.

2 Cook the pasta according to the package directions, until very al dente (about 3 minutes less than if you're serving immediately). Drain, reserving a cup of the cooking liquid.

3 When the zucchini are cool, place most of them in a blender, leaving a few pieces for garnish, and puree until smooth.

4 While the linguine is cooking, heat the remaining olive oil in a large sauté pan over medium heat. Add the garlic and cook until it releases its aroma, about 1 to 2 minutes.

5 Add the mussels, shrimp, and stock. Cover and cook over medium heat until all the mussels are open, about 2 to 5 minutes. Discard any broken or unopened mussels.

6 Add the linguine and zucchini cream to the seafood mixture and toss well with ¼ cup reserved pasta water. If sauce seems too thick, add additional pasta water, ¼ cup at a time, until you're happy with the sauce consistency. Cook for 1 to 2 minutes to allow the flavors to combine and the linguine to achieve desired tenderness.

7 Toss with tongs to combine. Place the pasta on a platter or individual plates and arrange the mussels around the pasta. Top with the remaining zucchini pieces and parsley and serve immediately with lemon wedges.

NOTE: Cooking seafood in EVOO protects the beneficial but heat-sensitive omega-3 fats. The EVOO has antioxidant effects that prevent the breakdown of these omega-3 fats.

NOTE: Check out the front cover for a photo of this recipe.

TIP: Refer to Figure 11-4 for cleaning and deveining shrimp.

TIP: Serve a green salad with this dish to increase the vegetable servings.

VARY IT! To make a vegetarian version, swap the mussels and shrimp for a cup of broccoli and a cup of fresh sliced vegetables.

PER SERVING: *Calories 567 (From Fat 139); Fat 15g (Saturated 3g); Cholesterol 150mg; Sodium 589mg; Carbohydrate 64g (Dietary Fiber 3g); Protein 41g; Sugars 4g.*

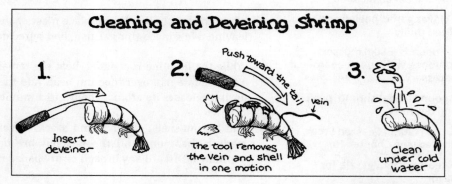

FIGURE 11-4: Cleaning and deveining shrimp.

Illustration by Liz Kurtzman

Tuscan Seafood Stew with Spinach Salad

PREP TIME: 15 MIN	COOK TIME: 30 MIN	YIELD: 4 SERVINGS

INGREDIENTS

¼ cup (60ml) Amy Riolo Selections or extra-virgin olive oil, plus 2 tablespoons (30 ml), divided

1 tablespoon (4g) minced parsley

1 tablespoon (4g) minced fresh sage leaves

5 garlic cloves, minced

12 ounces (340ml) calamari, cleaned and cut into 1-inch rings

1 tablespoon (16g) unsalted tomato paste

1 cup (240ml) dry white wine

2 cups (360g) chopped fresh tomatoes

¼ teaspoon (1.2g) salt

⅛ teaspoon (.6g) pepper

1 cup (240ml) Homemade Seafood Stock (see Chapter 10)

1 pound (454g) white fish, cut into large chunks

12 ounces (340g) large shrimp (fresh or frozen), peeled and deveined

4 thin slices whole-wheat bread, toasted

4 cups (120g) baby spinach

Juice of 1 lemon

1 cup (91g) broccoli florets, halved

½ cup (75g) cherry tomatoes, halved

DIRECTIONS

1 Heat the olive oil in a 6-quart saucepan over medium heat. Add the parsley, sage, and garlic. Cook until fragrant, about 1 minute.

2 Add the calamari and cook, stirring occasionally until the calamari is opaque, about 4 minutes. Add the tomato paste, stir well, and cook until the paste has darkened slightly, about 1 minute. Add the wine and cook, stirring often, until the liquid has evaporated, about 20 minutes.

3 Add the tomatoes along with their juice, season with salt and pepper, add the stock, and bring to a boil.

4 Add the fish and shrimp, stir, and cover. Cook, stirring occasionally until the seafood is tender, about 5 to 10 minutes. Ladle into spoons and serve hot with toasted bread.

5 Make the salad by combining the spinach, lemon juice, 2 tablespoons olive oil, broccoli, and tomatoes in a large bowl and toss to coat. Sprinkle with a pinch of salt and pepper if desired. Serve immediately.

NOTE: Calamari, or squid, is a source of omega-3 fatty acids that contributes to heart health; it contains taurine, an amino acid with potential anti-inflammatory effects, that supports overall health.

PER SERVING: *Calories 690 (From Fat 288); Fat 32g (Saturated 5g); Cholesterol 424mg; Sodium 798mg; Carbohydrate 31g (Dietary Fiber 5g); Protein 60g; Sugars 6g.*

Pan-Seared Shrimp with Barley Pilaf over Butternut Squash

PREP TIME: 15 MIN	COOK TIME: 30 MIN	YIELD: 4 SERVINGS

INGREDIENTS

2 cups (280g) butternut squash

¼ cup (60ml) Amy Riolo Selections or extra-virgin olive oil, divided

1 small eggplant, cubed

½ cup (90g) finely chopped fresh tomatoes

½ teaspoon (.5g) cinnamon

½ teaspoon (.5g) allspice

1 pound (454g) jumbo shrimp, peeled and deveined

½ teaspoon (2.4g) salt, divided

⅛ teaspoon (.6g) pepper

1 cup (157g) barley, cooked

Juice and zest of 1 lemon

DIRECTIONS

1 Preheat the oven to 425 degrees F. Line a baking sheet with parchment paper and place the squash on top. Drizzle with 1 tablespoon olive oil and turn to coat. Roast in the oven, about 25 to 35 minutes, or until tender. Remove and set aside.

2 Heat another tablespoon of olive oil in a large skillet over medium-high heat and add the eggplant. Turn to coat and cook for about 5 minutes, uncovered, until the eggplant becomes tender. Add the tomatoes, cinnamon, and allspice and stir to coat. Cover, reduce the heat to medium, and simmer until the tomatoes are tender. Transfer the squash to a blender or food processor and carefully puree until smooth.

3 Heat the remaining 2 tablespoons olive oil in another large skillet and add the shrimp. Season with ¼ teaspoon salt and pepper and cook 2 to 3 minutes or until the shrimp are golden. When the shrimp are finished, remove from the heat and top with lemon juice.

4 Taste the butternut squash and, if necessary, add the remaining ¼ teaspoon salt and stir.

5 To serve, toss the eggplant mixture into the barley and spoon into a serving bowl. Spoon the butternut squash puree onto another plate and top with the shrimp. Scatter the lemon zest over the shrimp and serve both dishes hot.

NOTE: Shrimp is a low-calorie seafood rich in astaxanthin, a powerful antioxidant that supports skin health, reduces inflammation, and may contribute to cardiovascular health. It also provides omega-3 fatty acids that promote heart health and potentially reduce the risk of chronic diseases. The selenium content in shrimp is essential for immune function and thyroid health, while the presence of astaxanthin and other carotenoids may support eye health and provide protection against oxidative stress.

PER SERVING: *Calories 357 (From Fat 144); Fat 16g (Saturated 2g); Cholesterol 172mg; Sodium 410mg; Carbohydrate 29g (Dietary Fiber 8g); Protein 26g; Sugars 5g.*

Italian Fish and Vegetable Kabobs with Green Salad

PREP TIME: 20 MIN	COOK TIME: 10 MIN	YIELD: 4 SERVINGS

INGREDIENTS

1¼ pounds (567g) fresh tuna, or your favorite firm fish, cut into 1-inch cubes

24 grape tomatoes

1 medium zucchini, cut into 24 rounds

1 medium green bell pepper, cut into 12 pieces

1 medium red bell pepper, cut into 12 pieces

1 clove garlic

4 tablespoons (60ml) Amy Riolo Selections or extra-virgin olive oil

Juice and zest of 1 lemon

⅛ teaspoon (.6g) salt

¼ teaspoon (1.2) pepper

1 cup (20g) mixed field greens

DIRECTIONS

1 Heat the grill or grill pan to high. Thread the tuna, tomatoes, zucchini, and peppers onto 8 skewers, leaving space between each one. Set the kabobs on a baking sheet. Repeat until you've used all the ingredients.

2 Place the garlic, 2 tablespoons olive oil, lemon juice and zest, salt, and pepper into a small blender and blend until emulsified. If you don't have a small blender, mince the garlic and add it and the other ingredients to a medium bowl. Whisk until emulsified.

3 Brush ½ of the mixture over the kabobs and reserve the other half.

4 Grill until the tuna is opaque and vegetables are tender, about 6 to 10 minutes, turning occasionally.

5 Place the mixed greens in a bowl and toss with the remaining dressing. Pour onto a platter. To serve, place the skewers on top of the greens. Drizzle with remaining 2 tablespoons olive oil and serve immediately.

NOTE: This recipe places the high-quality protein and fats of fish alongside high fiber, vitamins, and colorful polyphenol and carotenoid-rich, low glycemic vegetables — all with the added flavor and health benefits of high polyphenol EVOO. What's not to like!

TIP: You can also cook the fish under the broiler instead of roasting it if desired.

PER SERVING: Calories 316 (From Fat 138); Fat 15g (Saturated 2g); Cholesterol 64mg; Sodium 124mg; Carbohydrate 9g (Dietary Fiber 3g); Protein 35g; Sugars 6g.

Salmon Rolls Stuffed with Asparagus and Basil Cream

PREP TIME: 20 MIN | COOK TIME: 20 MIN | YIELD: 4 SERVINGS

INGREDIENTS

2 tablespoons (30ml) Amy Riolo Selections or extra-virgin olive oil, divided

1 bunch asparagus, ends trimmed

2 cloves garlic, minced

¼ teaspoon (1.2g) salt, divided

⅛ teaspoon (.6g) pepper, divided

¼ cup (11g) finely chopped fresh basil

½ cup (112g) Greek yogurt

4 salmon fillets (3.5 ounces each) (397g), skinned

Juice of 1 lemon

DIRECTIONS

1 Preheat oven to 425 degrees F. Drizzle 1 tablespoon olive oil onto a baking sheet. Top with the asparagus and garlic and toss to coat. Roast for 10 minutes, or until tender. Remove from the heat and season with half of salt and pepper.

2 When cooled slightly, carefully transfer ¾ of the asparagus to a blender or food processor with the fresh basil and yogurt.

3 Grease the bottom of a baking dish with the remaining 1 tablespoon of olive oil.

4 Place the salmon on a work service and cover with ¼ of the asparagus cream on each, then top with a few of the reserved cooked asparagus spears. Loosely roll up the fillets and place, seam side down, in the baking dish. Drizzle the lemon and season with the remaining salt and pepper. Cover with aluminum foil and bake for 15 to 20 minutes or until the salmon is cooked through.

NOTE: Salmon is a fatty fish rich in omega-3 fatty acids, which support heart health, brain function, and may reduce inflammation. Additionally, salmon contains astaxanthin, an antioxidant that may contribute to skin health and protects against oxidative stress. Asparagus is a low-calorie vegetable that contains rutin, a flavonoid with antioxidant properties that may support cardiovascular health. It also provides folate, which promotes DNA synthesis and cell repair, and fiber for digestive health.

TIP: Serve this recipe with ½ cup of cooked orzo, a whole-wheat dinner roll, or rice, if desired.

VARY IT! Swap the mixture for spinach and feta cheese.

PER SERVING: *Calories 243 (From Fat 130); Fat 14g (Saturated 3g); Cholesterol 55mg; Sodium 172mg; Carbohydrate 4g (Dietary Fiber 2g); Protein 24g; Sugars 2g.*

Pan-Roasted, Greek-Style Cod with Mixed Vegetables

| PREP TIME: 10 MIN | COOK TIME: 30 MIN | YIELD: 4 SERVINGS |

INGREDIENTS

¼ cup (60ml) plus 1 teaspoon (5ml) Amy Riolo Selections or extra-virgin olive oil, divided

1 bunch fresh parsley, chopped

1½ pound (680g) (about 4) medium Yukon Gold potatoes, cut into very thin (¼-inch) slices

1 pound (454g) fresh baby spinach

2 medium green bell peppers, sliced into rings

4 medium tomatoes, 1 diced and 1 halved and cut into ¼-inch slices

5 garlic cloves, roughly chopped

4 tablespoons (15g) fresh oregano, finely chopped

4 (⅓ pound each) (603g) fish fillets

¼ teaspoon (1.2g) salt

⅛ teaspoon (.6g) pepper

½ cup (120ml) water

DIRECTIONS

1 Preheat the oven to 425 degrees F. Grease the bottom of an 11 x 17-inch baking dish with 1 teaspoon olive oil. Place the parsley, potatoes, spinach, pepper, diced tomato, garlic, and oregano on the bottom of the pan, layering each one on top of the other. Season the fish with the salt and pepper and lay the fish on top of the vegetable mixture.

2 Pour 1 cup water over the vegetable mixture and on the sides of the pan. Place the tomato slices on top of the fish. Season with salt and pepper to taste. Bake for 20 to 30 minutes, or until the fish is opaque and flakes easily when pierced with a fork.

3 Carefully remove the fish and serve each plate with a bed of vegetables on the bottom and a fish fillet on top. Spoon the sauce over the top and sides to finish.

NOTE: Codfish is a lean source of high-quality protein, and it provides essential nutrients like vitamin B12 and selenium. The omega-3 fatty acids in cod and other white fish may also support heart health and reduce inflammation.

VARY IT! You can also prepare chicken legs this way.

PER SERVING: *Calories 466 (From Fat 163); Fat 18g (Saturated 3g); Cholesterol 42mg; Sodium 306mg; Carbohydrate 42g (Dietary Fiber 9g); Protein 39g; Sugars 6g.*

Roasted Fresh Tuna and Vegetable Tower

PREP TIME: 15 MIN	COOK TIME: 35 MIN	YIELD: 4 SERVINGS

INGREDIENTS

1 pound (454g) fresh tuna cut into 1-inch cubes

2 tablespoons (30ml) Amy Riolo Selections or extra-virgin olive oil, divided

¼ teaspoon (1.2g) salt

⅛ teaspoon (.6g) chili pepper

1 cup cucumber, diced into ¼-inch (.6cm) cubes

1 red bell pepper, diced into ¼-inch (.6cm) cubes

1 avocado, thinly sliced

1 cup (20g) microgreens

¼ cup (60ml) Amy Riolo Selections White Balsamic or balsamic vinegar

DIRECTIONS

1 Preheat oven to 425 degrees F. Place the tuna on a baking sheet and toss with 1 tablespoon olive oil, salt, and pepper. Roast for 5 to 10 minutes, or until your preferred doneness.

2 Place a 3-inch round ring mold in the center of each dinner plate and begin to build the tower by adding the cucumber to the bottom to form a solid layer, then layer the red pepper in the same way, followed by the avocado.

3 Follow with a layer of the tuna, dividing among the molds, one-quarter at a time.

4 Place the plates in the freezer for 20 minutes to chill.

5 Place the microgreens on top of the tuna and carefully remove the mold. Drizzle with vinegar and serve immediately.

NOTE: Tuna is rich in omega-3 fatty acids, which supports brain health and may reduce the risk of cardiovascular disease. Tuna also provides high-quality protein, vitamins B6 and B12, and selenium, which contribute to overall health.

TIP: This dish is normally served with raw tuna instead of roasted. If you prefer to eat your tuna raw, use the best quality tuna and check with your doctor to ensure that it's safe for you. If you don't have a 3-inch mold, you can use a clean, emptied-out can of tuna fish with the lid removed or a lined 3-inch ramekin to make the towers.

VARY IT! You can use smoked salmon instead of tuna.

PER SERVING: *Calories 287 (From Fat 139); Fat 15g (Saturated 2g); Cholesterol 51mg; Sodium 167mg; Carbohydrate 9g (Dietary Fiber 4g); Protein 28g; Sugars 3g.*

Making the Best of Poultry

The term poultry refers to fowl such as chicken, turkey, ducks, and geese. While each of these are eaten globally, chicken is by far the most popular today, and we focus on chicken meat in this section. Many people rely on chicken breast as a lean meat while trying to eat healthfully but can get stuck in an uninspired rut of everyday recipes. The dishes in this section focus on pleasing your palate and your blood glucose.

Americans currently consume an average of 60 pounds of chicken per year, making it the nation's protein of choice. Because it's so widely used, however, many people fall into chicken ruts — making the same dishes over and over again with dispirited results. Luckily, succulent time-honored recipes from all around the globe offer a multitude of savory, alluring, and healthful options to choose from.

Chicken contains high-quality protein and a relatively low amount of fat. In addition, the fat in chicken is mostly of the unsaturated type, which protects against heart disease. One 3-ounce serving contains just 1 gram of saturated fat and less than 4 grams of total fat, yet is packed with 31 grams of protein, which is more than half of the daily recommended allowance for adult females. Chicken meat contains a significant amount of B vitamins, which aid in metabolism, immune system and blood sugar level maintenance, cell growth, and nerve cell and red blood cell maintenance along with other immune-boosting ingredients.

Turkey is also a nutritious protein choice. Like chicken, it's a great source of protein, is lowfat, and rich in many minerals and vitamins. Niacin, B6, B12, and choline, in particular, are found in turkey meat. Like chicken, it's important to skip the skin when eating turkey.

REMEMBER

Skip the processed deli meat versions of poultry and opt for fresh pieces of roasted meat in 3- to 4-ounce servings at a time.

Citrus Chicken, Strawberry, and Avocado Salad

PREP TIME: 10 MIN	COOK TIME: 20 MIN	YIELD: 4 SERVINGS

INGREDIENTS

1 pound (454g) skinless, boneless chicken breasts, sliced into thin strips (about 2-inches (5cm) each)

¼ cup (60 ml) Amy Riolo Selections or extra-virgin olive oil, divided

Juice and zest of 1 orange

Juice and zest of 1 lemon

¼ teaspoon (1.2g) salt

⅛ teaspoon (.6g) pepper

4 cups (120g) baby kale or spinach

1 cup (166g) thinly sliced strawberries

1 avocado, deseeded and cut into 1-inch cubes

3 tablespoons (45ml) Amy Riolo Selections White Balsamic or balsamic vinegar

DIRECTIONS

1 Preheat oven to 425 degrees F. Combine the chicken, 2 tablespoons olive oil, orange and lemon juice and zest, salt, and pepper in a baking dish and turn to coat. Roast for 20 minutes, or until the chicken registers 160 degrees F on a meat thermometer and is cooked through. Remove from the oven and set aside.

2 Layer the kale, strawberries, and avocado on a serving platter.

3 Drizzle with the remaining olive oil and 2 tablespoons vinegar. Serve immediately.

NOTE: Chicken is a lean source of protein, providing essential amino acids for muscle health. It also contains vitamins such as niacin and B6 that support metabolism and minerals like phosphorus that support bone health.

TIP: Roast chicken in larger quantities to have for sandwiches and wraps during the week.

VARY IT! Use thinly sliced pieces of beef or shrimp instead of chicken.

PER SERVING: *Calories 372 (From Fat 217); Fat 24g (Saturated 4g); Cholesterol 73mg; Sodium 280mg; Carbohydrate 14g (Dietary Fiber 5g); Protein 26g; Sugars 6g.*

Beet Couscous with Orange–Glazed Chicken and Pecans

PREP TIME: 15 MIN	COOK TIME: 45 MIN	YIELD: 4 SERVINGS

INGREDIENTS

4 pieces chicken leg and thighs, skinless

¼ cup (60ml) Amy Riolo Selections or extra-virgin olive oil, divided

1 tablespoon (3g) sumac or poultry seasoning

2 teaspoons (2g) pure cinnamon, divided

1 orange, juiced and zested

⅛ teaspoon (.6g) pepper

4 cups (544g) medium red beets

DIRECTIONS

1 Preheat the oven to 425 degrees F. Place the chicken in a roasting pan or baking pan greased with 1 tablespoon olive oil. Sprinkle sumac and 1 teaspoon cinnamon over both sides and drizzle with orange juice. Scatter with pepper and bake, uncovered, for 30 minutes, or until chicken legs register 160 degrees F on a meat thermometer. Remove from the oven and set aside, covered with aluminum foil to cool.

2 To roast the beets, place them on a baking sheet and roast them alongside or underneath the chicken until tender, about 30 to 45 minutes. Remove from the oven, and when cool, carefully peel the skins and chop them into small dices. Wash your hands.

Couscous

INGREDIENTS

1½ cups (360ml) water

1 cup (224g) pearl couscous

1 lemon, juiced

1 orange, juiced

¼ teaspoon (1.2g) unrefined sea salt

⅓ cup (33g) pecan halves, toasted and chopped

DIRECTIONS

1 Bring 1 cup water to a boil in a medium saucepan over high heat. Add the couscous, stir, and cover with a tight-fitting lid. Reduce the heat and simmer for 8 to 10 minutes or until cooked through and tender.

2 Whisk the lemon juice, orange juice, 2 tablespoons of olive oil, and salt together to make a dressing and mix into the couscous, fluffing with a fork to separate the granules.

3 Immediately add the warm beets and mix well to combine to create a pink couscous.

4 Divide the couscous into 4 dinner plates. Top each with a chicken leg or thigh (drizzle with remaining pan juices to make it moist) and top with pecans.

NOTE: Couscous is a wheat-based grain that provides complex carbohydrates for sustained energy. It contains selenium that supports immune function and small amounts of B vitamins that contribute to overall metabolic health. Pearl couscous is also known as Israeli couscous or Moghrabiah.

TIP: You can prepare the beets in advance and store them in the fridge until you're ready.

NOTE: This dish is so pretty that you'll forget that it's good for you. The beautiful pink color makes it fun for special occasions. Check out the color insert for a photo.

VARY IT! Use turkey instead of chicken.

PER SERVING: *Calories 509 (From Fat 197); Fat 22g (Saturated 3g); Cholesterol 34mg; Sodium 259mg; Carbohydrate 61g (Dietary Fiber 9g); Protein 18g; Sugars 14g.*

THE BEAUTY OF BEETS

Beets are a great source of folate — a nutrient important for normal cell functions and especially valuable in pregnancy. A 3.5-ounce (100g) serving contains more than 20 percent of average daily recommended amounts (though in pregnancy, supplementation is always advised). They also are a great source of plant nitrates that help to lower blood pressure. Betalains are colored bioactive compounds that may have antioxidant, anti-inflammatory, and anticancer effects. We recommend roasting extra beets in advance and storing them in airtight containers in the fridge to use in salads, sliced onto toast, or in purees and dips when needed.

Roasted Spice–Dusted Chicken with Veggies

PREP TIME: 10 MIN	COOK TIME: 30 MIN	YIELD: 4 SERVINGS

INGREDIENTS

4 chicken legs (with thighs), skin on, bone in

2 tablespoons (30ml) Amy Riolo Selections olive oil or extra-virgin olive oil, divided

1 teaspoon (1g) sumac

2 cups (214g) cauliflower florets

2 cups (289g) grape tomatoes, halved

4 cups (364g) broccoli florets

⅛ teaspoons (.6g) pepper

¼ teaspoon (1.2g) salt

1 lemon, juiced and zested

DIRECTIONS

1 Preheat the oven to 425 degrees F. Place the chicken on a baking sheet and brush with 1 tablespoon olive oil and dust with sumac. Scatter the cauliflower, tomatoes, and broccoli around the chicken.

2 Sprinkle with salt and pepper, drizzle the vegetables with the remaining tablespoon of olive oil, and mix to coat.

3 Drizzle the lemon juice over the chicken and roast for 30 minutes, or until the chicken registers 160 degrees F and both the chicken and vegetables are cooked. Sprinkle with lemon zest and serve warm.

NOTE: Sumac is a spice rich in antioxidants, including flavonoids and tannins, which may have anti-inflammatory properties. It also contains vitamin C, which supports immune function and skin health.

TIP: Sumac is a ruby red spice that is tangy in flavor and hails from the Middle East. You can find it in international markets and specialty grocery stores. Substitute your favorite spice If desired.

VARY IT! Swap out chicken for fish.

PER SERVING: *Calories 383 (From Fat 203); Fat 23g (Saturated 5g); Cholesterol 104mg; Sodium 633mg; Carbohydrate 13g (Dietary Fiber 4g); Protein 34g; Sugars 5g.*

Oregano Chicken with Lemon Potatoes and Green Beans

PREP TIME: 10 MIN	COOK TIME: 30 MIN	YIELD: 4 SERVINGS

INGREDIENTS

4 chicken drumsticks, skin on

2 tablespoons (30ml) Amy Riolo Selections olive oil or extra-virgin olive oil

1 teaspoon (1g) dried oregano

2 Russet potatoes, peeled and cut into ¼-inch (.5cm) cubes

4 cups (400g) green beans, trimmed

⅛ teaspoon (.6g) pepper

¼ teaspoon (1.2g) salt

1 cup (180g) diced fresh tomatoes

1 lemon, juiced and zested

DIRECTIONS

1 Preheat the oven to 425 degrees F. Place the chicken on a baking sheet and brush with olive oil. Scatter the oregano, potatoes, and green beans around the sheet and toss to mix well.

2 Sprinkle with salt and pepper and scatter with the tomatoes. Mix to coat.

3 Drizzle the lemon juice over the chicken and roast for 30 minutes, or until the chicken registers 160 degrees F, stirring halfway through until both the chicken and vegetables are cooked. Sprinkle with zest and serve warm.

NOTE: The acidity of lemon juice reduces the rise in glucose from the potatoes so it not only adds flavor but also regulates glucose. Oregano is an herb that contains compounds like carvacrol and thymol, which have antimicrobial and antioxidant properties. It also provides vitamins A and K that contribute to immune and bone health.

TIP: Make this recipe in advance and serve the next day.

VARY IT! Swap out chicken for fish.

PER SERVING: *Calories 243 (From Fat 99); Fat 11g (Saturated 2g); Cholesterol 36mg; Sodium 166mg; Carbohydrate 26g (Dietary Fiber 5g); Protein 12g; Sugars 6g.*

Chapter **12**

Fruit, Cheese, Nuts, and Desserts

Even if you have diabetes, sugar doesn't have to be off limits. But it's no secret that the amount of sugar consumed globally today is out of control. Manufacturers sneak it into all kinds of products, including prepackaged rice pilaf mix, ketchup, and, of course, baked goods, under the names high-fructose corn syrup and malt syrup. Even though diabetes is a disease that involves impaired metabolism of carbohydrates, you can still enjoy desserts that contain starches and sugar. You just need to select your ingredients wisely and eat reasonably modest portions. But don't waste time feeling guilty because you can't stay away from sweets.

Sweet is one of the basic tastes, just like sour and salty, and craving sweet foods is normal. The difference between sweetness and the other tastes, however, is that it's the first flavor people perceive as infants when drinking their mothers' milk. Because breastmilk is sweet, infants immediately correlate it with feelings of nourishment, satisfaction, safety, and comfort. It's for that reason that sweets pick you up when you're down and consuming them is a way to feel comforted in the short term.

In this chapter, we show you how to create appealing desserts that feature nutritious ingredients while satisfying your sweet tooth. We help you look at dessert through a different lens, discover how to pair them with other items in your meal, and enjoy them wholeheartedly when you do consume them, including chocolate. By drawing upon traditional recipes that are naturally sweet and combining them with spices and nuts, many of the recipes in this chapter can do double duty as breakfast or snack items too. Be sure to read the Note in each recipe to find out about its nutritional values. Also refer to the book's Introduction for some recipe conventions we use.

DOCTOR SAYS

All carbohydrates contain sugars and are a necessary and nutrient-rich part of a healthy and balanced diet. Part 1 of this book as well as our books, the recent editions of *Diabetes For Dummies* and *Diabetes Meal Planning & Nutrition For Dummies*, are chock-full of information about the best types of carbohydrates to eat, especially for people with prediabetes and diabetes. Continuous blood glucose monitoring technologies help you to understand your specific body's response to sugars and sweeteners. When adding sugars, evidence is beginning to emerge to suggest that for most people unprocessed or raw honey, which retains natural antioxidant, anti-inflammatory and antimicrobial compounds, may be better at controlling blood glucose and insulin response than other added sugars.

Finding a New Take on Fruit

Fruit is the go-to daily dessert in many parts of the world. Eating fresh fruit for dessert is a great way to enjoy natural sweetness while increasing the fiber, vitamin, mineral, and antioxidant servings in your daily diet. When paired with a few healthful fats such as cheese and nuts, eating fresh fruit enables you to satisfy your sweet tooth while keeping your blood glucose levels in check.

Some fruits have a higher glycemic index than others, and each person may have a slightly different blood glucose response to one fruit or another. Wherever possible, monitor these effects and discover which fruit is best for you and your diabetes control.

These sections include recipes for fruit-based desserts and cheese and nut platters as an alternative.

Fruit-based desserts

In the Mediterranean region, people plan their desserts around fresh fruits in the same fashion that they plan their main meals around vegetables. Using seasonal fruits as a base for an after–dinner treat, you'll be sure to get the nutrients you need (remember to eat six to nine servings of fresh fruits and vegetables per day) while enjoying a wide variety of flavors and textures. Even if you don't have time to prepare anything, a piece of fruit and a few raw nuts is a great option.

IDEAL FRUITS FOR SOMEONE WITH DIABETES

People who eat a diet rich in whole fruits may be less likely to develop diabetes 2, according to a study in the October 2021 *Journal of Clinical Endocrinology & Metabolism*. Even though you can eat all fresh, natural, fruit in small quantities as part of a balanced meal without causing spikes in blood sugar, specific types are particularly suited to people with diabetes. Choosing fruits that are low in carbohydrates and low in glycemic index, but high in vitamins, minerals, fiber, and antioxidants is key.

Always remember to consume fruit in its whole, natural form and avoid fruit in syrups or processed varieties. Here are some of your best options:

- Blueberries
- Strawberries
- Blackberries
- Raspberries
- Tart cherries
- Peaches

- Apricots
- Apples
- Oranges
- Pears
- Kiwifruits

A single serving of these fruits makes an excellent snack, especially paired with a few plain, unsalted almonds or walnuts or a serving of plain, full-fat Greek yogurt. Try eating fruits in season as much as possible in order to obtain the most nutritional benefits.

Grape, Blueberry, and Goat Cheese Wreath

PREP TIME: 10 MIN	YIELD: 4 SERVINGS

INGREDIENTS

1 large bunch fresh green grapes, washed and halved

1 cup (148g) fresh blueberries

2 ounces (57g) goat cheese

1 tablespoon (15ml) water

Handful of fresh mint leaves

1 teaspoon (7g) raw honey

DIRECTIONS

1 Place the grape halves in a circular wreath shape on a white plate, leaving the center empty.

2 Scatter the blueberries around the top.

3 Mix the goat cheese with a tablespoon of water in a small bowl.

4 Using a small melon baller or your fingers, form small, pebble-sized balls with the goat cheese and place in various nooks around the wreath to resemble small flowers.

5 Arrange 2 to 3 mint leaves around the base of each goat cheese ball to resemble stems.

6 Drizzle the honey over the wreath and serve or refrigerate until serving.

NOTE: Blueberries are rich in anthocyanins, a type of flavonoid with potent antioxidant properties that support cognitive function, reduce inflammation, and may contribute to heart health. They also provide vitamin C and fiber, which support immune function and digestive health.

TIP: Serve this healthful festive recipe at holiday time.

VARY IT! In the summertime, swap out grapes for berries of your choice.

PER SERVING: *Calories 104 (From Fat 38); Fat 4g (Saturated 3g); Cholesterol 11mg; Sodium 59mg; Carbohydrate 14g (Dietary Fiber 1g); Protein 4g; Sugars 11g.*

Calabrian-Style Almond and Spice-Stuffed Figs

PREP TIME: 15 MIN	COOK TIME: 15 MIN	YIELD: 6 SERVINGS

INGREDIENTS

12 fresh, ripe figs or good-quality dried figs

¼ cup (27g) slivered almonds, chopped

Zest of 1 orange

1 teaspoon (1g) ground cinnamon

1 teaspoon (1g) ground cloves

2 ounces (57g) 80 percent or higher dark chocolate, fair trade if possible

DIRECTIONS

1 If using dried figs, preheat the oven to 350 degrees F. Line a baking sheet with parchment paper.

2 Hold the fig upright, make an incision halfway down if using dried figs and ¼ of the way down if using fresh figs. Insert your finger in the incision to open it a bit.

3 In a small bowl, combine the almonds, orange zest, cinnamon, and cloves. Stuff each fig with the filling. Press the figs closed and place them an inch apart on a baking sheet.

4 If using dried figs, bake until soften and darkened, about 5 to 8 minutes. If using fresh figs, you don't need to bake them.

5 Fill the bottom of a double boiler with enough water to almost touch the bottom of the top part. Place the chocolate in the top of the double boiler over low heat. Heat, stirring constantly, just until the chocolate is melted, about 2 to 3 minutes.

6 If using dried figs, remove them from the oven. Use tongs to hold the figs by the stem and dip them quickly into the warm chocolate leaving the top quarter exposed. Place on a cooling rack with wax or parchment paper and allow to cool. Allow to stand 20 minutes at room temperature before serving.

NOTE: Dark chocolate contains flavonoids, particularly cocoa flavanols, which have antioxidant properties and may support heart health by improving blood flow and reducing blood pressure. Additionally, dark chocolate may positively impact mood and cognitive function. Cloves are rich in antioxidants, particularly eugenol, which has anti-inflammatory and antimicrobial properties.

TIP: If using fresh figs, be sure to use firm ones. If they're too soft, they'll fall apart when covered with chocolate. Because this dish is typically served at Christmas time in Calabria, it's often made with the prized dried white local figs. If you can't find Calabrian or other good quality white figs, substitute other dried figs. If they're hard to the touch, soak them in water for an hour before proceeding with the recipe.

PER SERVING: *Calories 156 (From Fat 59); Fat 7g (Saturated 3g); Cholesterol 0mg; Sodium 3mg; Carbohydrate 24g (Dietary Fiber 4g); Protein 2g; Sugars 19g.*

Grape, Goat Cheese, and Almond Skewers

PREP TIME: 20 MIN	YIELD: 4 SERVINGS

INGREDIENTS

24 seedless green grapes (about ½ pound) (227g)

2 ounces (57g) goat cheese

3 tablespoons (45 ml) milk

½ cup (48g) blanched almonds, coarsely ground, plus extra for garnish

1 orange, halved, for serving

DIRECTIONS

1 Remove the grapes from the stem and wash well.

2 In a small bowl, combine the goat cheese and milk. Mix well until a creamy, icing-like consistency is formed. Transfer to a plate.

3 Place the almonds on another plate.

4 Thread 6 grapes onto an 8-inch skewer, leaving a little room between each and at least a 1-inch border from the point end. Roll each one onto the goat cheese mixture and use a brush or your fingers to create a thin, even coat over the grapes.

5 Dip each skewer into the almonds and turn to coat well several times. Shake off the excess almonds and set on a separate plate. Continue this process until all four skewers are complete.

6 Cut off the bottom of the orange so it can sit flat. Place the orange cut-side down on a large plate. Stick the pointed ends of the skewers into the orange so that the skewers look like a bouquet. Chill until serving.

NOTE: Goat cheese is a good source of calcium and protein, supporting bone health and muscle development. It contains healthier shorter chain fats that are thought to be better for cholesterol levels than other saturated fats, and it's often easier to digest than cow's milk cheese.

NOTE: In Spain people customarily eat 12 grapes at midnight on New Year's Eve for good luck. I (Amy) like to serve 2 of these skewers instead of 12 plain grapes on New Year's. This is a fun and elegant way to dress up fruit.

PER SERVING: *Calories 177 (From Fat 94); Fat 10g (Saturated 4g); Cholesterol 12mg; Sodium 64mg; Carbohydrate 16g (Dietary Fiber 3g); Protein 7g; Sugars 12g.*

⬤ Watermelon "Cake"

INGREDIENTS

1 medium seedless watermelon

1 kiwifruit

½ cup (74g) blueberries

½ cup (62g) raspberries

½ cup (72g) blackberries

½ cup (13g) fresh mint, divided

2 cups (452g) Greek yogurt

2 tablespoons (42g) raw honey

1 teaspoon (5ml) vanilla

DIRECTIONS

1 Cut the watermelon in half vertically down the center. Using a 9-inch round cake pan as a guide, slice a 9-inch round and 4-inch-deep circle out of the center of one of the watermelon sides and trim off the rind. Shape it into a circle by removing all of the white rind.

2 Using a 6-inch round cake pan or a 6-inch circular piece of paper as a guide, cut a 6-inch layer that's 4 inches deep out of the other side of the watermelon.

3 With the leftover watermelon, carve out a 3-inch round slice that's also 4 inches deep.

4 Peel the kiwifruit and cut it into four thick slices. Use a small cookie cutter or a cutout from a piece of paper to shape them into star shapes.

5 Place the largest layer of the watermelon on a serving platter. Insert a few toothpicks halfway into the middle of the piece. Add the 6-inch layer, pressing down on the toothpicks so that they adhere. Using the same technique with the toothpicks, layer the 3-inch piece on top.

6 Scatter the berries and kiwifruit stars around the sides and top of the watermelon, placing one star on top. Scatter half of the mint leaves around the watermelon cake. Refrigerate until serving.

7 Combine the remaining mint, yogurt, honey, and vanilla in a small bowl. Mix well to incorporate the ingredients, cover, and chill until serving. When ready to serve, slice the cake into eight equal size pieces and top with berries and a few tablespoons of the yogurt mixture.

NOTE: Watermelon is hydrating and contains the antioxidant lycopene, which may contribute to heart health and protect against certain cancers. It also provides vitamins A and C, which support immune function and skin health.

NOTE: This is now my favorite birthday and special-occasion cake to serve. Even if you offer a traditional cake, this one makes a fun addition to any celebratory table.

PER SERVING: *Calories 206 (From Fat 31); Fat 3g (Saturated 2g); Cholesterol 0mg; Sodium 25mg; Carbohydrate 41g (Dietary Fiber 3g); Protein 8g; Sugars 32g.*

Cheese and nut platters as an alternative

In Europe cheese and nut platters are often served at the end of a meal or in place of dessert. This elegant option also has a nutritional advantage for people with diabetes because it provides additional calcium, protein, and healthful fats to keep your palate happy and your body fueled throughout the evening. Here you can try some quick and tasty recipes that highlight the cheese and nuts.

TIP

If you tend to eat dinner early in the evening, a small serving of cheese and nuts can be a good evening snack choice.

CHOOSING CHEESE

Here are some types of cheese that are good choices for people with diabetes. Keep them on hand for a snack or in place of dessert when the mood strikes. Be sure to enjoy them in small amounts and buy the best quality possible.

Diabetes-friendly cheeses include, but aren't limited to the following:

- Plain feta
- Goat cheese
- Aged cheeses (such as Pecorino, Parmigiano, and Cabrales)
- Ricotta
- Mozzarella
- Cottage cheese

French Cheese Plate

INGREDIENTS

4 ounces (113g) goat cheese

4 ounces (113g) brie

20 raw almonds

¼ cup (72g) no-sugar-added raspberry or apricot preserves

2 apples, thinly sliced

4 slices thinly sliced whole-wheat bread

DIRECTIONS

1 Using a large decorative platter, cheese plate, or cutting board, arrange the goat cheese and brie opposite ends.

2 Place the almonds in a small ramekin and set it in the middle of the platter.

3 Place the preserves in another small ramekin and place it next to the almonds.

4 Arrange the apple slices and bread pieces on the open parts of the platter.

NOTE: Unprocessed cheeses are a great source of probiotics, which helps to maintain a healthy and diverse gut microbiome, important for many aspects of physical and mental health.

TIP: Individual portions of this fruit plate (minus the preserves) can be a great snack.

VARY IT! Use your favorite cheese and nut combinations to create your own cheese boards but remember to follow these proportions and choose cheese made from different kinds of milk and with different textures to make it more interesting.

PER SERVING: Calories 396 (From Fat 189); Fat 21g (Saturated 11g); Cholesterol 50mg; Sodium 410mg; Carbohydrate 38g (Dietary Fiber 5g); Protein 17g; Sugars 18g.

Seasonal Italian Fruit and Cheese Platter

PREP TIME: 5 TO 10 MIN	YIELD: 4 SERVINGS

INGREDIENTS

1 bunch red grapes

8 fresh or dried (unsweetened) figs

2 plums, sliced

1 cup (100g) walnuts

4 ounces (113g) Parmigiano-Reggiano cheese, sliced into thin pieces

4 teaspoons (28g) raw honey

DIRECTIONS

1 Arrange the grapes, figs, and plums on a large serving platter.

2 Place the walnuts in a small ramekin and set it on one end of the platter.

3 Arrange the Parmigiano–Reggiano slices in the middle of the platter and drizzle with honey.

NOTE: Parmigiano cheese is a rich source of calcium and protein, which supports bone health and muscle function. It also contains vitamin B12, which contributes to nerve function, and phosphorus, which supports energy metabolism. The aging process of Parmigiano enhances its umami flavor and makes it easier to digest for people with lactose sensitivity.

TIP: Make this platter in advance and drizzle the honey over the cheese before serving.

VARY IT! The fruit used in this recipe is usually ripe in late summer-early autumn in Italy; you can use whichever combination of fruit is seasonal in your area when preparing it.

PER SERVING: *Calories 422 (From Fat 224); Fat 25g (Saturated 7g); Cholesterol 25mg; Sodium 436mg; Carbohydrate 40g (Dietary Fiber 5g); Protein 16g; Sugars 32g.*

🍅 Crostini with Ricotta, Fig Preserves, and Walnuts

PREP TIME: 5 MIN	COOK TIME: 3 MIN	YIELD: 4 SERVINGS

INGREDIENTS

4 thin slices of Homemade Whole-Grain Bread (see Chapter 6) or 100 percent whole-grain bread

1 cup (246g) whole-milk ricotta, drained

¼ cup (72g) no-sugar added fig preserves, or sliced fresh figs

¼ cup (25g) walnuts, chopped

½ teaspoon (.5g) pure Ceylon cinnamon

DIRECTIONS

1 Preheat the broiler and toast the bread for 1 to 2 minutes or until hardened but barely golden. Using tongs, carefully turn over and toast for an additional 30 seconds. Remove from the broiler.

2 Place the ricotta in a food processor or blender and puree until smooth.

3 Slather the ricotta over the bread and top with a teaspoon of fig preserves and ¼ of the walnuts.

4 Sprinkle the cinnamon over the top and serve warm.

NOTE: Ricotta cheese is a good source of high-quality protein, calcium, and phosphorus, which supports bone health and muscle function. It also contains whey protein, which is easily digestible. Ricotta is lower in fat than many other cheeses, and the fats that it does contain are mainly unsaturated, contributing to heart health. Additionally, ricotta cheese provides essential amino acids, B vitamins, and minerals that contribute to overall nutritional balance.

TIP: This recipe also makes a delicious and satisfying breakfast.

VARY IT! Substitute plain Greek yogurt or goat cheese for the ricotta and swap out your favorite no-sugar-added preserves.

PER SERVING: *Calories 265 (From Fat 125); Fat 14g (Saturated 6g); Cholesterol 31mg; Sodium 166mg; Carbohydrate 26g (Dietary Fiber 3g); Protein 11g; Sugars 8g.*

Fruit salads and yogurt

Fruit salads and yogurt are the most healthful and easiest to prepare of desserts. Complete with all three micronutrients (carbohydrates, protein and fat), Greek yogurt is a powerful ally in blood glucose maintenance. Pairing fresh fruit with plain yogurt ensures that the fruit doesn't create a sudden spike in blood sugar levels. These recipes also make great breakfasts and snacks.

YOGURT AND FRUIT: A MATCH MADE IN HEAVEN

No matter the season, fresh fruit salads are always a welcome finale to a meal, snack, or breakfast. Combining the carbohydrates in fruit with the protein and fat in yogurt makes a light but balanced meal that can be enjoyed anytime.

Taking the time to prepare a fruit salad in advance and storing it in the refrigerator makes it easy to enjoy on a regular basis. By eating a serving of various types of fruits, you're also sure to get different nutrients while enjoying fruit. Macerating fruit in honey and in herbs such as fresh mint, basil, or lavender helps to amplify the flavors of the fruit.

When pairing fruit with yogurt, we always recommend plain, full-fat Greek or Greek-style yogurt because of its protein content. Authentic Greek yogurt that comes from Greece is made from a combination of sheep and goat milk, while the version sold in the United States is made from cow milk. Many American and international manufacturers sell so-called Greek-style yogurt even though the yogurt doesn't come from Greece or a Greek company.

Remember: When purchasing yogurt, be sure that it's plain and has no added sugars. Also check the protein content. Real Greek yogurt is higher in protein, which helps balance out blood sugar.

Summer Berry and Fresh Fig Salad

INGREDIENTS

4 fresh figs, halved

½ cup (74g) fresh blueberries

½ cup (62g) fresh raspberries

1 tablespoon (13g) sugar

Juice and zest of 1 lemon

1 cup (152g) fresh strawberries, hulled and halved

1 cup (226g) Greek yogurt

1 teaspoon (5ml) vanilla

1 teaspoon (3.4g) flaxseeds

2 teaspoons (14g) raw honey

DIRECTIONS

1 Combine the figs, blueberries, and raspberries with the sugar and lemon juice and zest in a medium bowl and mix well to incorporate sugar.

2 Place the strawberries, yogurt, vanilla, flaxseeds, and honey in a food processor or blender and puree until smooth.

3 Fill the bottom of 4 dessert bowls or decorative dessert cups with ¼ each of the strawberry mixture. Top with equal amounts of the fig and berry mixture. Serve immediately or refrigerate until serving.

NOTE: Berries are a great source of polyphenols, and figs are a good source of dietary fiber, potassium, and vitamins like vitamin K. They contain antioxidants, including phenols and flavonoids, which contribute to heart health and may have anti-inflammatory effects.

NOTE: This dish also makes a tasty summertime breakfast.

VARY IT! Omit the sugar and lemon juice and zest and combine all the ingredients in a blender to make four breakfast or recovery smoothies to enjoy after a workout.

PER SERVING: Calories 154 (From Fat 31); Fat 3g (Saturated 2g); Cholesterol 0mg; Sodium 22mg; Carbohydrate 27g (Dietary Fiber 4g); Protein 6g; Sugars 21g.

Cardamom-Scented Apricots with Honey, Yogurt, and Pistachios

INGREDIENTS

2 cups (453g) Greek yogurt

1 teaspoon (1g) ground cardamom

3 tablespoons (63g) raw honey, divided

1 tablespoon (15ml) Amy Riolo Selections or extra-virgin olive oil

1 cup (250g) dried no-sugar-added apricots

Juice and zest 1 orange

2 tablespoons (17g) raw pistachios, finely chopped

DIRECTIONS

1 In a medium bowl, combine the yogurt and cardamom, stirring until incorporated. Stir in a tablespoon of the honey.

2 Heat the olive oil in a medium skillet over medium-high heat. Add the apricots and toss to coat. Add the remaining 2 tablespoons of honey, stir, and reduce the heat to medium-low. Cook, stirring occasionally until the apricots begin to caramelize and plump up, 6 to 8 minutes.

3 Divide the yogurt into 4 serving glasses.

4 When the apricots are ready, deglaze the skillet with the orange juice. When the liquid's almost evaporated, after 2 to 3 minutes, stir in the orange zest.

5 Spoon the apricot mixture on top of the yogurt in equal amounts in the serving glasses. Top each with ½ tablespoon of pistachios. Serve immediately or refrigerate.

NOTE: Cardamom is rich in antioxidants, particularly compounds called cineole and limonene, which may have anti-inflammatory and digestive benefits. It also contains minerals like potassium and magnesium that support heart health.

TIP: Leftover portions of this dish make a delicious breakfast.

VARY IT! Use dates, raisins, dried figs, and your favorite nuts instead of apricots and pistachios.

PER SERVING: *Calories 271 (From Fat 97); Fat 11g (Saturated 4g); Cholesterol 0mg; Sodium 56mg; Carbohydrate 36g (Dietary Fiber 2g); Protein 12g; Sugars 31g.*

Enjoying Sweet Indulgences

In addition to your body's natural sugar cravings, you may also crave sugar for psychological and emotional reasons. Sometimes your day literally lacks sweetness. Whether you're experiencing chronic illness or stress, another rough patch in life, or simply don't receive the affection you desire, you may crave sweet foods even more. These recipes provide the sweetness that everyone craves in a healthful way that also provides nutritional benefits to the body. They're not only nutritious and easy enough to enjoy often but also special enough to serve to guests.

In addition to swapping out healthful desserts for heavy, sugar-laden ones, we recommend searching for the sweetness in life wherever possible. Here are some ways to do so:

>> Listen to relaxing music.

>> Walk in nature.

>> Read a note from a loved one or write sweet poetry.

>> Smell comforting scents or aromas.

>> Make a gratitude list.

>> Watch a touching movie.

>> Hug someone.

Fresh fruit-inspired treats

You'll want to share the impressive and scrumptious desserts in this section with others. Grilled pineapple is satisfying in the summer, and it also adds an unexpected tropical touch to a winter meal as well. Panna Cotta is a cooked Italian cream dessert that's served in the finest Italian restaurants in the world. This diabetes-friendly version is as attractive as it is tasty. Save the Cantaloupe in Coconut Cream recipe for the warmer months when melons are plentiful.

Grilled Pineapple with Ricotta and Raw Honey

PREP TIME: 10 MIN	COOK TIME: 8 MIN	YIELD: 4 SERVINGS

INGREDIENTS

8 fresh pineapple wedges, about 2 inches (5cm) round

3 tablespoons (63g) raw honey, divided

½ cup (123g) whole-milk ricotta

1 teaspoon (1g) pure Ceylon cinnamon

1 tablespoon (1.6g) finely chopped fresh mint

DIRECTIONS

1 Preheat your grill or grill pan to medium-high heat. If broiling, preheat your broiler to the highest position.

2 Place the pineapple chunks on the grill, grill pan, or baking sheet if you're broiling. Watching carefully, broil or grill, for 2 to 3 minutes, or until they begin to caramelize and turn color. Remove from the oven, drizzle with 1 tablespoon honey, turn to coat, and set aside.

3 Combine 1 tablespoon of honey with the ricotta and cinnamon in a blender and pulse until a smooth cream.

4 To serve, place 2 pineapple rings on individual dessert plates. Top each plate with ¼ of the ricotta mixture, drizzle with the remaining tablespoon of honey, and garnish with the fresh mint.

NOTE: Pineapple is a good source of vitamin C and manganese that contributes to immune health and bone formation. It contains *bromelain,* an enzyme with anti-inflammatory properties that may aid in digestion. Cinnamon contains *cinnamaldehyde,* a compound with antioxidant and anti-inflammatory properties. It may help regulate blood sugar levels and contribute to heart health.

VARY IT! You can prepare fresh peach and apricot halves in the same manner as the pineapple.

PER SERVING: *Calories 122 (From Fat 36); Fat 4g (Saturated 3g); Cholesterol 16mg; Sodium 27mg; Carbohydrate 19g (Dietary Fiber 1g); Protein 4g; Sugars 17g.*

🍓 Strawberry Almond Panna Cotta

INGREDIENTS

2 tablespoons (30ml) water

2 teaspoons (4.6g) powdered gelatin

2 cups (480ml) unsweetened vanilla almond milk

3 tablespoons (63g) pure honey, divided

2 teaspoons (8g) vanilla extract, divided

⅛ cup (30ml) Amy Riolo Selections White Balsamic or balsamic vinegar

1 cup (152g) hulled strawberries, thinly sliced, plus 2 extra, halved, for garnish

2 teaspoons (5ml) fresh lemon juice

Pinch salt

DIRECTIONS

1 Place two tablespoons water in a medium bowl. Sprinkle the gelatin over the surface and stir with a fork. Allow to rehydrate for 5 to 10 minutes until the gelatin has softened.

2 In a large liquid measuring cup, add the almond milk, 2 tablespoons honey, and 1 teaspoon vanilla and whisk to combine. Pour the sweetened almond milk into a medium saucepan over medium heat, stirring occasionally. Remove from the heat when the milk is steaming hot and is about to boil. Add a few tablespoons of milk mixture to the gelatin to temper it while stirring. Whisk until the gelatin is completely dissolved.

3 Place 4 small ramekins, teacups, or heat-proof clear glasses on a small, rimmed baking tray. Ladle the milk in even quantities into the containers.

4 Allow to cool to room temperature, and then cover the containers and the tray with plastic wrap. Place the entire tray in the fridge and chill for at least 4 hours or up to a few days.

5 Heat the balsamic vinegar in a small saucepan over high heat. Add the strawberries along with remaining honey, vanilla, lemon juice, and salt, stirring, and reduce to low heat. Allow the mixture to simmer until the strawberries break down into a thick compote, stirring occasionally, approximately 10 minutes. Remove from heat and cool or store in the refrigerator until serving.

6 When ready to serve, place the strawberry mixture on top of the panna cotta and top with a slice of a fresh strawberry half.

VARY IT! Swap the strawberries for blueberries, blackberries, or raspberries if you prefer.

NOTE: Refer to the color insert for a photo of this recipe.

PER SERVING: *Calories 85 (From Fat 12); Fat 1g (Saturated 0g); Cholesterol 0mg; Sodium 2mg; Carbohydrate 17g (Dietary Fiber 1g); Protein 2g; Sugars 15g.*

☙ Cantaloupe in Coconut Rose Cream

PREP TIME: 15 MIN	YIELD: 8 SERVINGS

INGREDIENTS

1 small cantaloupe

1 cup (296g) coconut cream

1 teaspoon (1g) ground cardamom

2 teaspoons (10ml) rose water

2 tablespoons (42g) raw honey

¼ cup (23g) dried coconut

¼ cup (31g) plain pistachios, chopped

DIRECTIONS

1 Halve the cantaloupe, remove the seeds, and use a melon baller to form the fruit into balls. Chill if not serving immediately.

2 Combine the coconut cream, cardamom, rose water, honey, and dried coconut in a small bowl. Stir to combine, cover, and chill if not serving immediately.

3 To serve, layer even amounts of coconut and cream in 8 dessert cups. Divide the cantaloupe balls into each dessert cup.

4 Garnish with the pistachios and serve.

NOTE: Coconut is rich in medium-chain triglycerides (MCTs), which can be a quick source of energy. It also provides essential minerals like iron and zinc that support immune function and metabolism.

TIP: This dish tastes best when the melon is in season and is served chilled.

VARY IT! Swap apricot for the cantaloupe and almonds for the pistachios, if desired.

PER SERVING: *Calories 202 (From Fat 78); Fat 9g (Saturated 7g); Cholesterol 0mg; Sodium 31mg; Carbohydrate 31g (Dietary Fiber 1g); Protein 2g; Sugars 29g.*

Puddings and creamy treats

Puddings and creamy treats can be the most satisfying and comforting of desserts. The texture alone evokes happy memories for many. In these recipes, wholesome grains, fresh fruit, and milk combine to make delicious desserts that you can also enjoy for breakfast.

When you think of puddings, you probably tend to think of gelatin-based desserts, but that's only the beginning! Puddings have been made for millennia by thickening fruit juices, simmering whole grains with sweeteners, and in additional ways.

These recipes refer to what chefs often call "spoon desserts," those that are easiest to prepare because they don't need to be baked. Despite their quickness to prepare, they add the same comforting touch to the end of a meal as a slow-cooked dessert would.

The Wheat Berry and Pomegranate Pudding with Pistachios conjures up ancient flavors from the Fertile Crescent. Wheat berry puddings, in various forms, are used to celebrate the birth of a child, the Spring Equinox, Easter, and many other holidays because wheat was traditionally associated with wealth and birth. The Chocolate Chia Pudding is a much more modern invention — and still a tasty and nutrition option.

Wheat Berry Pomegranate Pudding with Pistachios

INGREDIENTS

1¼ cups (225g) wheat berries

3 cups (720ml) 2 percent milk or almond milk

2 tablespoons (42g) agave nectar

½ cup (87g) pomegranate arils

½ cup (62g) plain shelled pistachios, finely chopped

DIRECTIONS

1 Bring a large saucepan ¾ full of water to boil over high heat. Add the wheat berries and cook for 45 minutes, or until tender.

2 Combine the cooked wheat berries with the milk in a medium saucepan and stir. Cover and cook the mixture over low heat for 1 hour, until most of the milk has evaporated and the wheat berries are creamy, stirring every 15 minutes or so. Allow to cool to almost room temperature.

3 Stir in the pomegranate arils, agave nectar, and most of the pistachios. Place the pudding in small dessert bowls and garnish with the remaining pistachios.

NOTE: Wheat berries, which are traditional in Mediterranean breakfasts and desserts, are a whole grain rich in fiber, B vitamins, and minerals like iron and magnesium. The fiber content supports digestive health, while the nutrients contribute to overall energy metabolism and red blood cell formation.

VARY IT! Use rice or barley instead of wheat berries, if desired. Swap pomegranate for your favorite fruit.

PER SERVING: Calories 306 (From Fat 87); Fat 10g (Saturated 3g); Cholesterol 12mg; Sodium 53mg; Carbohydrate 48g (Dietary Fiber 9g); Protein 12g; Sugars 15g.

🍅 Chocolate Chia Pudding

PREP TIME: 5 MIN PLUS 45 MIN TO 1 HR REFRIGERATION TIME	YIELD: 4 SERVINGS

INGREDIENTS

3 cups (720 ml) unsweetened almond milk

1 teaspoon (5ml) pure vanilla

½ cup (48g) unsweetened cocoa

Pinch of salt

1 cup (161g) chia seeds

1 ounce (28g) dark chocolate (80 percent or higher)

DIRECTIONS

1 Whisk the almond milk, vanilla, cocoa, and salt until combined.

2 Place the chia seeds in a large bowl and pour the mixture over it and stir well to combine.

3 Cover the pudding and refrigerate for about 45 minutes to 1 hour, or until it reaches the desired consistency whisking every 10 minutes to prevent clumps from forming. When pudding is thick and chilled, it's ready to serve.

4 Spoon into 4 dessert bowls and grate the dark chocolate over the top to serve.

NOTE: Chia seeds are rich in omega-3 fatty acids, fiber, and antioxidants. The high fiber content supports digestive health, and the omega-3s contribute to heart health and may have anti-inflammatory effects.

TIP: You can also enjoy this pudding at breakfast time.

VARY IT! Use vanilla protein powder to make vanilla chia pudding.

PER SERVING: Calories 285 (From Fat 164); Fat 18g (Saturated 3g); Cholesterol 0mg; Sodium 48mg; Carbohydrate 29g (Dietary Fiber 21g); Protein 10g; Sugars 2g.

Frozen desserts

Most people appreciate sorbet, granita, and ice cream in warmer months. The best thing about serving frozen desserts to guests is that you can make them in advance and have them ready when needed. These desserts have a sweet spot in everyone's heart, whether they have diabetes or not.

One of the challenges for people who are trying to eat healthfully is the desire for a large, sweet dessert. By keeping healthier versions on hand in the freezer, you don't have to deprive yourself of anything, and you're more likely to steer clear of the high-fat and high-sugar desserts that cause a spike in blood sugar.

Granita is an Italian warm weather classic. During the hot months in Italy, Coffee Granita can also be enjoyed with breakfast or as a pick-me-up in the afternoon.

Frozen Peanut Butter Cups are great to have on hand for when you crave something sweet. The Raspberry Sorbet is as beautiful to look at as it is luscious to eat. Whichever frozen dessert you decide to make, it will be worth the effort.

◌ Coffee Granita

INGREDIENTS

1¼ cups (300ml) cold espresso

½ cup (100g) sugar

1¾ cup (415ml) water

½ cup (120ml) heavy cream

1 teaspoon (5ml) vanilla

DIRECTIONS

1 Place the cold espresso in a medium bowl and set aside.

2 In a medium saucepan, combine the sugar and water. Make a syrup by heating the mixture until it starts to boil. Remove from the heat and add the sugar–water mixture to the espresso. Stir and let cool for about 30 min. Pour the mixture into a freezer–proof container. Place flat in the freezer.

3 Remove from the freezer every hour and whisk to break up the larger ice crystals until all the liquid is frozen, about 2 to 3 hours, depending on your freezer temperature. If you continue to stir every hour, until frozen, it shouldn't freeze solid. If you run into that problem, however, you can pulse the coffee ice in the food processor.

4 Make the whipped cream by placing the heavy cream in a blender with the vanilla and whipping until fluffy. Otherwise place in a bowl and whisk by hand until you reach the desired consistency.

5 To serve, scoop the frozen granita into old-fashioned glasses. Store covered in the freezer.

NOTE: Coffee contains antioxidants, such as chlorogenic acid, and caffeine, which may have cognitive and mood-enhancing effects. Moderate coffee consumption has been associated with a reduced risk of certain diseases, including Parkinson's and Alzheimer's.

TIP: This recipe is an Italian summertime classic. When it's too hot to enjoy traditional espresso at breakfast or at the end of the meal, most people opt for granita, often served with a dollop of fresh whipped cream.

VARY IT! Swap the espresso for lemon or strawberry juice to make a fruit-flavored granita.

PER SERVING: *Calories 201 (From Fat 101); Fat 11g (Saturated 7g); Cholesterol 41mg; Sodium 24mg; Carbohydrate 26g (Dietary Fiber 0g); Protein 1g; Sugars 25g.*

Frozen Peanut Butter and Vanilla Cups

PREP TIME: 10 MIN PLUS FREEZING	YIELD: 5 SERVINGS

INGREDIENTS

12 ounces (340g) dark chocolate (80 percent or more), chopped

1 tablespoon (13g) coconut oil

½ cup (112g) Greek yogurt

½ cup (128g) organic creamy peanut butter

1 tablespoon (15ml) pure vanilla extract

¼ cup (85g) raw honey

DIRECTIONS

1 Line a cupcake pan with 10 paper liners.

2 In a medium saucepan, melt the chocolate and coconut oil over low heat, stirring with a wooden spoon.

3 Spoon 1 tablespoon of melted chocolate into each liner and freeze for 10 minutes.

4 Mix the yogurt, peanut butter, vanilla, and honey in a medium bowl.

5 When the chocolate is frozen, spoon the yogurt/peanut butter mixture evenly over the top of each chocolate base. If you have leftover chocolate, you can drizzle that over top. Freeze until firm, about 1 hour. Keep covered in the freezer or refrigerator until serving. Allow to rest at room temperature 5 minutes before serving. Serve 2 cups per person.

NOTE: Peanut butter is a good source of protein, healthy fats, and essential nutrients like vitamin E, magnesium, and potassium. The monounsaturated fats contribute to heart health, and the protein supports muscle development.

TIP: Make this fun and tasty recipe with your kids.

VARY IT! Swap almond butter or pistachio cream for the peanut butter.

PER SERVING: Calories 654 (From Fat 411); Fat 46g (Saturated 22g); Cholesterol 2mg; Sodium 140mg; Carbohydrate 51g (Dietary Fiber 9g); Protein 14g; Sugars 33g.

🍅 Raspberry Sorbet with Blueberries and Blackberries

| PREP TIME: 10 MIN PLUS FREEZING | YIELD: 4 SERVINGS |

INGREDIENTS

12 ounces (340g) fresh raspberries

Juice and zest of 1 lemon

¼ cup (60ml) no-sugar-added white grape juice

1 tablespoon (21g) raw honey

½ cup (74g) blueberries

½ cup (72g) blackberries

DIRECTIONS

1 Wash the raspberries and place them in a blender or food processor. Puree until smooth. Add the lemon juice, grape juice, and honey. Puree for another minute.

2 Pass the mixture through a fine-mesh sieve, stirring and pushing the raspberry pulp into the sieve to separate the seeds. Place the strained mixture in a large plastic container and put in the freezer for 1 hour.

3 Remove the sorbet from the freezer and spoon it back into the blender. Puree to break down the ice crystals that have formed. Freeze for another 2 to 3 hours or until the mixture is frozen.

4 Toss the blueberries and blackberries together in a small bowl. To serve, distribute the sorbet in fruit glasses and top with ¼ cup berries and lemon zest.

NOTE: Raspberries are rich in antioxidants, including quercetin and ellagic acid, which may have anti-inflammatory and anticancer properties. They also provide vitamin C, fiber, and manganese. Blackberries are high in vitamins C and K, fiber, and antioxidants like anthocyanins. They contribute to immune health, support bone health, and may have anti-inflammatory effects.

NOTE: Sorbets are an elegant way to finish a meal, especially in the summer. If you have an ice cream maker and want a smoother consistency, you can use it to make this sorbet.

VARY IT! Use blackberries instead of raspberries. You can also swap out the grape juice for prosecco or champagne.

PER SERVING: *Calories 91 (From Fat 7); Fat 1g (Saturated 0g); Cholesterol 0mg; Sodium 2mg; Carbohydrate 22g (Dietary Fiber 7g); Protein 2g; Sugars 13g.*

🍓 Strawberry Swirl Ice Cream

INGREDIENTS

2 cups (304g) fresh strawberries, cleaned, hulled, and divided in half

2 tablespoons (30ml) water

¼ cup (85g) pure honey, divided

1 cup (226g) Greek yogurt, drained

1¼ cups (300ml) whole milk

2 teaspoons (10ml) vanilla extract

1 pinch salt

DIRECTIONS

1 Puree 1 cup strawberries and 2 tablespoons water in a blender or food processor until smooth. Add 2 tablespoons of the honey. Cover and place in refrigerator.

2 Finely chop the remaining cup of strawberries.

3 In a medium bowl, whisk the yogurt, milk, vanilla, remaining 2 tablespoons of honey, and salt. Stir in the chopped strawberries and refrigerate 1 to 2 hours or overnight.

4 Turn on the ice cream maker, pour the mixture into the frozen freezer bowl, and let the maker run until a soft, creamy consistency is achieved, about 20 minutes.

5 Slowly pour in the strawberry puree from the refrigerator. Turn off as soon as the puree is swirled in but not blended — this takes only a few seconds.

6 Transfer the ice cream to an airtight container and freeze for at least 3 hours, or until it achieves the desired consistency. Serve in dessert bowls.

NOTE: Strawberries are rich in vitamin C, manganese, and antioxidants, such as quercetin and anthocyanins, which contribute to immune health, support skin health, and may have anti-inflammatory effects. The high fiber content also promotes digestive health.

NOTE: Check out a photo of this recipe in the color insert.

TIP: Keep this recipe on hand when you need delicious treats within reach.

VAR IT! Swap strawberries for blueberries.

PER SERVING: *Calories 95 (From Fat 26); Fat 3g (Saturated 2g); Cholesterol 5mg; Sodium 49mg; Carbohydrate 15g (Dietary Fiber 1g); Protein 4g; Sugars 11g.*

Cookies and biscotti

The Italian word "biscotti" is also the Italian word for "cookies," but English uses biscotti exclusively for twice-baked cookies. Here we offer authentic recipes for both types.

Even though the Italian tradition has several desserts and cookie recipes that aren't too sweet, people with sweet tooths can still be satisfied. These recipes are my (Amy) family recipes. The Pine Nut Cookies were traditionally served at weddings and during the holidays. Luckily, they're easy to make, and you can store them in the freezer in an airtight container for months.

The Calabrian Orange and Almond Biscotti is a delicious and nutritious recipe to have on hand. In Italy, people eat these cookies with caffe latte or cappuccino at breakfast as well as serve them after a meal or in the mid afternoon with espresso. Baking these cookies is as rewarding as eating them. In no time, your kitchen will be wafting in the warm Mediterranean aromas. They also make wonderful edible gifts.

🍑 Italian Pine Nut Cookies

PREP TIME: 15 MIN	COOK TIME: 12 TO 14 MIN	YIELD: 18 SERVINGS

INGREDIENTS

1 cup (200g) sugar

1 cup (339g) raw honey

¼ teaspoon (1.2g) salt

3 eggs

2¼ cups (281g) unbleached, all-purpose flour

½ teaspoon (2.3g) baking powder

2 teaspoons (10ml) almond extract

6 tablespoons (50g) pine nuts

DIRECTIONS

1 Preheat the oven to 375 degrees F.

2 Place the sugar, honey, salt, and eggs in a large bowl. Beat the mixture with a whisk, about 2 to 3 minutes, or use an electric mixer until the eggs are foamy.

3 With a wooden spoon, fold in the flour, baking powder, and almond extract. The batter should be the consistency of chocolate chip cookie dough. If it's too thin, add a bit more flour, 1 tablespoon at a time, until it reaches the right consistency.

4 Line 2 baking sheets with parchment paper. Drop rounded teaspoons full of dough about 2 inches apart on the baking sheets. Sprinkle each cookie with 6 to 8 pine nuts and bake for 10 minutes or until light golden in color. Remove the cookies from the oven and cool to serve.

NOTE: Pine nuts are a good source of monounsaturated fats, protein, and essential minerals like magnesium and zinc. The fats contribute to heart health, while magnesium supports bone health and zinc plays a role in immune function.

NOTE: This classic Italian cookie is traditionally served at holidays and weddings.

TIP: You can make these cookies in advance and store in airtight containers (with wax paper in between layers) in the freezer for a few months. Remove and thaw for a few hours before serving.

VARY IT! Swap the all-purpose flour for almond flour to make a gluten-free version.

PER SERVING (2 COOKIES): *Calories 188 (From Fat 26); Fat 3g (Saturated 0g); Cholesterol 35mg; Sodium 52mg; Carbohydrate 39g (Dietary Fiber 1g); Protein 3g; Sugars 27g.*

🍅 Almond and Orange Biscotti

PREP TIME: 15 MIN	COOK TIME: 30 TO 45 MIN PLUS COOLING TIME	YIELD: 14 SERVINGS

INGREDIENTS

3¼ cups (364g) almond flour

½ cup (100g) sugar

2 teaspoons (9g) baking powder

¼ teaspoon (1.2g) salt

4 eggs

2 tablespoons (42g) pure honey

2 tablespoons (30ml) orange juice

2 tablespoons (12g) orange zest

1 teaspoon (5ml) vanilla extract

1 teaspoon (5ml) almond extract

½ cup (72g) whole almonds, toasted, and sliced in half

DIRECTIONS

1 Preheat the oven to 375 degrees F. Line a baking sheet with parchment paper or silicon mats.

2 Stir the flour, sugar, baking powder, and salt in a large bowl with a wooden spoon to combine.

3 In another large bowl, mix and combine the eggs, honey, orange juice, orange zest, and vanilla and almond extracts.

4 Pour the egg mixture into the flour mixture. When done mixing, stir in the opposite direction to make sure that all ingredients have been incorporated.

5 Stir in the almonds. Drop the dough onto the baking sheet to form 2 (14 x 4-inch) logs that are spaced 2 to 3 inches apart.

6 Wet your fingertips and smooth out the logs into even shapes. Bake for 20 minutes, until the logs are golden. Remove from the oven and allow to cool 10 minutes.

7 Reduce the temperature to 325 degrees. Carefully transfer the logs to your work surface, and using a serrated knife, cut them into ½-inch thick slices. Reline the baking sheet and arrange slices on the sheet. Bake again for 10 minutes, or until golden. Cool completely and store in an airtight container. Serve with espresso or coffee for dunking.

NOTE: Almonds are packed with healthy monounsaturated fats, vitamin E, and magnesium, which support heart health, skin health, and muscle function. Almonds also provide a good source of protein, fiber, and antioxidants, which contribute to overall well-being.

TIP: You can enjoy this classic recipe from Calabria, Italy at breakfast. Be sure to serve it with espresso, cappuccino, or caffe latte for dunking.

NOTE: Refer to the color insert for a photo of this recipe.

PER SERVING: *Calories 238 (From Fat 153); Fat 17g (Saturated 0g); Cholesterol 60mg; Sodium 124mg; Carbohydrate 17g (Dietary Fiber 4g); Protein 8g; Sugars 11g.*

3
Eating Healthfully Away from Home

Chapter **13**

Overcoming Barriers to Healthy Eating

Whether they're physical or perceived, obstacles to healthy eating are the main reason why people don't stick to new lifestyle plans. Fortunately, many of the obstacles are misconceptions that can be easily overcome with a few strategies. In this chapter we give you the tools that you need to succeed in eating healthful food, including when you're traveling.

Noting Potential Obstacles

Eating well has challenges. One of the best ways to see where you are when you face these challenges is to keep a journal of what you eat for a few weeks. Include everything that you eat, what your schedule looks like, and any emotional or psychological factors you're dealing with. After you're done tracking your results, take note of any trends that you can spot.

Here are a few common obstacles you may relate with along with ways to overcome them:

>> **You feel that certain emotions lead you to make unhealthful food choices.** If emotional triggers cause you to eat more sugar, fat, or salt than you should — or you just make poor food choices in general — you aren't alone. Most people experience this situation. The first step to overcoming this barrier is awareness. If you know that you eat ice cream in copious amounts when you're sad, for example, or consume more salt when you're stressed, you can use your cravings as an indicator to check in with your emotions before eating those particular foods.

Work to identify the trend and then replace the food with a healthier version, such as some of the recipes in Part 2, or use other methods such as practicing yoga, mindfulness, and meditation, exercising, and getting fresh air to help you feel better. If you can, you'll be well along on the road to success. If you can't do this on your own, however, seek a certified health coach, spiritual guide, or another type of mental therapist who can help you deal with the unwanted emotions and give you tools to avoid falling into this trap when eating.

>> **You're too busy to eat foods that are good for you.** In the modern societies around the globe, the fast-food industry is often to blame for unhealthful eating. If that's your reason, then make an extra commitment to wanting to feel your best in order to be motivated and inspired to plan accordingly.

The following can help you overcome this barrier:

- Batch cooking once a week, simpler, healthful foods, and maybe even enlist the help of friends and family.

- Identify which activities in your life are less important than your health and spend less time doing them so that you have more time to prepare healthy meals for yourself.

>> **You think traveling prevents you from eating well.** If you're always on the road, consistently eating healthfully is difficult. The good news: These days many places offer few healthful options, but you may not like what they have. Refer to the next section for more helpful information when you're away from home.

>> **You dine with certain people who only eat junk food or unhealthy food.** If your friends and family members make poor food choices, more than likely you'll do the same. To avoid falling into this pitfall is to come to the table prepared. Decide in advance which of the foods that they're preparing or serving are good for you. If there aren't any, bring your own food to the gathering or ask them to include one of the recipes from Part 2 as one of their

offerings. Explain how important this is to your health, and you may find that others are dealing with similar diagnosis and appreciate your attention to detail.

TIP

» **You believe that eating healthfully is difficult.** If you were raised on a diet that wasn't good for you, you may have a negative attitude around food. Even though that's completely normal, it won't help you live your best life. Prior to the invention of fast and processed foods people around the globe ate healthfully without a fancy degree.

If this is your obstacle, you first have to believe that eating healthfully can be easy, take away some tips from this Part 1 of book, and commit to putting them into practice.

» **You believe that eating healthfully is too expensive.** This myth is difficult to debunk, especially in the United States. Medical and nutrition professionals hear this obstacle from many people and in the media. That's because ultraprocessed food is usually cheap and readily available. The truth is, however, if you're eating unhealthful food, you're not filling up on it, it doesn't provide the nutrients to get you through your day, and it will harm your health.

A little bit of nutritious, fiber-filled food, such as legumes, green leafy vegetables, and grains, go a long way. You can fill up faster with less of them, stay full longer, and heal your body instead of harming it. The recipes in Part 2 can put this strategy to good use.

» **You lack cooking skills.** You don't know how to prepare healthful food, you don't like not being able to cook, or you don't want to cook for others. Luckily, today you can find healthful recipes in many places. This book is a great place to begin.

We always encourage people to try cooking a little bit at a time when they aren't pressured to prepare a meal for others. Allow yourself to get lost in the sensory aspect of it. You may be surprised at how therapeutic cooking is as well as the money you can save preparing delicious and nutritious meals for yourself at a fraction of the cost compared to eating out at restaurants.

» **You believe that good-for-you food tastes bad.** When grown and prepared properly, healthful foods can and should taste great. The recipes in Part 2 serve that purpose. You can find many online sources that also offer additional resources.

» **You live in an area that's considered a food desert.** A *food desert* refers to areas that don't have access to fresh fruits, produce, and healthful ingredients. Overcoming this obstacle is extremely difficult because food deserts exist often because of political and societal factors out of your control. Food deserts usually are in undeveloped and low-income areas, and residents often suffer from discrepancies in healthcare as well.

That said, some public policy interventions focus on making healthful food accessible to people in food deserts. Consult with your local social service departments in your area if you live in a food desert and have difficulty shopping at stores that sell healthful foods. Furthermore, some nonprofit organizations provide healthful foods to people who live in these areas. Building a pantry of shelf-stable whole grains, legumes, and healthful oils is especially important if you live in a food desert. You can supplement fresh foods and frozen vegetables and fish when available to avoid frequent trips to a faraway farmers' market or supermarket.

>> **You don't know how to pair foods together to create a complete, nutritious meal.** Another obstacle is lack of knowledge of nutrition, which many people share. Chapter 3 provides the basics that you need to make healthful choices.

Planning for When You Can't Eat at Home

Preparedness is key when eating out. Whether you're eating at a fast-casual restaurant, a food truck, a friend's home, or a fine dining restaurant, here are a few tips that can help you make the most out of your experience from a nutritional standpoint:

>> **Know your weaknesses.** If you love to eat fatty or sugary foods at restaurants or tend to overeat in restaurants, make a plan. Identify eating establishments that serve food you enjoy, is good for you, and start frequenting them more often. If portions are large, ask the server to serve half the portion and place the other half wrapped to go before they bring your food to the table.

>> **Identify places that offer diabetes-friendly foods.** Any type of restaurant that offers lots of fresh vegetables and lean proteins is a good place to start. See the next section for more tips.

>> **Always carry water and snacks.** Having unsalted nuts, a piece of fresh fruit, fresh vegetables with hummus, or plain Greek yogurt and water on hand can help you avoid the blood sugar imbalances that increase hunger before eating out. Oftentimes arriving at a restaurant hungry can lead to bad food choices.

>> **If going to someone's home, bring a dish to share that you can enjoy if everything else is unhealthful.** Doing so may seem awkward at first, but many hosts find it helpful if you bring something that is a part of your meal plan. Bringing enough for everyone to taste may help them also eat healthier. Always let your host know ahead of time so that they can plan accordingly and so you can avoid the need to explain yourself during the meal.

Preparing When Eating Out

No matter where you dine, some menu items lend themselves to being more nutritious. You can enjoy old favorites once in a while, but making good choices on a daily basis will have you looking and feeling your best. Always remember to include the three macronutrients in your meals no matter where you're eating. Focus on these foods:

>> A portion of lean protein (fish, chicken, meat, beans, and lentils)

>> Complex carbohydrates (quinoa, brown rice, millet, barley, whole wheat, amaranth, potatoes, and sweet potatoes)

>> Healthful fats (avocado, EVOO, and plain Greek yogurt)

The following sections delve deeper into eating out and provide numerous tips to help you choose the eating establishment and also you order diabetes-friendly foods.

Selecting restaurants that offer diabetes-friendly food

Before you eat out, making sure you take the time to plan ahead and locate a restaurant that serves diabetes-friendly foods is imperative so you can partake in the food with your dining friends or family. If you don't make plans, you may end up going hungry or eating unhealthy food that can have serious implications with your health.

These tips can lead you to making wise choices:

>> **Seek restaurants that offer a good selection of fresh vegetables and good-quality ingredients.**

>> **Choose restaurants that provide simple, nutritious, preparations of lean protein, namely fish and chicken.**

>> **Try restaurants from different cultures that are known for wholesome food and fresh preparations.** Examples include Ethiopian, Indian, Mediterranean, and so on. These diets flavor foods with lots of herbs and spices in order to create the most tasty and delicious recipes that enhance the health.

No particular kind of food is better or worse than any other, with the exception of fast food (we discuss this issue in Chapter 14). You may think that vegetarian food is better than animal sources, but a dish of pasta in a creamy sauce is no better than a piece of fatty steak. Often, restaurants have several menu items that fit into your nutrition plan.

>> **Consider choosing a restaurant that you can walk to and from.** The exercise you get will offset the extra calories you may consume.

>> **Check out the restaurant's menu online.** Before deciding to visit a particular restaurant, go to the establishment's website and make sure that it serves food you can eat.

>> **Call ahead and find out whether you can substitute items on the menu.** Nonfranchise and non-fast-food restaurants are much more likely to let you substitute menu items. Fast-food restaurants are able to serve large numbers of people at lower prices by making the food entirely uniform. On the other hand, as Chapter 14 explains, this uniformity makes it easier to know the exact ingredients and methods of preparation.

You need to ask only a few questions to know whether a restaurant will be accommodating. For example, ask whether the staff will do the following:

- Offer EVOO and lemon juice or vinegar instead of heavy salad dressings.

- Reduce the amount of butter and sugar in a dish.

- Serve gravies, salad dressings, and sauces on the side.

- Bake, broil, and poach instead of frying or sautéing.

>> **Choose a restaurant with history.** An older restaurant often has the advantage of having experienced and well-trained waitstaff who know what the kitchen staff is willing to do for you, based on what has been done before.

>> **Find out whether the restaurant already has special meals or entrees for people with chronic diseases such as heart or celiac disease.** They're much more likely to be health conscious in their cooking.

>> **Consider what you've already eaten that day.** For example, if you've already eaten your daily limit of carbohydrate, then the choice of a restaurant where pasta or rice is the major ingredient may not be a good one. People often choose a restaurant days in advance, so if you know ahead where you'll be dining, you can plan to modify your eating accordingly earlier in the day, especially if the restaurant specializes in foods you should eat in small quantities.

>> **Drink water or have a vegetable snack before you go to the restaurant.** Doing so prevents you making poor choices because you're hungry.

>> **Skip restaurants known for large portions.** If you know that the restaurant serves huge portions of everything, don't go there unless you plan to share your meal or take part of your meal home.

Ordering when you eat out

Your strategy for ordering from the menu should include the following:

>> **Plan to leave some food or take home half your order because the portions are usually too large.** You can also order a dish to share with another person.

>> **If you decide to have wine, order it by the glass.** Diners almost always finish a bottle of wine, and unless eight of you share the bottle, you'll drink too much.

>> **Consider using an appetizer as your entree.** In many restaurants, the entree portions are large enough to feed at least two people, so unless you're planning on taking half of it home, an ample appetizer may be a more appropriately sized main course. Enjoy it with a garden salad dressed with EVOO and lemon juice or vinegar.

>> **Get as much information about the dish as you can from the server.** Feel free to get a complete description, including portion size, of an appetizer or entree from the server so that you aren't surprised when the food arrives. Pay particular attention to how the food is cooked — in fat or butter, for example. Avoid those dishes and opt for dishes that are prepared more simply with EVOO, herbs, and lemon. Grilled items are also a great choice.

>> **Consider a meal of soup and salad.** This combination can be delicious and filling and is low in calories and carbohydrates.

>> **Order clear soups rather than cream soups.** Minestrone, bean soups, chicken soup, or vegetables soups that are served in clear or tomato broth are better choices for someone with diabetes compared to chowders or cream of broccoli, cheese, and mushroom soups that usually contain butter, flour, and sometimes cream.

>> **Ask for salad dressings and sauces on the side if possible.** This way, you're in control of the amount you consume.

>> **Stick to the seas.** You're probably wise to choose fish more often than meat, both to avoid fat and to take advantage of the cholesterol-lowering properties of fish. Remember, however, that fried fish can be as fat-laden as steak.

>> **Let your server know that you need to eat soon.** If your food will be delayed because the kitchen is slow or busy, ask that vegetable snacks be brought to the table.

DOCTOR SAYS

Deciphering menus can be difficult. The medical community used to assume that cooking in any fat at all was harmful, but now we know that it isn't so. Cooking in fat is good for you if it's with EVOO. If you're eating out, find out whether or not the restaurant uses EVOO before ordering. In addition, retaining the healthful fats of fish is good for you. We don't advocate lowfat cooking in general or the need to lose good fats — so-called good fats are the monounsaturated and polyunsaturated fats found in natural foods. Even though they need to be eaten in moderation, they are part of a healthful diet. Avoid the industrial-made trans fats.

Traveling and Eating Well

Whether you're preparing or purchasing foods to go, having a few flavor profiles and recipes in the back of your mind or on a list can help you stay on track when you're traveling. Chapter 8 focuses on putting together small plates on the go. These sections identify some example meal plans when you're traveling and other traveling and cost-savings tips.

Creating sample to-go meal plans

If time and availability permits, make these items at home prior to traveling. If not, you can purchase similar items from many supermarkets and food at to-go restaurants at airports and in major urban areas.

In addition to the recipes in Part 2 of this book, here are some safe options to enjoy while traveling:

Breakfast ideas

Fresh fruit salad with granola and seeds

Black coffee, espresso, herbal, black or green tea

Glass of water

Plain Greek yogurt and fresh fruit smoothie

Black coffee, espresso, herbal or black tea

Glass of water

Warm quinoa or oatmeal with almond milk, berries, and sesame seeds

Black coffee, espresso, herbal or black tea

Glass of water

Blueberry almond yogurt bowl with honey, cinnamon, and chia seeds

Black coffee, espresso, herbal or black tea

Glass of water

Lunch ideas

Homemade hummus and whole-wheat pita with fresh vegetables

Salad with green leafy vegetables, EVOO, lemon juice, or vinegar

Glass of water

Baba Ghanouj with Crudites with Spiced Edamame and Chickpeas

Glass of water

Cream of Broccoli and Celery Soup

1 hardboiled egg

Glass of water

Snack ideas

Handful of almonds

Glass of water

1 serving of 85 percent dark chocolate

5 walnuts

Glass of water

1 serving unsweetened Greek yogurt with a handful of blueberries

Glass of water

1 serving hummus, baba ghanouj, or tzatziki with crudites

Dinner ideas

Citrus marinated salmon, or other fish, with sautéed greens, a sweet potato, and salad

Glass of water

Asparagus, or broccoli and other assorted vegetables and tofu or tempeh stir-fry with soba noodles or brown rice

Glass of water

Grilled, marinated chicken with brown rice and green vegetables

Glass of water

Vegetable-based soup or stew

Mixed green salad tossed with extra-virgin olive oil and lemon juice or vinegar

Glass of water

Nighttime snack ideas

½ cup unsweetened Greek yogurt with ¼ cup fresh berries or vegetable crudites

Glass of water

1 pear or apple

5 almonds

Glass of water

¼ cup hummus or other bean puree with celery and carrot sticks

Glass of water

Knowing what you can do when traveling

Consider these tips when traveling:

>> Outline your travel routes ahead of time and choose restaurants where you can comfortably eat at.

>> Bring as much of your own food as possible.

>> When possible, opt for healthier to-go options at health food stores and supermarkets instead of fast-food options.

>> Decide in advance which items you'll eat at restaurants along the way.

Storing food on the go and saving money and time

In order to enjoy food on the go that you prepare, we suggest having these few items to keep food fresh:

>> A thermos

>> An insulated lunch bag and larger food bag

>> A cooler when appropriate

>> Ice packs

>> Disposable silverware

>> Food storage containers with tight-fitting lids

With these items on hand, you can prep ahead of time for trips or a long day away from home.

Chapter **14**

Making Eating Out a Nourishing Experience

Anourishing meal experience begins long before you ever arrive at a restaurant or decide what to eat. In addition to physical sustenance, nourishing the mind, emotions, and spirit helps you to get the most out of your meals and your life. Without a conscious effort to keep your mental, emotional, and spiritual health fulfilled, you may turn to food in order to fill in the gaps.

Reading a good book, listening to music that you love, staying mindful, and practicing gratitude are all ways to nourish your spirits. Adopting the attitude that good food is your friend is important — a true ally in your health journey that can help transform the way that you feel. When choosing a restaurant, you can make a conscious decision to select those that offer the best foods for you. This chapter discusses how to prepare for a restaurant visit, how to check the menu in different kinds of restaurants, and how to consider dessert.

Preparing for Restaurant Dining

The concept of eating out means different things in different places in the world and is always evolving. Whether you're eating at open air markets, in a casual establishment, or at a fine dining restaurant, the same rules for choosing healthful meals still apply.

Because a lot of people eat many of their meals in restaurants these days, integrating restaurant eating into a nutritional plan is essential for a person with diabetes. The restaurant business is booming, and creative chefs have the same celebrity status as famous sports stars. And they deserve it. They use fresh ingredients to produce some of the most delicious and unique tastes imaginable. Unfortunately, nutrition isn't always uppermost in their minds. People's experience with the food and restaurant industry proves that interest in good nutrition is increasing, but you're still on your own most of the time when selecting healthy foods. The reason for this isn't because restaurants don't want to offer healthy foods, but because consumer demand is often for less nutritious items. In addition, in order to cut food costs and remain profitable, many restaurants need to use fillers and rely on salt and sugar to flavor their foods. This chapter helps you ensure that your restaurant eating fits well into your nutritional plan as well as what to eat when you're there.

REMEMBER

You're ultimately responsible to ensure that you know what's in the food you order and make healthy choices. Restaurant chefs may be health conscious and try to keep the fat and the sugar low. But they have to respond to what they perceive to be their customers' needs. They think that one of the main needs is for a lot of food, so your portions will almost always be larger than necessary.

TIP

You have to evaluate the food you order by questioning your server. Even if the balance of macronutrients is right, you'll probably receive too much food and should take some home or leave some on your plate. When dining in restaurants that typically serve large portions, we recommend asking for half of the food to be wrapped to be taken home before being served to you at the dinner table — doing so makes it easier to not overeat.

Even though bringing restaurant food home in the United States is common practice, that's not the case in many places in the world. If you live in an area where it's culturally frowned upon to take food home from a restaurant, try ordering less to begin with and ask for an extra plate when the food is served. Serve yourself the proper amount of food on the empty plate and leave the excess or share it with another person in your dining party.

TIP

You may often find yourself having to choose a restaurant where you don't know the ingredients in the food or whether the menu items are healthy or not. Here are a few suggestions about choosing a restaurant in this situation:

>> No particular kind of food is better or worse than any other, with the exception of fast food. In fact, we promote heritage diets from various places around the globe. Whether you're interested in the eating patterns inspired by the rich culinary histories of the Mediterranean, Africa, or Asia, you're in luck (refer to Chapter 2). These traditional diets are inspired by many plant-based foods, tasty recipes, and a foundation of ingredients such as fruits, vegetables, whole grains, beans and legumes, nuts and seeds, and herbs and spices. Meat, seafood, and dairy are consumed less frequently but still an important part of the diets. Therefore, you can enjoy all cuisines on a diabetes-friendly diet. The trick, however, is finding the rich traditions in restaurants.

>> Much of what is touted as Italian, Indian, Chinese, or Mexican isn't authentic. In order to amplify flavor and please local palates, restaurateurs have to often add more sugar, sodium, and sauces to their classic recipes. With that in mind, you can search out more authentic restaurants and/or traditional recipes even in those whose menus have been tweaked to please other palates. Refer to the section "Planning at Each Meal and in Specific Kinds of Restaurants" later in this chapter for more information.

Starting the Meal

As you sit down to enjoy your meal, you can take many steps to make the experience of eating out the pleasure that it ought to be. A few simple considerations at this point allow you to enjoy the meal free of the concern that you are wrecking your nutritional program.

TIP

Among the steps that you can take are the following:

>> If you arrive early, avoid sitting in the bar with cocktails (which are all sugar and carbohydrate) before you move to your table to eat your meal.

>> Ask the host to seat you promptly so you don't have to wait and get too hungry or even hypoglycemic.

>> Ask your server not to bring bread or to take it off the table if it's there already. That goes for chips and crackers as well.

>> Ask for raw vegetables, what the restaurant menus call *crudites,* with dips such as tzatziki, extra-virgin olive oil (EVOO), hummus, or baba ghanouj, so you can munch on something before you order.

>> Check your blood glucose before you order so you'll know how much carbohydrate is appropriate at that time.

>> Wait to administer your short-acting insulin until you can be sure of the food delivery time. Alternatively if you have an automated system of administration of insulin, seeing how meals affect your blood sugar and the insulin dosing can be helpful.

Checking Out the Menu

Menus are often designed in a way to make diners order more and draw attention to the most profitable items on the menu. The regular menu and the specials of the day or season are arranged to encourage you to order a big meal. One of the more interesting things that we learned is how much food they had to put on each plate to satisfy U.S. tastes. When you order meat, fish, or poultry, you often get at least twice as much as the recommended serving.

Considering how frequently people eat out in the United States, it's no wonder the population is becoming increasingly obese and that diet is the No. 1 killer in the United States. The concept of getting more for your money when dining out should refer to more nutrients, not bigger portions.

Your strategy for ordering from the menu should include the following:

>> Peruse the menu online or call the restaurant before entering so that you know which safe items you can order and enjoy.

>> Immediately identify those items on the menu and close it — the longer you look at the menu, the more you'll be tempted to eat what you shouldn't.

>> Include a green salad with EEVO and vinegar or a side order of greens whenever possible.

>> Skip the fat-laden salad dressings.

   Not just the fat in these kinds of dressings matter and can be a problem. The likely ingredients including additives and preservatives of processed dressings are also important. In many cases restaurants buy them in bulk from an outside producer, and they aren't prepared from scratch.

REMEMBER

When you're eating at a restaurant, the best combination is as follows (flavor these three items with fresh herbs and spice for taste):

>> Lean protein (fish, chicken, meat, beans, and lentils)

>> Complex carbohydrates (quinoa, brown rice, millet, barley, whole wheat, amaranth, potatoes, and sweet potatoes)

>> Healthful fats (avocado, EVOO, and plain Greek yogurt)

Planning at Each Meal and in Specific Kinds of Restaurants

You can make good choices at every meal, whether it's breakfast, lunch, or dinner. Every kind of food offers you the opportunity to select a lowfat, low-salt alternative. You just need to think about it and be aware of the possibilities. Helping you choose healthy meals is the purpose of this section.

Breakfast

The good choices at breakfast are fresh foods, which usually contain plenty of fiber. Here are some ways to start your day:

>> Fresh fruit such as apples, oranges, or berries is a good way to begin the meal, followed by hot cereals such as oatmeal or quinoa with protein such as unsalted almonds and seeds.

>> Another good option is plain Greek yogurt with a piece of fresh fruit and a drizzle of honey.

>> Green, herbal, and black tea or black coffee and water are your best drink choices at breakfast.

Less desirable choices are foods such as quiche, bacon, fried or hash brown potatoes, croissants, pastries, and doughnuts. And be careful of the high-calorie coffees.

Appetizers, salads, and soups

Raw and fresh foods sautéed in EVOO and flavored with herbs and spices beat those cooked and covered with butter or sour cream, and that rule applies to appetizers, salads, and soups, too.

Here are some of our suggestions:

REMEMBER

>> Raw carrots and celery can be enjoyed at any time and to almost any extent.

>> Clear soups are always healthier.

>> Salsa has become a popular accompaniment for crackers and chips instead of a high-fat dip.

>> A delicious green salad is nutritious and filling.

>> Plain almonds eaten prior to a meal can help you digest your food better, and they're a great source of nutrients.

>> Even though they contain fat, avocados are a zero-cholesterol food and can be considered the healthful fat portion of the three macronutrients (protein, carbohydrate, and fat) in a balanced meal.

Steer clear of salty nuts, chips, and cheese before dinner because they add lots of calories, sodium, and fat. Fried appetizers are currently very popular, and they're often dripping with fat. Watch out for the sour cream dips and the mayonnaise dips because they, too, are full of fat, additives, and preservatives.

Vegetarian food

With obesity on the rise, there has been a trend to go to vegetarian restaurants. What is called *vegetarian* varies from no animal products at all, which is referred to as *vegan*, to eating eggs and/or dairy. Vegan diets can provide all the nutritional needs of a patient but must be carefully planned to do so. However, some people on a vegan diet may not get enough of certain nutrients and may need to take supplements of calcium, iodine, vitamin B12, and vitamin D.

Lacto vegetarians eat dairy but not eggs while *lacto-ovo vegetarians* eat eggs and milk. *Semi-vegetarians* eat some fish and poultry as well.

Wherever you fit in the continuum of vegetarians, you should know that your choice is a good one. In general, vegetarians are lighter in weight than nonvegetarians. If you have diabetes, being a vegetarian means your diabetes is easier to control, and if you're at risk for diabetes, you're less likely to get it if you eat veg-etarian. Vegetarian eating is also associated with fewer incidents of cancer, strokes, and heart attacks.

REMEMBER

You still have to make good choices in the vegetarian restaurant. A true vegetarian diet is heavy on fresh vegetables, beans, legumes, and quality complex carbohy-drates. If you call yourself a vegetarian but are mainly consuming simple carbs and little vegetables and legumes, your meal plan isn't diabetes-friendly or balanced.

Keep these tips in mind:

>> Stay away from the creamy, buttery foods and enjoy the lighter dishes made with grains like quinoa.

>> Use beans, seeds, and lentils to get your protein without the accompanying fat of meat.

WARNING

Vegetarian or vegan dishes sometimes pretend to be something they aren't, such as meat or fish, and may be highly processed with numerous added artificial fla-vorings and stabilizers. For example, a soy product that looks and tastes like king prawns is likely to have reached that state with a great deal of processing.

Seafood

Most fish are relatively low in fat, other than healthy omega-3 fats, and can be a great choice. But even the best fish can compromise your nutrition plan when they're fried in poor quality vegetable oils. Fish that stand out are cod, bass, hal-ibut, swordfish, fresh tuna or canned tuna, or sardines in water or EVOO. Most of the shellfish varieties are also lowfat.

Chinese food

You can eat some great Chinese food and not have to worry about upsetting your diet plan. Any of the soups on the menu will be delicious and fill you up. Stick to vegetable dishes with small amounts of meat in them. Avoid fried dishes, whether they're meats, tofu, or rice and noodles because they're likely to be fried in low quality oils. Steamed dishes and brown rice on the side are a much better choice.

Potstickers, an appetizer often found on the menu, and sweet-and-sour pork will really throw off your calorie count and your fat intake. Stay away from the almond cookies that often follow Chinese meals.

French food

While the old style of preparing French food promotes a lot of cream and rich sauces, a new style, called *nouvelle cuisine*, emphasizes the freshest ingredients, usually cooked in their own sauce. This style has revolutionized French restaurants. Still, some French chefs cling to the old ways, and their food isn't for you, unless you're prepared to share your meal or ask for the sauces on the side.

Most desserts in French restaurants are high in carbohydrates. Limit yourself to a taste or, better yet, don't tempt yourself by ordering the cake or custard in the first place. See if the pastry chef has a fruit dish, like a poached pear, that's both delicious and good for you.

Indian food

Rice and pita bread are good carbohydrate choices when paired with lean protein and healthful fats, but avoid foods made with coconut milk because of its fat content. Meat, fish, and poultry cooked in the tandoori manner (baked in an oven) are good options. Be sure to keep the fried foods to a minimum because they're likely prepared in poor quality oils.

Curries are fine as long as they're not made with coconut milk. Avoid ghee, which is aged clarified butter. Fried appetizers like samosas and creamy dishes don't help your blood glucose. Chicken tikka and chapatti are fine — they're made with delicious spices (for taste) but little unhealthy fat. Indian restaurants also serve lentils and greens, which are great options.

Italian food

As with all other international cuisines, not all is authentic. Due to the fact that Italian cuisine is currently ranked No. 1 in the world, a lot of restaurateurs call their restaurant chains Italian when they truly don't deserve that title.

Consider these suggestions:

>> For first courses, stick to small quantities of whole-grain or homemade pasta with fresh tomato-based sauces and avoid the creamy, buttery, cheesy sauces. Minestrone or other vegetable-based soups are hearty and low in fat.

>> For your second course, or as a main if you skip the first course, choose a chicken or fish dish with vegetable sides and a green salad.

> » Always ask for a good quality EVOO. If the restaurant staff is delighted that you've made this request and they proudly present an oil from their home region, you'll know that they care about your health as well as the quality of their food.

Mexican food

Mexican food has become increasingly popular globally, but most Mexican restaurants are actually Tex-Mex and not authentically Mexican. They may offer you many temptations to slip from your healthy eating plan. They often start with chips, nachos, and cheese. Tell your server to keep them off the table. Have salsa or guacamole as an appetizer. You can call ahead to see if they can give you fresh vegetables to dip into them instead of chips.

In addition, remember the following:

> » Chicken with rice, grilled fish, and grilled chicken are excellent choices, as are the chicken and seafood soups and various salad options.

> » Tortillas, burritos, and tostadas are delicious and can be good for you — just choose bean (not fried) and chicken varieties with vegetables as long as you avoid the addition of a lot of cheese and sour cream.

WARNING

Stay away from anything refried; it means just what the word says. Avoid all dishes laden with cheese, as well as dishes heavy in sausage. And keep in mind the importance of moderation. Mexican restaurants are known for large servings, so take some home.

Thai food

The creative use of spices, emphasis on fish, and use of fresh vegetables make this cuisine a good choice for you. Steer clear of the sauces sweetened with Thai palm sugar and large quantities of noodles in Pad Thai and other dishes.

Korean food

Korean cuisine is known for its healthy balance of flavors and ingredients as well as fermented foods. Kimchi, tofu stews, as well as the many vegetable, rice, and egg dishes are good choices.

Japanese food

Lots of fresh fish, vegetables, and whole grains make Japanese food a favorite for many. Stick with sushi, sashimi, miso soup, and skip the fried tempura.

North African food

Authentic North African cuisine is a rich mosaic of flavors, colors, and textures. Increasingly available around the globe, North African foods include healthful lentil and vegetables soups and a wide variety of cooked and raw vegetable salads to start the meal. Grilled and stewed fish and chicken with additional vegetables and a small amount of rice round out the meal. Stay away from fried dishes.

Greek and Levantine food

The cuisine of the Eastern Mediterranean is full of healthful vegetable and bean-based appetizers, wholesome bread, Greek yogurt, vegetable stews, and fresh fish dishes to choose from. Save the hearty dishes for a holiday.

Taking Pleasure in Your Food

If you've been conscientious in planning a delicious restaurant meal ahead of time, you deserve to enjoy the food. But you need to continue thinking about healthy eating (and drinking) habits even as you sit down to the meal. All the great planning can come undone if you're careless at this point. Think about the following advice as you eat:

>> If you have a glass of wine, make sure it's a small one. Restaurants commonly offer a glass that's a third of a standard bottle of wine.

>> Try using some behavior modification to prolong the meal and give your brain a chance to know that you've eaten: Eat slowly, chew each bite thoroughly, and put your fork down between each bite.

>> Remember that the meal is a social occasion. Spend more time talking to your companions and less time concentrating on the food.

>> Remove the skin if you're eating poultry and allow the sauce to drip off the morsel of food on your fork if you're eating a dish cooked in a sauce.

>> After you've carefully controlled the intake of food on your plate, don't add significant calories by tasting or finishing the food on your companion's plate.

Concluding with Dessert

For many people, the early parts of a meal are just a prelude to their favorite part, which is dessert. Most people have a sweet tooth, and dessert is often the way that they satisfy that need. The Italians don't call the part of the menu that features the desserts the *dolci* (which means "sweets") without reason. Dessert, in many restaurants, has become a showpiece. The pastry chef tries to show how sweet they can make the dessert while creating a culinary work of art. The term *decadent* is often used in describing the richness of these desserts.

Does this mean that you can't have any dessert at all? No. Making a wise choice simply requires a certain amount of awareness on your part. You need to ask yourself the question, "Is the taste of this dessert worth the potential damage it will do to my blood glucose and calorie intake?" If you can answer this question with a "yes," then have the dessert, but check your blood glucose and adjust your medications as needed after eating it. Then return to your nutritional plan without spending a lot of time regretting your lapse. You might even do a little extra exercise to counteract the calories.

On the other hand, if you answer no, ask yourself these questions to help you avoid temptation:

>> Do I really need or want the dessert?

>> Will I remember it ten minutes later when I'm at the theater?

>> Can I share the dessert or just taste it?

>> Is a fruit dessert or a small amount of high-quality cheese available that I could enjoy instead?

>> Because I really want a bit of dessert, can I forgo the carbohydrate portion of my meal and eat only a lean protein with cruciferous vegetables and leafy greens during the meal?

REMEMBER

To help you avoid that high-calorie dessert even further, think in terms of the number of minutes of active aerobic exercise you must do to account for the calories you consume in a dessert. If your exercise is walking, double these times. Here are some examples:

>> Boston cream pie: 32 minutes

>> Brownie: 32 minutes

>> Apple pie: 34 minutes

>> Hot fudge sundae: 38 minutes

>> Cheesecake: 40 minutes

>> Ice cream cone: 44 minutes

>> Strawberry milkshake: 47 minutes

You may conclude that dessert is worth your time, but we'll leave that decision up to you.

4

The Part of Tens

Make simple changes that pack a powerful punch.

Find out how to switch to a Mediterranean diet and lifestyle.

See what helps keep your blood glucose normal.

Get your kids to enjoy healthful eating habits.

Chapter **15**

Ten Simple Steps to Change Your Eating Habits

Following a nutritional plan sometimes seems so complicated. But really, if you follow the few simple rules outlined in this chapter, you can make the process much easier. This chapter provides you with ten simple things you can do today. None of them cost anything other than time. Adding one after another makes the results huge. Your weight, blood pressure, and blood glucose all fall, and you may well begin to feel the beneficial effects in other ways like feeling happier and more energetic. Who could ask for anything more?

Enjoying a Good Breakfast

People often think that the path to weight loss is to skip meals, and breakfast is often the first to go. However, the successful losers in the National Weight Loss Registry would disagree — 78 percent of them eat a good breakfast and only 4 percent skip breakfast. Eating a healthy breakfast prevents much greater eating later in the day.

TIP

So, what's a healthy breakfast? An easy option is mixed fruits or whole-grain cereal with Greek yogurt. Some other suggestions include steel cut oats with flax-seed, walnuts and fruit, or eggs with whole-wheat toast and fruit.

WARNING

Avoid heavy breakfasts like pancakes, French toast, or waffles with processed meats like bacon or sausage.

Still not convinced breakfast is for you? People who eat breakfast:

>> Are better able to concentrate at work or in school

>> Are stronger and can last longer doing physical activity

>> Tend to eat a more nutritionally complete diet overall

>> Have an easier time controlling their weight

>> Have lower cholesterol

>> Tend not to binge

>> Tend to have a better mood

Limiting Quantities and Making Substitutions

In the typical Western diet, many foods are high in sugar, fat, salt, and calories, but low in nutrition. We're thinking here of alcohol, cakes, candies, low cacao chocolate, cookies, doughnuts, energy drinks, french fries, fruit-flavored drinks, granola bars (yes, even supposedly so-called healthy granola bars), ice cream and other frozen desserts, muffins, nachos, pastries, potato chips, soft drinks, sports drinks, and more.

If you want to lose weight and/or improve your health, you have to severely limit or avoid these processed foods altogether. "What," you say, "Impossible!" But what if we guaranteed you'd live an additional three to five years. Well, we can't do that — there are no guarantees in life. But we can promise that you'll lose weight and feel better than you do now.

REMEMBER

You can substitute a healthier food for just about any not-so-healthy food. Here are some examples:

Instead of . . .	Try . . .
Cakes or pastries	Fruit with yogurt or a baked apple
Low cacao chocolate, candies, cookies, granola, or potato chips	Home baked popcorn with herbs, high cacao chocolate
Doughnuts or muffins	High-fiber, whole-grain muffins
French fries	Potato strips baked with a little extra-virgin olive oil
Fruit-flavored drinks and soft drinks	Carbonated water with lemon or lime
Ice cream	Frozen yogurt
Nachos	Artisanal cheese or hummus with whole-grain toast
Energy drinks, sports drinks	Water with lemon or lime

Eating Every Meal

When you miss meals, you become hungry. If you have type 1 diabetes, you can't safely miss meals, especially if you give yourself insulin. Instead of letting yourself become hungry, eat your meals at regular times so that you don't overcompensate at the next meal (or at a snack shortly after the meal you missed) when you're suffering from low blood glucose. Many people overtreat low blood glucose by eating too many sugar calories, resulting in high blood glucose later on.

WARNING

You shouldn't miss meals as a weight-loss method, particularly if you take a drug that lowers blood glucose into hypoglycemic levels. A pregnant woman with diabetes especially shouldn't miss meals. She must make up for the fact that her baby extracts large amounts of glucose from her blood. Both mother and growing baby are adversely affected if the mother's body must turn to stored fat for energy.

TIP

Eating smaller meals and having snacks in between is probably the best way to eat because doing so raises blood glucose the least, provides a constant source of energy, and allows control of the blood glucose using the least amount of external or internal insulin.

Setting Specific Goals

If you planned to climb Mt. Everest, your itinerary wouldn't read, "Arrive at the base, arrive at the top." In just the same way, the goals you set for losing weight and switching to the Mediterranean diet need to be achievable and very specific. For example, don't just set a goal to "Lose 40 pounds." You may be able to do it, eventually, but it's much more likely that you'll lose 5 pounds, and that should be your initial goal. After you've done that, you can plan to lose another 5 pounds, and so forth.

Goals should be very specific. For example, "I will eat fruit rather than cake for dessert" is a much better goal than "I will stop eating cake."

TIP

Choose goals that you have real control over. You're much more likely to succeed in choosing healthful foods than lowering your cholesterol, although improving your diet may cause your cholesterol to go down. It's also helpful to choose goals you can easily measure, like your weight and the number of steps you walk each day.

Your goals should be forgiving. Don't beat yourself up if you don't succeed the first time around.

Here are some specific goals to get you started:

>> I will enjoy delicious foods which I enjoy and that do my body the most good.

>> I will recognize that food can be a positive therapy in my life and plan meals with the most nutritious foods possible.

>> I will express gratitude toward the food that I'm eating and those who prepare and grow it.

>> I will eat with others as often as possible.

>> When I must eat alone, I will make it as pleasurable as possible.

>> I will listen to pleasant music or engage in pleasant conversation or mindfulness when I eat.

>> I will chew my food thoroughly to reduce the pace of eating.

>> When preparing food, I will be sure to use the proper portions for my size and lifestyle.

>> If eating in a restaurant or where portions are greatly distorted, I will reduce my portions by one-third.

- » I will eliminate second servings.

- » I will make healthful substitutions.

- » I will wear a pedometer and increase my daily steps by 100 until I reach 10,000 steps at least five days a week.

- » I will give myself specific rewards for achieving my goals, but those rewards will never be unhealthy food.

- » I will use yoga, meditation, or some other technique to manage the stress that leads to overeating.

Drinking Water throughout the Day

Seventy percent of your body is water, and all your many organs and cells require water to function properly. Most people, especially older people, don't get enough water. Older people often have the additional disadvantage of losing their ability to sense when they're thirsty. The consequences may include weakness and fatigue, not to mention constipation.

Water can replace all the sodas and juice drinks that add unwanted sugar and processed ingredients to your day. You soon lose your taste for those drinks and discover that you don't need (or miss) the aftertaste of soda and juice that you took for granted. Those drinks also raise the blood glucose very rapidly and are often used to treat low blood glucose.

TIP

Make drinking water a part of your daily habits. Drink some when you brush your teeth. Drink more with meals and snacks. Many people don't want to drink much water close to bedtime because if they do, they'll have to get up during the night to go to the bathroom — all the more reason to make sure you get your daily water ration.

Reinforcing Your Behavior Change

One of the most supportive ways to change your behavior is with reinforcement. Reinforcement may be *intrinsic* (a pleasurable state of mind like happiness or satisfaction) or *extrinsic* (a reward or encouragement, for example). You need to figure out which reinforcements work best for you. Here are some key intrinsic motivators:

>> **Curiosity:** You want to know the things that make you healthy.

>> **Independence:** You want to believe that you can succeed on your own.

>> **Power:** You want to feel that you have control over your own body.

Intrinsic motivators may be the force that gets you to follow a dietary program and do the necessary exercise. On the other hand, you may need tangible evidence of your success as well. Some of the strongest extrinsic motivators include the following:

>> Encouragement from friends and family

>> Gifts to yourself

>> Activities that you enjoy

Obviously, food can't be an extrinsic motivator unless and until you realize that fruits or vegetables are the things that should give you the most pleasure and not the desserts you may have enjoyed in the past.

Eliminating Processed Foods and Unwanted Ingredients

You can usually identify industrialized, highly processed foods by a long list of ingredients that are unrecognizable as something you'd naturally eat. These refined foods are often sold as convenience meals, which are formulated to appeal to people's taste for high salt and sugar and are very profitable for the multinational corporations that produce them. Some of the chemicals that have been used in the past have now been listed as hazardous for health, increasing the risk of weight gain, heart disease, or cancers, and laws in many countries limit or ban their use.

Other ingredients that are still widely used are coming under scrutiny and the subject of debate. For example, research has shown a possible relationship between some artificial sweeteners and weight gain and type 2 diabetes. Preservatives in processed meats may increase the risk of certain cancers. Some ingredients that are listed as stabilizers may be harmful to your gut microbiome. Chapter 5 discusses these processed and unnatural ingredients in greater detail.

Leaving Out Salt

Most Americans like a lot of salt in their food. Consequently, these people taste mostly salt and not much of the food. Try getting rid of the salt in your recipes. You can always add it later if you miss the flavor that salt adds. At first, you may think that the food tastes bland. Then you'll begin to discover the subtle tastes that were in the food but were overpowered by the salt.

Why do we emphasize cutting salt levels? Salt raises blood pressure in some people and that high blood pressure and type 2 diabetes combine to significantly raise the risks of heart disease, stroke, and kidney disease.

TIP

You can try the approach of slowly removing salt from the recipe. If the recipe calls for a teaspoon of salt, add only ¾ teaspoon. You won't notice the difference. Next time, try ½ teaspoon. And so on. In the recipes in Part 2, we use less salt wherever possible. Herbs and spices add much more interesting flavors and are rich in polyphenols, which may have positive effects on health.

Fresh dill, in particular, has a high amount of mineral salts that lends a salty flavor to recipes without the need for much sodium. Swap out traditional table salt for unrefined sea salt, if possible, to ensure that you're getting all the trace minerals from the salt that you're using with no additives. You can always add in an iodine supplement if your doctor or nutrition professional deems it necessary.

Tracking Food with a Diary

Try this little diversion: For the next two days, write down everything you eat and drink. Before you go to bed on the evening of the second day, take a separate piece of paper and try to reconstruct what you've eaten for the past two days without looking at your original list. Then compare the two lists. The differences in the lists will startle you. The point of this exercise is to show you that you're doing a lot of mindless eating. Trying to follow a nutritional plan from memory doesn't work.

The opposite is *mindful eating.* Thinking about what you eat can make meals much more healthy and also more enjoyable. You'll take more time and possibly eat a smaller portion. Some cultures and religions give thanks for a meal before eating. Another approach is to remember to thank the person (this may be yourself) who prepared the meal, which isn't only a positive affirmation but also a way to focus on enjoying what you're about to eat.

REMEMBER

A food diary not only shows you what you're eating all the time but also makes it easy to select items to reduce in portion size or eliminate altogether. To really have an effect, a food diary must be complete. The more complete your diary, the more likely it will help you and any caregiver to understand when you succeed and when you don't. Here's the information that's most important in your food diary:

>> All the foods and beverages you consumed during the day and night

>> The amount in ounces, grams, or portions of each food

>> How hungry you were when you ate the food (assign a number from 1, meaning stuffed, to 5, meaning extremely hungry)

>> The time of day when you ate

>> How you felt emotionally when you ate the food

>> Your exercise for the day

>> Your strategies for the following day

After you have all this information written down, you can begin to use the motivators in the "Reinforcing Your Behavior Change" section earlier in this chapter to reinforce your helpful eating and exercise behaviors. With this level of detail, you can calculate exactly how much you're eating and cut back if necessary. Finally, you can figure out if emotion plays a role.

Cooking from Scratch

Cooking from scratch is the best way to take control of your diet and be sure that what you're eating is good for you. By cooking for yourself you can also make sure that you're preparing the nutritious foods that you enjoy the most, personalizing the recipes and dishes to have them suit your palate and dietary needs. One way to make sure you don't eat additives and preservatives with long names or numbers is to create meals from foods with which you're familiar.

You can follow the recipes in Part 2 or make up your own more simple combinations of ingredients. Oftentimes it's possible to have a meal on the table in the same time as it takes for a convenience-ready meal to be cooked in its packaging in the oven. By cooking the meal from scratch you get to enjoy all the nutrients, none of the additives, while giving yourself the opportunity to explore new, healthy ways to prepare foods.

Here are some additional tips to help you cook from scratch:

>> Start with the freshest produce in season, and pick recipes based on that.

>> Choose a high-quality protein source such as poultry, fish, meat, or legumes

>> For roasting or baking add extra-virgin olive oil (EVOO) and herbs and spices for flavor.

>> Enjoy plentiful, colored vegetables, perhaps sautéed or roasted in the oven with a generous amount of EVOO as a salad.

>> Consider whole grains such as quinoa, brown rice, couscous, bulgur, barley, millet, and whole-wheat pasta.

>> Make up your own sauces with ingredients like tomatoes, garlic, onions and peppers instead of buying jarred versions.

>> Make your own stocks, so you know that they contain healthy amounts of seasoning.

>> Make your own salad dressings or drizzle a bit of EVOO and fresh lemon juice and/or a quality vinegar on top.

» Switching to whole grains and legumes

» Substituting fish and poultry for meat

» Using extra-virgin olive oil in place of butter and drizzling it everywhere

» Enjoying vegetables throughout the day

» Switching to fruits instead of cakes

Chapter **16**

Ten Simple Ways to Adopt a Mediterranean Diet

The Mediterranean diet is one that pleases both food lovers and health buffs simultaneously. Focusing on lifestyle instead of just eating, it provides the complete framework for feeling your best and maintaining a healthful eating pattern. Perhaps the single-most attractive feature of the Mediterranean diet is that you don't have to completely give up anything — splurges on occasion are part of the diet. On a daily basis, however, it encourages mouthwatering combinations of the best quality produce, herbs, legumes, lean protein, seafood, and dairy that are so satisfying that they'll change your perception of what eating healthy looks like.

If you're not already following a Mediterranean diet and lifestyle, you may think that giving up the lifestyle you've followed before may be difficult, but it isn't. Sometimes change can be enjoyable if you set out to embrace the process. You'll find that the substitutes that we suggest in this chapter enrich your life and enhance your palate if you allow it to.

After you start, you can enjoy the fact that you can eat specific foods to heal your body. When combined with physical activity and increased opportunities for socialization, your blood glucose, blood pressure, cholesterol, and weight will all take a turn for the better. The Mediterranean diet is sustainable for you because it's delicious and sustainable for planet Earth because it's plant-based. In this chapter, you find ten ways to go from your current eating style to the Mediterranean diet, no matter where you live.

Enjoying the Social Implications of Eating

Eating with others offers positive emotional responses and a deep sense of security that improves your daily life. Studies have demonstrated that children who eat at least one meal a day with parents do better in school and tend to eat less when they eat communally. If you can't meet in person, video chats are your next best bet to taking advantage of this free opportunity to improve your health.

TIP

When you're making your daily/weekly/monthly schedules, be sure to schedule times to eat with others. Plan on eating at least one meal a day with someone else — whether in person or virtually — so you can enjoy the mental, emotional, and physical benefits of communal eating daily.

If you have the opportunity to eat often with some of the same people, you have the additional benefit, and another key to longevity of having close confidants, which also sets you up for better physical and emotional health.

Discovering More about Culinary Medicine

When embarking on the Mediterranean diet, one of the best things that you can do is adopt the mentality that food is supposed to be good for you and taste good and vow to use that criteria when thinking about food.

The Mediterranean diet is based on an ancient eating plan that has kept communities relatively free from disease and enabled them to live long, healthy, and productive lives much longer than average for millennia. Those in the region traditionally ate natural, in-season foods. The local cultures knew which foods helped to prevent and heal certain conditions, and the diet was developed with both the desire to extract the most nutrients out of the least amount of food as well as to create the most delicious expressions of each food possible.

By planning daily meals with recipes like those in Part 2 and choosing the foods you love from those that are best for you, you can get the most out of what you consume and enjoy yourself in the process. Check out Chapter 5 and choose from the foods that you like when deciding what to eat.

Favoring Herbs and Spices

On the Mediterranean diet you have the variety of flavors, aromas, and textures that fresh herbs and spices provide. Plus, each one offers specific bioactive compounds — many of them listed in Chapter 4 — which can improve your mood and health, all while seasoning your food in exciting ways. I (Amy) rely heavily on special combinations of spices that are known not only for their great taste, but also for having a positive, anti-inflammatory effect on the body.

People in the Mediterranean region use copious amounts of fresh herbs. In fact, in many North African and Eastern Mediterranean countries, fresh herbs are the base for salad — instead of regular lettuce. There, fresh parsley and cilantro, which add wonderful flavors and offer many nutrients, are chopped up finely and served with diced fresh cucumbers, tomatoes, and peppers daily.

REMEMBER

Most people eat too much processed table salt. Although reducing the salt in your diet can help to bring down your blood pressure, you may complain about the loss of that salty flavor you're used to. Herbs and spices give you even more flavor than salt with positive side effects. See Chapter 5 for details.

We could write an entire book about the benefits of herbs and spices alone. The more that you can research their health benefits, discover the tastes that you like, and incorporate them into your cooking, the better off that you'll be. Also check out Chapter 5 for my (Amy's) anti-inflammatory spice mix.

Switching to Whole Grains

Grains (also called cereals) are the seeds of grasses that are cultivated for foods. They come in all sizes, from popcorn to teff, a grain that is so small that when it falls on the ground it's lost. The parts of a grain include

>> **Germ:** The small reproductive part of the grain, making up 3 percent of the grain by weight. The germ is rich in nutrients.

>> **Endosperm:** The tissue surrounding the germ, providing nutrition for the germ, making up 83 percent of the grain by weight. The endosperm is loaded with vitamins and minerals but especially starch (carbohydrate) and protein.

>> **Bran:** The hard outer layer of the grain, making up 14 percent of the grain by weight. The bran is rich in fiber.

Whole grains have all three parts. When grains are refined (milled), they lose the germ and the bran. Refining was developed to give grains a longer shelf life and better texture. White flour, for example, is all endosperm. Whole grains (not refined grains) are important sources of fiber, selenium, potassium, and magnesium. Food manufacturers enrich grains to add back some of the lost B vitamins but not the fiber.

REMEMBER

The traditional Mediterranean diet uses only whole grains such as barley, brown rice, buckwheat, bulgur, millet, farro, whole-wheat bread, whole-wheat pasta, whole-wheat crackers, and wild rice. Here are ways to enjoy whole grains:

>> Eat only the best quality whole-grain bread from bakeries, not the supermarket, where the emphasis is on shelf life, not taste.

>> Until your family enjoys whole grains, mix white and whole wheat together (for example, in pasta).

>> Use some of the spices in Chapter 5 to add more taste.

>> Use brown rice, wild rice, bulgur, and other new tastes.

>> Substitute rolled oaks or crushed bran cereal for refined cereals.

>> Add wild rice to soups, stews, and salads.

>> Add some sweetening if you want in the form of overripe bananas or a little honey.

Enjoying Fish or Poultry More Often

Many people in the United States and Europe eat some red meat most every day. Studies have shown that reducing red meat consumption is better for health and the environment. At least twice a week, substitute fish or poultry for meat. Or try a vegetarian day or two. You don't have to completely cut out steaks, hamburgers, sausages, hot dogs, pork, and lamb; just limit them to once a week, or better yet, once a month if possible.

That's how people view meat in the Mediterranean — by saving it for holidays and special occasions. By doing this, you significantly reduce the saturated fat and cholesterol in your diet. But you don't need to lose anything in the taste of your protein source.

TIP

If you do choose to eat red meat, avoid processed meats, always marinade or cook with EVOO, and reduce the portion size. Four ounces is a serving size.

Making EVOO Part of Every Meal

Including EVOO a part of every meal is key if you want to adopt the Mediterranean diet. All the countries that border the Mediterranean Sea, especially Spain, Italy, and Greece, grow enormous quantities of olives. When the olives are pressed, they produce olive oil. People in the Mediterranean have eaten olive for more than 6,500 years. Inhabitants of the Greek island of Ikaria and the Italian island of Sardinia reach the age of 90 at two and a half times the rate that Americans do, and they live a decade longer and enjoy a healthy, active old age.

The local diets, like that of others around the Mediterranean, are rich in olive oil and vegetables, with legumes, fruits, nuts, herbs, and spices, with moderate yogurt and cheese consumption especially from goat milk, low in meat products, with no processed foods, and may include modest amounts of wine with a meal. They emphasizes homegrown potatoes, beans (garbanzo, black-eyed peas, and lentils), wild greens, and locally produced goat milk and honey.

EVOO alone isn't responsible for the increased longevity — the whole lifestyle accounts for that — but EVOO has numerous benefits, which we discuss in Chapter 4.

Enjoying a few or even several tablespoons of EVOO each day is ideal in order to gain its benefits in cooking, flavoring, drizzling, and even replacing butter or margarine. You can safely cook at all normal temperatures with EEVO, exactly as they do in the Mediterranean — the antioxidant compounds protect the oil from burning or degrading and combine healthily with other nutrients in the foods you're cooking. Having a large container of EVOO in the kitchen is economical. Just store it away from light and heat and seal it after you use it. You may want a smaller bottle of fine EVOO for finishing dishes with delicious flavors and health-ful polyphenols. The more delightfully peppery and subtly bitter, the more likely it is that the oil is high in polyphenols.

Avoiding Highly Processed and Fast Foods

Highly processed and fast foods are loaded with unhealthy fat and salt as well as other added chemicals, and people who eat a lot of fast foods are heavier and less healthy than those who don't. In order to adopt the Mediterranean diet, steer clear of highly processed and fast foods.

Fast foods are never a part of the diet of people like those described in the previous section who live a long, healthy life. What can you do to break the fast-food habit? Here are some suggestions:

>> Figure out how much you spend on fast food and begin to cut back.

>> Keep a journal of why and when you eat fast food. If there are certain stimulants that promote fast-food eating, try to respond with a different behavior like exercise or cooking a delicious Mediterranean meal.

>> Use fast-food nutrition charts to calculate all the extra calories, fat, and salt you're consuming. Start cutting back.

>> Eliminate low-nutrition, high-calorie foods one at a time. Start with soda (including diet ones). Don't bring fast foods into your house.

>> Replace fast food with healthy food.

>> Make a habit of reading the ingredient list on food packets; if you can't recognize the ingredients as food, they're probably not doing you any good.

>> Make it harder to eat fast foods. Plan to walk to any fast-food restaurant, for example.

Consuming Vegetables throughout the Day

An easy way to embrace the Mediterranean diet is to eat more vegetables. The Mediterranean diet includes meals that are plant-based around seasonal vegetables, not protein. For example in English, when describing a meat stew, we'd say "Meat Stew with Green Beans." People in the Mediterranean say a "Green Bean Stew" or a "Green Bean Stew with Meat." This detail to semantics is important because it underlines the important role of the vegetable, as well as using a larger quantity in proportion to the meat.

REMEMBER

You can't eat too many vegetables. To eat a significant amount of calories through vegetables, you would have to eat so much that you wouldn't be able to eat much of anything else. That's not a bad thing; six to nine servings of fresh fruit and vegetables a day should be a minimum guideline.

Here some ways to increase your vegetable intake:

>> Enjoy small, interesting salads with lunch and dinner.

>> Eat vegetable crudites with dips as snacks.

>> Add vegetables to omelets, soups, stews, and pasta dishes.

>> Discover tasty vegetarian dishes.

You can find so many different kinds of vegetables in the grocery store, but most people limit themselves to just a few of them. Your whole meal can consist of vegetables with a small amount of protein thrown in just as a garnish. Try a vegetarian restaurant or vegetarian dishes in globally inspired restaurants to see for yourself how delicious freshly prepared vegetables can be!

TIP

Plant foods that are high in fiber are often great prebiotics and act as food for the microbiome. Probiotics such as fermented foods including yogurt, cheeses and pickles add specific beneficial species to your microbiome. Try to include these in every meal.

Snacking on Dried Fruit or Unsalted Nuts

An apple, 4 apricots, a banana, ¾ cup blueberries, 12 cherries, 15 grapes, an orange, 1 pear, 2 plums, 1¼ cups strawberries, 1½ cups watermelon . . . all these represent just 60 kilocalories. Compare that to typical pieces of yellow cake with vanilla frosting (239 kilocalories), pound cake (116 kilocalories), pineapple upside-down cake (367 kilocalories), Boston cream pie (232 kilocalories), strawberry shortcake (428 kilocalories), or apple crumb cake (540 kilocalories). Even the cake with the fewest kilocalories has twice that of a fruit choice!

But how can you give up cakes in favor of fruits? Make it easy to eat a fruit and hard to eat cake. Don't keep cake in the house. Do keep bowls of fruit visible and in easy reach. If you must have that occasional piece of cake, don't buy a whole cake — just buy one piece and cut it in four pieces so you eat one-quarter piece each time.

Alternately, you can eat some nuts for a snack, but make sure they're unsalted and preferable with edible skins on. The following selections are about the same kilocalories as that piece of fruit:

- >> 6 almonds
- >> 1 tablespoon cashews
- >> 2 whole pecans
- >> 10 large peanuts
- >> 2 whole walnuts
- >> 2 teaspoons pumpkin seeds

This simple but profound change in your eating habits will reveal itself on the scale very rapidly. You'll be eating almost two-thirds of a pound fewer calories per week — a three-pound weight loss each month in addition to all the other changes you're making.

REMEMBER

A handful of mixed unsalted nuts provides filling fiber, healthy fats, vitamins, minerals and polyphenol antioxidant and anti-inflammatory compounds and is part of the Mediterranean diet.

Sipping a Little Wine and a Lot of Water

When you're adopting a Mediterranean diet, water should be your main drink throughout the day and at mealtimes. A serving of wine (especially red) if you enjoy it with a balanced meal is preferred over soft drinks and sugary juices.

The first thing that you'll to do is to cut out sodas and sugary or artificially sweetened drinks and focus on the main beverages of the Mediterranean diet — lots of water and wine in moderation. Wine, especially red wine, is a fixture of the Mediterranean diet in many countries. People enjoy it in small amounts, always with meals. Alcohol consumption is related to an increased risk of diseases like cancer, but wine seems to have some protective compounds, and the Mediterranean diet as a whole probably mitigates those risks.

TECHNICAL STUFF

We don't know exactly what it is in wine that might help, but we suspect it's the substance resveratrol or other polyphenols called procyanidins. Yet taking resveratrol separate from wine doesn't seem to help. Wine in moderation reduces bad cholesterol and increases good cholesterol and has been shown to reduce the risk of heart disease, especially in men. So when you raise a small glass "to your health," it may have some basis in fact, but if you choose to, always remember to drink wine in moderation.

TIP

Water should be your main beverage. You don't have to waste your money on fancy bottled waters, especially if they use plastic bottles that pollute the planet. If you're in a country where the tap water isn't potable, or in a place such as the United States where the tap water contains chemical substances, consider a home water filtration system or water pitcher which contains a filter.

REMEMBER

If you have diabetes and are taking certain medications, you may need more water than others. Unless your doctor has asked you to limit water intake, try to drink at least two liters – if not more, of clean, spring or purified water each day.

The old rule of eight 8-ounce glasses of water a day isn't based on scientific evidence. Some of the main functions of water are as follows:

>> To replace all the water you lose each day through urination, evaporation, breathing, and defecation

>> To help you feel full so you don't eat more

>> To maintain cleansing the body through kidney function

>> To maintain normal bowel function

Filling Up on Legumes

Legumes are the food of the future and include beans, peas, and lentils. They have little fat and no cholesterol, and they provide folic acid, potassium, iron, magnesium, and several other nutrients. The fats they do contain are good for you, and legumes are loaded with fiber. Their high protein content makes them a very good substitute for meat, fish, or poultry. They include black beans, black-eyed peas, chickpeas, edamame, fava beans, lentils, lima beans, kidney beans, and over 13,000 other varieties. They can be used in soups, salads, stews, as snacks, to make hummus (chickpeas), and anywhere you feel like throwing in a few legumes.

The dried legumes need to be soaked to rehydrate them before you cook them. Then you cook them in water to soften them. They can be made into dips or eaten directly as snacks. To reduce the production of intestinal gas, don't cook them in the soaking water — use canned beans or cook them very slowly.

Legumes make you feel full, a very definite benefit. If you combine legumes with whole grains, you'll be getting all nine essential amino acids, the building blocks for protein in your body. Soybeans alone have all the essential amino acids. Like berries, legumes contain lots of antioxidants, healthful substances that protect the eyes, the skin, the immune system, and the brain.

Legumes are used in crop rotation cycles in grape orchards in the Mediterranean. Growing them enriches the soil while using very little land, so they're as good for the environment as they are for your body.

Chapter **17**

Ten Keys to a Normal Blood Glucose

I n the most recent edition of *Diabetes For Dummies,* we describe the management of diabetes in detail. In this chapter, you find the highlights of that extensive discussion. Although this book is about eating, controlling your blood glucose requires much more from you. Everything we suggest is directed toward normalizing your blood glucose.

REMEMBER

Doctors consider your blood glucose *normal* when it's less than 100 mg/dl (5.5 mmol/L) if you've eaten nothing for 8 to 12 hours. If you've eaten, your blood glucose is normal if it's less than 140 mg/dl (7.8 mmol/L) two hours after eating. If you never see a blood glucose level higher than 140, you're doing very well, indeed. See Chapter 1 for a full explanation of mg/dl (milligrams per deciliter) and mmol/L (millimoles per liter).

Knowing Your Blood Glucose

No excuse is adequate for you to not know your blood glucose at all times, although we've heard some pretty far-out excuses over the years — close to "The dog ate my glucose meter." The capability to measure blood glucose accurately and rapidly is the greatest advance in diabetes care since the discovery of insulin. Yet many people don't track their blood glucose.

Sure, sticking your finger hurts, but laser devices now make it painless, and even the needles are so fine that you barely feel them. How can you know what to do about your blood glucose if you don't know what it is in the first place?

The number of glucose meters you can choose is vast, and they're all good. Your insurance company may prefer one type of meter, or your doctor may have computer hardware and software for only one type. Other than those limitations, the choice is yours.

TIP

If you have very stable blood glucose levels, test once a day — some days in the morning before breakfast, other days in the evening before supper. Varying the time of day you test your blood glucose gives you and your doctor a clearer picture of your control under different circumstances. If your diabetes requires insulin or is unstable, you need to test at least before meals and at bedtime in order to select your insulin dose.

Painless devices, including continuous monitoring and even closed-loop systems for delivering insulin to those who need it in a real-time response to blood glucose measurements, are now much more widely available in many parts of the world. These devices are revolutionizing the way many people are able to control their diabetes.

Using Exercise to Control Your Glucose

When people are asked how much exercise they do, about a third say that they do nothing at all. If you're a person with diabetes and consider yourself a part of that group that doesn't exercise, then you aren't taking advantage of a major tool — not just for controlling your blood glucose but also for improving your physical and mental state in general. When a large group of people who were expected to develop diabetes because both parents had diabetes participated in a regular exercise program in one recent study, 80 percent who stayed on the program didn't develop diabetes.

Don't think that exercise means hours of exhaustion followed by a period of recovery. We're talking about a brisk walk, lasting no more than 60 minutes, every day, and not necessarily all at once. If you want to do more, that's fine, but most people can do this much. People who can't walk for some reason can get their exercise by moving their arms. To lose weight as a result of exercise, you need to do 90 minutes a day, every day.

REMEMBER

Exercise can provide several benefits to your overall health. Exercise does the following:

>> Lowers the blood glucose by using it for energy

>> Helps with weight loss

>> Lowers bad cholesterol and triglyceride fats and raises good cholesterol

>> Lowers blood pressure

>> Reduces stress levels

>> Improves mood

>> Reduces the need for drugs and insulin shots

Taking Your Medications

Some people who are diagnosed with type 2 diabetes are able to reverse or put their diabetes into remission by embracing the lifestyle changes we describe in this book. For others it may be necessary to add one or more of the many available drugs. Now, with the right combination of medications (and by using some of the other tools in this chapter), just about any patient can achieve excellent control. But no medication works if you don't take it.

REMEMBER

The word *compliance* applies here. Compliance refers to the willingness of people to follow instructions — specifically, taking their medications. People tend to be very compliant at the beginning of treatment, but as they improve, compliance falls off. Diabetic control falls off along with it.

The fact is, as you get older, the forces that contribute to a worsening of your blood glucose tend to get stronger. You want to do all you can to reverse that tendency. Taking your medications is an essential part of your overall program.

If you're confused by all the medications you take, get yourself a medication box that holds each day's medications in separate compartments so you make sure the compartment for each day is empty by the next day. Any doctor who prescribes more than two medicines to you should be able to get one for you, and you can definitely get them in drugstores.

Seeking Immediate Help for Foot Problems

One error that leads to a lot of grief in diabetes is failure to seek immediate help for any foot problems. Your doctor may see you and examine your feet only once in two or three months. You need to look at your feet every day. At the first sign of any skin breakdown or other abnormality (such as discoloration), you must see your doctor. In diabetes, foot problems can go from minor to major in a very brief time. We don't pull punches in this area, because seeing your doctor is so important — major problems may mean amputation of toes or more.

You can reverse most foot problems if you catch and treat them early. You may require a different shoe or need to keep weight off the foot for a time — minor inconveniences compared to an amputation.

Besides inspecting your feet daily, here are some other actions you can take:

>> Testing bath water with your hands to check its temperature, because numb feet can't sense if the water is scalding hot

>> Ensuring that nothing is inside your shoe before you put it on

>> Wearing new shoes only a short time before checking for damage

Taking immediate action goes for any infection you develop as a diabetic. Infections raise the blood glucose while you're sick. Try to avoid taking steroids for anything if you possibly can. Steroids really make the glucose shoot up.

Brushing Off Dental Problems

Keeping your teeth in excellent condition is important, but especially if you have diabetes. *Excellent condition* means brushing them twice a day and using dental floss at the end of the day to reach where the toothbrush never goes. It also means visits to the dentist on a regular basis for cleaning and examination.

We've seen many people with diabetes have dental problems as a result of poor dental hygiene. As a side effect, controlling the blood glucose is much harder. After patients cure their teeth, they require much less medication.

REMEMBER

People with diabetes don't have more cavities than people without diabetes, but they do have more gum disease if their glucose isn't under control. Gum disease results from the high glucose that bathes the mouth — a perfect medium for bacteria. Keeping your glucose under control helps you avoid losing teeth as a result of gum disease, as well as the further deterioration in glucose control.

Maintaining a Positive Attitude

Your mental approach to your diabetes plays a major role in determining your success in controlling the disease. Think of diabetes as a challenge — like high school math or asking out your first date. As you overcome challenges in one area of your life, the skills you master help you in other areas. Looking at something as a challenge allows you to use all your creativity.

When you approach something with pessimism and negativity, you tend to not see all the possible ways you can succeed. You may take the attitude that "It doesn't matter what I do." That attitude leads to failure to take medications, failure to eat properly, failure to exercise, and so forth.

Simply understanding the workings of your body, which comes with treating your diabetes, probably makes you healthier than the couch potato who understands little more than the most recent sitcom.

TIP

Some people do get depressed when they find out they have diabetes. If you're depressed and your depression isn't improving after several weeks, consider seeking professional help.

Planning for the Unexpected

Life is full of surprises — like when you were told you have diabetes. You probably weren't ready to hear that news. But you can make yourself ready to deal with surprises that may damage your glucose control.

Most of those surprises have to do with food. You may be offered the wrong kind of food, too much food, or too little food, or the timing of food doesn't correspond to the requirements of your medication. You need to have plans for all these situations before they occur.

You can always reduce your portions when the food is the wrong kind or excessive, and you can carry portable calories (like glucose tablets) when food is insufficient or delayed. Other surprises have to do with your medication, like leaving it in your luggage — which is on its way to Europe while you're headed to Hawaii.

TIP

Keep your important medications with you in your carry-on luggage, not in checked luggage. Again, your ability to think ahead can prevent you from ever being separated from your medication.

Not everything is going to go right all the time. However, you can minimize the damage by planning ahead.

Becoming Aware of New Developments

The pace of new discoveries in diabetes is so rapid that keeping on top of the field is difficult even for us, the experts. How much more difficult must it be for you? You don't have access to all the publications and the medical journals that we see every day.

TIP

However, you can keep current in a number of ways. The following tips can help you stay up-to-date on all the advances:

>> Begin by taking a course in diabetes from a certified diabetes educator. Such a course gives you a basis for a future understanding of advances in diabetes.

>> Get a copy of our book, the most recent edition of *Diabetes For Dummies* (John Wiley & Sons, Inc.), which explains every aspect of diabetes for the nonprofessional.

>> Join a diabetes organization, particularly the American Diabetes Association or your country specific equivalent. You'll start to receive excellent publications, which often contains the cutting edge of diabetes research as well as available treatments.

>> Don't hesitate to question your doctor or ask to see a diabetes specialist if your doctor's answers don't satisfy you.

The cure for diabetes may be in next week's newspaper. Give yourself every opportunity to find and understand it.

Utilizing the Experts

The available knowledge about diabetes is huge and growing rapidly.

Fortunately, you can turn to multiple people for help. Take advantage of them all at one time or another, including the following people:

>> Your primary physician, who takes care of diabetes and all your other medical concerns

>> A diabetes specialist, who is aware of the latest and greatest in diabetes treatment

>> An eye doctor, who must examine you at least once a year

>> A foot doctor, to trim your toenails and treat foot problems

>> A dietitian, to help you plan your nutritional program

>> A diabetes educator, to teach you a basic understanding of this disease

>> A pharmacist, who can help you understand your medications

>> A mental health worker, if you run into adjustment problems

Take advantage of any or all of these people when you need them. Most insurance companies are enlightened enough to pay for them if you use them and in many countries they can be accessed free of charge in a state-funded system.

Avoiding What Doesn't Work

Not wasting your time and money on worthless treatments is important. When you consider the almost half a billion people living with diabetes in the world today, they provide a huge potential market for people with the latest wonder cure for diabetes. Before you waste your money, check out the claims of these scammers with your diabetes experts.

You can find plenty of treatments for diabetes advertised online. It is always important to make sure you are taking advice from reliable sources. There are government public health sites and reputable international or national diabetes resources. It is always a good idea to discuss and check out the reliability of information with your professionally qualified, regulated and respected health care professional.

Don't make any substantial changes in your diabetes management without first discussing them with your physician.

» **Selecting the right recipes**

» **Making healthful substitutions**

Chapter **18**

Ten (Plus One) Strategies for Teaching Kids Healthy Eating Habits

hildren can be naturally cautious about trying new foods, which is something you're grateful for if your toddler wanders off in the garden and picks up a horse chestnut or a wild mushroom. Evolution has provided some protective instincts to help children avoid poisonous foods and a tendency for children to enjoy tastes such as the sweetness of sugars from energy dense fruits. But ultimately it's what you teach them that determines their feelings about food. In fact, in countries where adults eat the most healthful diets, children commonly do the same. We've seen children in the Mediterranean happily deboning and enjoying whole fish at the dinner table and others asking for olives.

You can do numerous things to encourage your children to eat vegetables. This chapter provides eleven ideas to help your children consume more veggies. We're sure you can come up with a few others.

REMEMBER

If your child has been diagnosed with type 1 diabetes, you need to help them understand the effect of foods and insulin on their diabetes, in collaboration with their healthcare professionals. Furthermore, make sure they know about the complications of their diabetes, especially the risks of serious loss of control of blood glucose. If your child has been diagnosed with type 2 diabetes, you also need access to specialist professional advice. Ensure that your child is allowed to develop a positive relationship with healthy food to optimize their blood glucose levels and, where appropriate, lose weight. The advice in this chapter can help all children, with or without diabetes, to have a truly healthful diet.

Modeling Behavior

If you show your children (and nieces and nephews and grandkids) to love vegetables and consider them delicious, then more than likely they'll feel the same about vegetables. Nowadays advertisers spend a lot of time and money enticing children to eat poorly. You need to present an equally appealing case for nutritious food. Kids love to follow your example, learning that many mildly bitter and pungent flavors are healthy, healing, and enjoyable.

TIP

The best time to model this behavior is at family meals. Be patient, gentle, and encouraging, and most kids will learn to explore interesting flavors in vegetables, herbs, and spices. Set the example. Let them see you eating and enjoying the vegetables. The message will come through loud and clear. And remember, that many adults have been raised on processed foods with excessive added sugars, fats, and salt, and perhaps have some learning to do as well.

Here's an example of how with a little effort, I made vegetables appealing to kids. I (Amy) believe in romancing healthful food to feed children much in the same way that large fast-food chains entice them with trinkets and toys that come inside colorful boxes. Once when I adopted an elementary school class in Washington, D.C., I was tasked with the responsibility of teaching third graders how to cook kale and collard greens that they had recently harvested in their urban garden with their teacher. Knowing that the kids probably didn't have a natural affinity toward those particular leafy greens, I thought back to the most flavorful versions of them I'd ever had.

I immediately remembered an Ethiopian recipe where the greens were sautéed with ginger, onions, garlic, and red peppers before being served on injera bread. I first taught them about Ethiopia and kids there harvesting the greens with pictures of ingredients before demonstrating the recipe. I asked one of the students' mothers who was from Ethiopia to bring injera bread to accompany the recipe. The kids were so excited that they enjoyed the recipe and asked for seconds. Some asked to take it home to their parents who never had the chance to eat kale. The recipe went on to find a permanent place in the school's cafeteria.

Starting Early

Children learn their eating habits at a very young age, age 2 or even younger. From the time they can eat solid or even semi-solid food, they should be given choices of vegetables. We don't recommend using canned vegetables, because they're often filled with salt and sugar, but rather making the vegetables into small portions yourself.

Give the child the vegetable to eat by itself, not with a choice of fatty things or sweet things that they'll gravitate toward. Don't threaten that the "good stuff" comes only after the vegetables are eaten. Vegetables must be seen as part of the good stuff.

REMEMBER

Concealing vegetables from children in recipes such as sauces and soups should be a last resort. If you've tried everything and really have a hard time getting them to enjoy produce, then consider using smoothies, soups, and sauces as a way to help them.

Allowing Children to Pick

Children love to feel that they have power. When at home, show them how much you and those around you love produce. Get excited about them and tell them what vegetables do for their bodies. Prepare the most tasty vegetable recipes possible, and then give them the power to choose the vegetables in the market that they and you will eat.

TIP

Move around to the different colors, explaining that the reason for the different colors is that each color represents a different kind of food that they need in their body. Get a rainbow of vegetables and present them in an interesting way, such as in the Swiss Chard with Vegetable Confetti "Tacos" in in Part 2. You can even use pieces of fruits and vegetables to make animal and other shapes with really young kids as a fun way to get them interested. Let them flip through this book's color insert and pick a dish you can make and eat together.

Try to know what the vegetables contain so you can explain to the child (much of that information is in Part 1). This vegetable gives you this vitamin and mineral. That vegetable gives you that one. Your body uses them all to create a healthy person.

Involving Children in Food Preparation

When you ask children to describe their earliest memories, they often talk happily about helping their grandmother make some kind of food. That's exactly how I (Amy) learned to love cooking. Nonna Angela taught me about the importance of preparing and sharing food, which began a life dedicated to teaching and inspiring others to enjoy a healthy and delicious lifestyle.

REMEMBER

Preparing food together can be a great bonding experience between you and your child, and it also provides you with the opportunity to model good nutrition. Both cooking and baking from scratch are great forms of therapy for children. The communal time spent doing tasks such as kneading, rolling, stirring, and sautéing often cause kids to feel safe and secure, which also fosters everyone involved to open up and talk. If you ask your teenager how their day was, they'll probably respond with "okay," but if you spend 15 minutes kneading dough with them, they'll be more likely to open up and tell you what's on their mind without you ever having to ask.

If your child helps you to prepare fresh food including vegetables, they'll want to try what they've prepared. Have your child create their own nutrition plan for a day and discuss every part of it, pointing out what is carbohydrate, protein, fat, the balance among those foods, and how they affect their diabetes. Use illustrations such as the Mediterranean diet pyramid in Chapter 2 or the child's nutrition plan as a guide for planning, showing the important role that vegetables play in the plan.

REMEMBER

Never prepare one meal for your child with diabetes and another for the rest of the family. Everyone can benefit from the better choices you make with your child's nutritious food. The child also realizes that eating isn't punishment for a person with diabetes because the whole family eats the same way.

Keeping Problem Foods Out of Sight and Good Foods in Easy View

If potato chips or creamy cookies sit on the kitchen counter, can you blame your child (or yourself) for grabbing a handful every time they go by? Don't buy these foods in the first place. If you do, keep them out of sight. You know what happens when you walk up to a buffet table. You can more easily avoid what you don't see.

TIP

On the other hand, keep fruits and vegetables in plain sight. Have carrot sticks and celery sticks easily available. Keep some cooked broccoli and cauliflower in the refrigerator.

Again, your child follows your example. If you raid the freezer for ice cream, don't be surprised to see your child do the same thing. If you raid the refrigerator for broccoli or asparagus, that's what your child will do as well. The great benefit to you when you set an example for your child is the excellent nutrition that you get.

Growing a Garden

By growing your own garden, even if all you have is a small box, you can show your child where vegetables come from, how they grow, when to pick them, and the fun of eating what you grow. Plus, foods that you grow and pick yourself, just at the peak of taste, are a different experience from what you get at the supermarket. Only the farmers' market can come close. So if you can't possibly grow your own, take your child to a farmers' market.

TIP

If you do have a little space, here are a few recommendations from an old farmer (Dr. Rubin, author of previous editions in the *Diabetes For Dummies* series):

>> Grow some bush beans from seeds for the beautiful flowers that precede the delicious and plentiful beans and to demonstrate what can come from a tiny seed. They don't require staking up like pole beans.

>> Grow some beets and carrots, also from seeds, to show that foods grow under the earth as well as above the earth, and they get pretty sweet at that.

>> Grow some tomatoes and zucchini from plants to show how things can grow in abundance from only one or two plants that start very tiny.

Let your child do the picking. The thrill of picking your own food isn't to be missed. If you can't pick in your own garden, pick where you can pay for the produce in another garden.

Finding Vegetable Recipes They Like

Children tend to prefer some vegetables over others because those veggies are naturally sweeter, but they can still be full of fiber, vitamins, minerals, and bioactive compounds. Peas, sweetcorn, sweet potatoes and tomatoes (which is a fruit rather than a vegetable) are easiest to introduce first, with green leafy vegetables, broccoli, garlic, herbs, and spices sometimes being tastes that are acquired later.

TIP

Although a shot of good quality extra-virgin olive oil (EVOO) can be pleasantly bitter and peppery for adults familiar with these flavors, preparing and cooking vegetables with it softens and mellows the tastes of the oil and the vegetables, making the combination very enjoyable for most kids. Children in the Mediterranean region are brought up on this nutritious and healthy diet, from pureed vegetables at an early age to roasts and stews as they grow.

Stir-Frying Veggies

One of the best ways to cook vegetables ending with a delicious dish without adding a lot of fat is to stir-fry. The natural tastes of the vegetables are sealed in. The Chinese have been doing it this way for generations. Until they adopted Western styles of cooking and eating, diabetes wasn't much of a problem among the Chinese. And in the Mediterranean, sautéing vegetables in EVOO is very much on the menu.

Stir-fry many different kinds of vegetables together to make a vegetable medley. Some may take a little longer or a little shorter to fry so put the ones together that take the same time. A meal made up just with stir-fried vegetables can be all your child needs to realize how delicious vegetables can be. You don't have to throw in any chicken or beef — that's an important message to send your child. A meal can be complete without animal protein. Eating vegetarian is a very healthful way to go.

Using a Dip

Sometimes dipping the vegetables into a delicious dip that you prepare can make the vegetables and legumes even more delicious, desirable, and easy to eat. Chapter 10 offers several dip recipes, including one that is a complete meal from a nutritional standpoint and that kids can enjoy at any time of the day.

Knowing the Right Sized Portion

A 2-year-old child requires a lot less than a 20-year old adult. The recommended serving size of vegetables for a toddler is a tablespoon per year of age. If you want to get your 2-year-old to eat five of his servings of vegetables, all you have to do is get them to eat 10 tablespoons during the course of the day. That's a lot easier than you thought. If your child wants more, don't stop them!

With so little that has to be eaten to reach the daily goal, it may be easier to stick to just one or two vegetables on any given day. Today is carrot and bean day while tomorrow is beet and zucchini day. Vegetables can be fun!

Giving 100 Percent Fruit Juice

If you want to get some more fruit into your child and they won't eat enough solid fruit, give them 100 percent fruit juice. Remember that these natural sugars in juices will raise blood glucose levels more than if they were in the whole fruit, so dilute with water and keep to a few drinks a day. You can get juice from just about any fruit and many vegetables.

You can also make delicious fruit smoothies with lots of fruit, some juice, and a little yogurt to slow the absorption of the sugars. Kids love them!

TIP

Don't buy the canned variety, which always has too much salt in it for some dumb reason. Get a juicer and make your own. The wonderful possibilities of putting together all kinds of fruit flavors is easily available if you make your own.

Appendix A
Metric Conversion Guide

The recipes in this book weren't developed or tested using metric measurements. There may be some variation in quality when converting to metric units.

TABLE A-1

Common Abbreviations

Abbreviation(s)	What It Stands For
cm	Centimeter
G, g	Gram
kg	Kilogram
L, l	Liter
lb.	Pound
mL, ml	Milliliter

TABLE A-2

Volume

U.S. Units	Canadian Metric	Australian Metric
¼ teaspoon	1 milliliter	1 milliliter
½ teaspoon	2 milliliters	2 milliliters
1 teaspoon	5 milliliters	5 milliliters
1 tablespoon	15 milliliters	20 milliliters
¼ cup	50 milliliters	60 milliliters
⅓ cup	75 milliliters	80 milliliters
½ cup	125 milliliters	125 milliliters
⅔ cup	150 milliliters	170 milliliters
¾ cup	175 milliliters	190 milliliters
1 cup	250 milliliters	250 milliliters
1 quart	1 liter	1 liter
1½ quarts	1.5 liters	1.5 liters
2 quarts	2 liters	2 liters
2½ quarts	2.5 liters	2.5 liters
3 quarts	3 liters	3 liters
4 quarts (1 gallon)	4 liters	4 liters

TABLE A-3

Weight

U.S. Units	Canadian Metric	Australian Metric
1 ounce	30 grams	30 grams
2 ounces	55 grams	60 grams
3 ounces	85 grams	90 grams
4 ounces (¼ pound)	115 grams	125 grams
8 ounces (½ pound)	225 grams	225 grams
16 ounces (1 pound)	455 grams	500 grams (½ kilogram)

Length

Inches	Centimeters
0.5	1.5
1	2.5
2	5.0
3	7.5
4	10.0
5	12.5
6	15.0
7	17.5
8	20.5
9	23.0
10	25.5
11	28.0
12	30.5

Temperature (Degrees)

Fahrenheit	Celsius
32	0
212	100
250	120
275	140
300	150
325	160
350	180
375	190
400	200
425	220
450	230
475	240
500	260

Index

About the Authors

Dr. Simon Poole, MBBS DRCOG FBMA MIANE, has been a primary care physician in Cambridge, England for more than 30 years with a particular interest in lifestyle medicine and nutrition as well as the management of long-term medical conditions. He has taught and undertaken research with Cambridge University and is a founding member of the British and European Associations of Lifestyle Medicine.

Simon is a council member of the U.S. True Health Initiative, an International Senior Collaborator with the Global Centre for Nutrition and Health in Cambridge, and was awarded Fellowship of the British Medical Association for services to the profession in 2018, which included longstanding membership of Council of the Royal College of General Practitioners and Public Health Medicine Committee. Simon is a recognized international authority and speaker on lifestyle medicine, chairing the Food Values Conference series at the Pontifical Academy of Science of The Vatican, and the author of the award-winning book *The Olive Oil Diet* (Hachette), *The Real Mediterranean Diet* (Cambridge Academic), and the latest editions of *Diabetes For Dummies* and *Diabetes Meal Planning & Nutrition For Dummies* (John Wiley & Sons, Inc.).

Best-selling author **Amy Riolo** is also an award-winning chef, television host, and Mediterranean diet ambassador. The author of 16 books (this is No. 17), she has been named Knight of the Order of the Star of Italy by the Italian government, "The Ambassador of Italian Cuisine in the US" by the Italian International Agency for Foreign Press, "Ambassador of the Italian Mediterranean Diet 2022-2024" by the International Academy of the Italian Mediterranean Diet in her ancestral homeland of Calabria, Italy, and "Ambassador of Mediterranean Cuisine in the World" by the Rome-based media agency *We The Italians*. In 2019, she launched her own private label collection of premium Italian imported culinary ingredients called Amy Riolo Selections and include extra-virgin olive oil, balsamic vinegar, and pesto sauce from award-winning artisan companies.

Dedication

Simon Poole: I dedicate this book to my sister, Penny, for her constant encouragement and support.

Amy Riolo: I dedicate my contributions to this book to my parents, Faith and Rick Riolo, for their love and support.

Authors' Acknowledgments

The authors want to thank Dr. Alan L. Rubin and Cait James, MS, for their comprehensive original editions of this book. At Wiley, we want to thank Tracy Boggier for being so enthusiastic, efficient, and great to work with. We truly appreciate the expert and efficient editorial support and guidance of Chad Sievers and thank Kristie Pyles for all of their support as well. Many thanks to Rachel Nix for her meticulous recipe testing and nutritional analysis, and to Wendy Jo Paterson, Grace Geri Goodale, and Reminisce with Us for their photographs and styling.

Dr. Simon Poole: When I reflect on my career path, which has led me to encourage my patients in consultations and a wider audience in my writing to enjoy a healthier lifestyle, I realize how many people have inspired and enlightened me on that journey. Patients, medical colleagues, and communities have always provided encouragement and feedback on the books that I've written and the public presentations I've given. Farmers and chefs have taught me a great deal about how to produce and prepare food for life. Researchers have generously invited me to conferences to speak, to listen, and to learn. I'm particularly grateful to all those at the Global Institute for Health and Nutrition based at Cambridge and Parma Universities, especially Professors Ray and Del Rio for the welcome, support, and the privilege of membership of such an esteemed organization. I feel passionately that is the responsibility of those of us who are privileged to have been trained to seek, interpret, and discern credible and reliable knowledge and to share it in a manageable, understandable, and motivational way to support people to live their best lives. With this in mind, I'm especially grateful to the editors at Wiley for indulging me in telling stories of smart plants, bioactive compounds, and African antelopes in this series of *Diabetes For Dummies* books, to engage the imagination and excitement of readers, and I hope to inspire a different view of the world. And of course, I'll always be deeply indebted to my co-author Amy Riolo for bringing her patience, profound wisdom, culinary skills, and so much more to our books.

Amy Riolo: My earliest memories of cooking were with my mother, Faith Riolo, who taught me that food was not just something we eat to nourish ourselves, but an edible gift that could be given to express love. When she was later diagnosed with diabetes, it was my love for her and desire to create delicious and nutritious meals for my parents that eventually led me to write books on the topic. I owe much of my professional culinary success to my father, Rick Riolo, for always believing in my talent and supporting my career goals. To my beloved little brother, Jeremy, you are my why, and I'm grateful to be able to pass our family's knowledge down to you.

My nonna, Angela Magnone Foti, taught me to cook and bake, as well as valuable lessons that served me outside of the kitchen. My Yia Yia, Mary Michos Riolo, shared her beloved Greek traditions with me as well. I would probably never have published a cookbook if it weren't for my mentor, Sheilah Kaufman, who patiently taught me much more than I ever planned on learning. I'm proud to pass her knowledge on to others. Without the assistance and guidance of my late friend, spirit sister, and healer Kathleen Ammalee Rogers, I'd never have been able to realize my professional writing goals. I'm very thankful to Chef Luigi Diotaiuti, for always believing in me and for encouraging me to foster my dreams and goals.

There are dozens of people whom I'm proud to call friends and colleagues that I interact with daily and whom each indirectly enable me to achieve my goals. I'm grateful to each of you. I want to thank Italian President Matarella, Misistro Gonzalez of the Embassy of Italy in the United States, and Counselor Michela Carboniero of the Italian Cultural Institute for giving me the honor of being titled Knight of the Order of the Star of Italy. I also thank my dear friends and importers of Amy Riolo Selections products, Stefano and Davide Ferrari and Vince Di Piazza of DITALIA for distributing them. Many thanks to all my wonderful producers: Tenute Cristiano, Olio Anfosso, Pasta Marella, and Acetaia Castelli for their partnerships. In Calabria, Italy, I thank my cousins, Angela Riolo, Pina and Franco Riolo, Tonia Riolo, and Mario Riolo for increasing my knowledge and for their support. I thank Chefs Salvatore Murano and Enzo Murano of Max Trattoria Enoteca for including me in their culinary-cultural pursuits in Italy and for naming me an honorary member of ARCP (the Regional Association of Pythagorean Cooks). I thank Alessandro Cuomo for naming me Director of A.N.I.T.A. (The Italian Academy of Traditional Italian Foods). I am very grateful to the Italian Trade Agency in New York and the Embassy of Italy in Washington, D.C., for the opportunities and honors that they have bestowed upon me. Mille grazie to Dr. Battista Liserre for his inspirational work on nourishing both the mind and the soul and to Silvestro Parisee for including me in projects which promote Calabria. To my dear friends Jonathan Bardzik, Gail Broeckel, Ann Hotung, Sharon Wolpoff, Jeff Fritz, Paul Kolze, Stu Hershey, Maria Fusco, and Kim Foley, you're my spirit family and I'm blessed to have you in my life. Many thanks to Melissa's Produce for their generous donation of produce for recipe development. Many thanks to my tour partner Alex Safos of Indigo Gazelle Tours for the fantastic opportunities to cook and write in Morocco and Greece. And finally, I thank my co-author, Dr. Simon Poole, for his tremendous knowledge and commitment to the cause of promoting health and happiness, for always inspiring me, and for valuing my voice. It's a pleasure and an honor to collaborate with you.

Publisher's Acknowledgments

Senior Acquisitions Editor: Tracy Boggier

Project Editor and Copy Editor: Chad R. Sievers

Technical Editor: Elizabeth Lipski, PhD, CNS

Recipe Tester and Nutritional Analyst: Rachel Nix

Production Editor: Tamilmani Varadharaj

Photographers & Stylists: Wendy Jo Peterson and Grace Geri Goodale

Cover photo: Linguine with Seafood and Zucchini Cream Sauce by Wendy Jo Peterson and Grace Geri Goodale

Back cover photo: Pink Beet Hummus and Avocado Toast by Wendy Jo Peterson and Grace Geri Goodale